Transgender and Gender Diverse Children and Adolescents

Editors

NATALIA RAMOS
SERENA CHANG
SCOTT LEIBOWITZ

CHILD AND ADOLESCENT PSYCHIATRIC CLINICS OF NORTH AMERICA

www.childpsych.theclinics.com

Consulting Editor
JUSTINE LARSON

October 2023 • Volume 32 • Number 4

ELSEVIER

1600 John F. Kennedy Boulevard • Suite 1800 • Philadelphia, Pennsylvania, 19103-2899

http://www.theclinics.com

CHILD AND ADOLESCENT PSYCHIATRIC CLINICS OF NORTH AMERICA Volume 32, Number 4
October 2023 ISSN 1056–4993, ISBN-13: 978-0-323-93861-7

Editor: Megan Ashdown
Developmental Editor: Shivank Joshi

Child and Adolescent Psychiatric Clinics of North America (ISSN 1056-4993) is published quarterly by Elsevier Inc., 360 Park Avenue South, New York, NY 10010-1710. Months of issue are January, April, July, and October. Business and Editorial Offices: 1600 John F. Kennedy Boulevard, Suite 1800, Philadelphia, PA 19103-2899. Periodicals postage paid at New York, NY and additional mailing offices. Subscription prices are $369.00 per year (US individuals), $709.00 per year (US institutions), $100.00 per year (US & Canadian students), $411.00 per year (Canadian individuals), $862.00 per year (Canadian institutions), $473.00 per year (international individuals), $709.00 per year (international institutions), and $200.00 per year (international students). International air speed delivery is included in all *Clinics* subscription prices. All prices are subject to change without notice. **POSTMASTER:** Send address changes to *Child and Adolescent Psychiatric Clinics of North America*, Elsevier Health Sciences Division, Subscription Customer Service, 3251 Riverport Lane, Maryland Heights, MO 63043. **Customer Service: 1-800-654-2452 (U.S. and Canada); 314-447-8871 (outside U.S. and Canada). Fax: 314-447-8029. E-mail:** JournalsCustomer Service-usa@elsevier.com **(for print support) or** journalsonlinesupport-usa@elsevier.com **(for online support).**

Reprints. For copies of 100 or more of articles in this publication, please contact the Commercial Reprints Department, Elsevier Inc., 360 Park Avenue South, New York, New York 10010-1710 Tel.: 212-633-3874; Fax: 212-633-3820, E-mail: reprints@elsevier.com.

Child and Adolescent Psychiatric Clinics of North America is covered in *MEDLINE/PubMed (Index Medicus), ISI, SSCI, Research Alert, Social Search, Current Contents,* and *EMBASE/Excerpta Medica.*

Contributors

CONSULTING EDITOR

JUSTINE LARSON, MD, MPH, DFAACAP
Medical Director, Schools and Residential Treatment, Consulting Editor, *Child and Adolescent Psychiatric Clinics of North America*, Adjunct Assistant Professor, University of Maryland Department of Psychiatry, Sheppard Pratt, Rockville, Maryland, USA

EDITORS

NATALIA RAMOS, MD, MPH
Assistant Clinical Professor, Department of Psychiatry and Biobehavioral Sciences, University of California, Los Angeles David Geffen School of Medicine, Jane & Terry Semel Institute for Neuroscience, Los Angeles, California, USA

SERENA CHANG, MD
Director of Psychiatry, Callen-Lorde Community Health Center, Clinical Assistant Professor, Departments of Psychiatry and Child and Adolescent Psychiatry, New York University, New York, New York, USA

SCOTT LEIBOWITZ, MD, DFAACAP
World Professional Association of Transgender Health, Standard of Care 8th Edition Adolescent Chapter Lead, Department of Psychiatry, Nationwide Children's Hospital, The Ohio State University College of Medicine, Columbus, Ohio, USA

AUTHORS

DALIA N. BALSAMO, MD
Department of Psychiatry and Neuroscience, University of California, Riverside School of Medicine, Riverside, California, USA

ANTONIA BARBA, LCSW
Inform Transform, Bronxville, New York, USA

ERIN L. BELFORT, MD, DFAACAP
Maine Medical Center, Associate Professor of Psychiatry, Tufts University School of Medicine, Portland, Maine, USA

BRANDY BROWN, DSW, LCSW
Maine Medical Center, Tufts University School of Medicine, The Gender Clinic, Portland, Maine, USA

SERENA CHANG, MD
Director of Psychiatry, Callen-Lorde Community Health Center, Clinical Assistant Professor, Departments of Psychiatry and Child and Adolescent Psychiatry, New York University, New York, New York, USA

JUDITH A. COHEN, MD
Allegheny Health Network, Drexel University College of Medicine, Pittsburgh, Pennsylvania, USA

AMY CURTIS, MD
Assistant Professor, Department of Psychiatry and Behavioral Sciences, University of Washington School of Medicine, Seattle Children's Hospital, Seattle, Washington, USA

PETER T. DANIOLOS, MD, DFAACAP
Member of the Faculty, Harvard Medical School Child and Adolescent Psychiatry, Cambridge Health Alliance/Cambridge Hospital, Boston, Massachusetts, USA

BRETT DOLOTINA, BS
Department of Epidemiology, Mailman School of Public Health, Columbia University, New York, New York, USA

LAURA ERICKSON-SCHROTH, MD, MA
Chief Medical Officer, The Jed Foundation, Psychiatrist, Hetrick Martin Institute for LGBTQ Youth, Assistant Professor of Psychiatry, Columbia University Medical Center, New York, New York, USA

ABIGAIL L. FISCHBACH, BA
Research Coordinator, Gender and Autism Program, Division of Pediatric Neuropsychology, Children's National Hospital, Washington, DC, USA

GEORGE GIANAKAKOS, MD
Pritzker Department of Psychiatry and Behavioral Health, Ann and Robert H. Lurie Children's Hospital of Chicago, Chicago, Illinois, USA

MARVEL C. HARRIS
Private Consultant, Hilversum, the Netherlands

TERENCE L. HOWARD, MD, MS
Rising Third-Year Resident Physician, University of California, San Francisco Department of Psychiatry and Behavioral Sciences, San Francisco, California, USA

KAI J. HUANG, MD Candidate
Program in Medical Education - Urban Underserved, University of California, San Francisco School of Medicine, Medical Student Experience, San Francisco, California, USA

ARON JANSSEN, MD
Vice Chair of Clinical Affairs, The Pritzker Department of Psychiatry and Behavioral Health, Associate Professor of Psychiatry and Behavioral Sciences, Northwestern University Feinberg School of Medicine, Chicago, Illinois, USA

BRANDON JOHNSON, MD
Assistant Professor, Department of Psychiatry, Icahn School of Medicine at Mount Sinai, New York, New York, USA

MARIJA KAMCEVA, MD
Resident, Department of Psychiatry, Massachusetts General Hospital, McLean Hospital, Somerville, Massachusetts, USA

SASCHA E. KLOMP, BA
Private Consultant, Utrecht, the Netherlands

JUSTINE LARSON, MD, MPH, DFAACAP
Medical Director, Schools and Residential Treatment, Consulting Editor, *Child and Adolescent Psychiatric Clinics of North America*, Adjunct Assistant Professor, University of Maryland Department of Psychiatry, Sheppard Pratt, Rockville, Maryland, USA

SCOTT LEIBOWITZ, MD, DFAACAP
World Professional Association of Transgender Health, Standard of Care 8th Edition Adolescent Chapter Lead, Department of Psychiatry, Nationwide Children's Hospital, The Ohio State University College of Medicine, Columbus, Ohio, USA

XIMENA LOPEZ, MD
Associate Professor of Pediatrics, Pediatric Endocrinology Division, UT Southwestern Medical Center, Dallas, Texas, USA

MOLLIE C. MARR, PhD, MD
Candidate, Medical Scientist Training Program, Oregon Health & Science University, Portland, Oregon, USA

AUSTIN NGUY, BA
Department of Psychiatry and Neuroscience, University of California, Riverside School of Medicine, Riverside, California, USA

NATALIA RAMOS, MD, MPH
Assistant Clinical Professor, Department of Psychiatry and Biobehavioral Sciences, University of California, Los Angeles David Geffen School of Medicine, Jane & Terry Semel Institute for Neuroscience, Los Angeles, California, USA

G. NIC RIDER, PhD
Assistant Professor, Department of Family Medicine and Community Health, Institute for Sexual and Gender Health, University of Minnesota Medical School, Minneapolis, Minnesota, USA

CAITLIN RYAN, PhD, ACSW
Director, Family Acceptance Project, San Francisco State University, San Francisco, California, USA

PUJA SINGH, MD
Pediatric Endocrinology Division, UT Southwestern Medical Center, Dallas, Texas, USA

JAIME STEVENS, MD, MPH
Affirming Psychiatry LLC, University of Hawaii, Honolulu, Hawaii, USA

JOHN F. STRANG, PsyD
Director, Gender and Autism Program, Division of Pediatric Neuropsychology, Neuropsychologist, Center for Neuroscience, Children's National Research Institute, Children's National Hospital, Associate Professor, Departments of Pediatrics, Psychiatry and Behavioral Sciences, George Washington University School of Medicine, Washington, DC, USA

SHANNA SWARINGEN, DO
Assistant Clinical Professor, Division of Psychiatry and Behavioral Health, The Ohio State University College of Medicine, Nationwide Children's Hospital, Columbus, Ohio, USA

NATHALIE SZILAGYI, MD
Instructor, Yale Child Study Center, Yale School of Medicine, New Haven, Connecticut, USA; Director, Aurora Psychiatric Associates, Greenwich, Connecticut, USA

AMY TISHELMAN, PhD
Research Associate Professor, Department of Psychology and Neuroscience, Boston College, Chestnut Hill, Massachusetts, USA

ANNA I. R. VAN DER MIESEN, MD, PhD
Medical Doctor in Child and Adolescent Psychiatry and Post-Doctoral Researcher, Department of Child and Adolescent Psychiatry, Center of Expertise on Gender Dysphoria, Amsterdam University Medical Centers, Location Vrije Universiteit, Amsterdam, the Netherlands; Visiting Researcher, Margaret and Wallace McCain Centre for Child, Youth and Family Mental Health, Campbell Family Mental Health Research Institute, Centre for Addiction and Mental Health, Toronto, Ontario, Canada

JONATHON W. WANTA, MD
Pritzker Department of Psychiatry and Behavioral Health, Ann and Robert H. Lurie Children's Hospital of Chicago, Chicago, Illinois, USA

MILANA WOLFF, BS
Doctoral Candidate, College of Engineering and Physical Sciences, University of Wyoming, Laramie, Wyoming, USA

A. NING ZHOU, MD
Sr. Psychiatric Physician Specialist, San Francisco Department of Public Health Behavioral Health Services, Clinical Instructor - Volunteer, University of California, San Francisco, Department of Psychiatry and Behavioral Sciences, San Francisco, California, USA

Contents

> Gender–once an afterthought despite its significant yet unspoken role in the average American's daily life (public restrooms, clothes shopping, grooming, sports teams)–has become a fraught sociopolitical issue. The concept of gender as a construct, once relegated to the realm of Women's and Gender Studies courses, went mainstream while, concurrently, gender reveal parties have experienced a surge in popularity. Meanwhile, youth (and adults) have become increasingly comfortable exploring their gender identities and expression, which has led to an increase in inquiries regarding gender-affirming care–along with an accompanying backlash resulting in an increasing number–of states attempting to enact restrictions and bans, effectively turning healthcare for transgender youth into the latest political battlefield. This section will define and provide an overview of common gender- and sexual orientation-related terminology and basic topics in order to establish an understanding for the remainder of the articles in this edition.

> Traumatic stress increases the risk for mental health conditions and adversely impacts health, academic performance, and coping. Transgender and gender diverse (TGD) youth experience higher rates of abuse and maltreatment and interpersonal and community-embedded discrimination than their cisgender peers. Neurobiologic stress responses and social stress theory provide useful frameworks for understanding the effects of discrimination, stigma, and rejection. Despite facing higher rates of interpersonal trauma, TGD youth are quite resilient when able to access supports and affirming trauma-informed services. Clinicians play an important role in identifying and addressing traumatic stress impacting TGD youth and bolstering resilience.

> This article explores how race, sex, and gender are better thought of as a continuum rather than binary categories. Starting with a discussion of intersectionality, we examine the importance of ethnic-racial identity and explore unique cultural considerations for working with Black, Latinx, and AAPI transgender and nonbinary youth. We then examine intersex youth

and variations of sex development, as well as specific challenges they face. Finally, we explore nonbinary gender identities and the importance of individually tailoring affirming interventions. For all sections, we highlight the strengths and resilience of the youth and offer clinical recommendations for child and adolescent providers.

This article provides an overview of the World Professional Association of Transgender Health (WPATH) Standard of Care 8th edition (SOC8) recommendations for adolescents seeking gender-affirming care. SOC8 was the first iteration of the guidelines to employ a Delphi consensus process that required 75% agreement of 120 multidisciplinary international transgender health experts for approval of its recommendations. While the evidence base for adolescent care is evolving, gender-affirming treatment is medically necessary and promotes long-term psychological wellbeing. The guidelines emphasize the importance of an assessment to determine maturity and decision-making capacity for treatments that have long-term body implications.

This article provides an overview of the World Professional Association of Transgender Health (WPATH) Standard of Care 8th edition (SOC8) chapter on transgender and gender diverse (TGD) prepubescent children. This is the first WPATH SOC chapter in history specifically devoted to children, acknowledging that the developmental needs and experiences of these youth can be distinguished from those of TGD adolescents. The child standards are based on the consensus of a range of expert authors and a broader consensus derived from a Delphi process involving the entire international interdisciplinary SOC8 authorship. The child SOC draw upon general developmental literature and employ an ecological framework to establish practice recommendations, including an assessment framework that engages family members and community outreach as warranted.

Transgender and gender diverse (TGD) individuals face higher rates of stressors driving disproportionate health risks. Although psychiatric conditions are important to consider in the context of greater health-promoting efforts for TGD youth, any mental health concerns may or may not be related to gender identity or associated dysphoria. Nevertheless, it is essential to consider the impact of complex mental health factors on decisional capacity and gender care discussions. Psychiatric care of TGD youth includes stratifying risk factors through a minority stress lens, balancing acute needs with patient and caregiver priorities, and bolstering resilience using affirming care principles.

John F. Strang, Anna I.R. van der Miesen, Abigail L. Fischbach, Milana Wolff, Marvel C. Harris, and Sascha E. Klomp

Autism and gender diversity often intersect. Many transgender youth seeking gender-related medical interventions are autistic. Clinicians serving these youth lack an autism-specific evidence base to guide gender care decisions. At present, care decisions are based on extrapolation of care models from transgender youth samples, generally. At this point, there is no evidence to suggest that autistic youth are likely to experience shifts in gender or gender-related medical requests, although this has been insufficiently studied. This article, cowritten by expert clinicians and autistic gender-diverse collaborators, provides an overview of clinical care considerations and the current evidence base.

Erin L. Belfort and Brandy Brown

Clinicians working with youth encounter transgender and gender diverse youth and play a role in supporting the psychological and social well-being of youth and their families. Mental health clinicians start with a thorough assessment, development of a biopsychosocial formulation of the youth, and a collaborative treatment plan. Determining if the youth meets diagnostic criteria for Gender Dysphoria and identifying co-occurring mental health diagnoses inform recommendations for psychiatric medication management, individual and/or family therapy interventions, and/or referrals to medical colleagues. Supporting development of a coherent identity narrative and healthy interpersonal attachments with others is an important goal of treatment.

Caitlin Ryan, Antonia Barba, and Judith A. Cohen

Parental and caregiver inclusion is critical in providing psychosocial care for transgender and gender diverse (TGD) children and adolescents. High levels of trauma among TGD youth call for the use of evidence-based models and resources to decrease family rejection and increase affirmation and support while healing trauma that is both related to and unrelated to the child's gender identity and expression. The integrated Family Acceptance Project-Trauma-Focused Cognitive Behavioral Therapy treatment model provides a structured and effective approach to engaging TGD youth with trauma and their parents.

Puja Singh and Ximena Lopez

Individuals with gender dysphoria (as defined by the Diagnostic and Statistical Manual of Mental Disorders experience a marked incongruence between their sex assigned at birth and experienced gender resulting in significant distress or impairment in social, occupational, or other important areas of functioning. For transgender and gender diverse minors, the Endocrine Society recommends a multidisciplinary approach to gender-affirming medical treatment that involves a physician and a mental health provider, also consistent with the World Professional Association for Transgender Health Standard of Care 8th Edition recommendations. This article outlines the role of medical providers in implementing safe and effective gender-affirming medical treatments for youth.

For some transgender and gender diverse (TGD) youth, exploration of gender identity and expression may be non-linear. Some TGD youth elect to detransition, broadly defined as the cessation or reversal of an already-initiated social and/or medical gender affirmation process. Youths' experiences with detransition appear to be highly heterogeneous, and rates of detransition appear to be quite low. Nevertheless, it is essential that providers facilitate non-judgmental, open-ended discussions about the possibilities of gender identity and gender expression evolution, with a focus on how clinicians will support young people and their families regardless of how their gender trajectory may evolve.

Transgender children and adolescents are at an elevated risk for negative mental health outcomes due to exposure to stigma and discrimination regarding their identity. While various environments may perpetuate this stigma, many supports also exist that can bolster safety, affirmation, and resilience in this population. Opportunities for support exist within schools, broader communities, religious organizations, and with medical professionals who practice gender-affirming care. Clinicians who are familiar with resources in their communities can effectively guide transgender youth and their families to these affirming spaces.

Transgender and gender diverse (TGD) youth are overrepresented in legal and social support systems intended to protect and support youth along their developmental journeys. However, these systems often fall short for TGD youth and further stigmatize an already vulnerable population. This article provides an overview of the experience, care, and treatment of systems-involved TGD youth. Working with systems-involved transgender and gender diverse youth necessitates a high level of compassion and advocacy in pursuit of more equitable care and access.

Jaime Stevens

Inpatient and other residential care environments require special consider-ations for safety and unique opportunities to provide affirming care to TGD youth. Gender-positive policies, staff training, communication, placement, programming, and discharge planning are imperative; however, data and literature are limited in regard to affirming care for TGD youth in such en-vironments. This chapter draws from published research and best practice to support the wellness of TGD individuals in inpatient and similar settings. It offers clinical guidance for clinicians, administrators, educators, and ad-vocates to provide safer and more effective care for TGD youth in such fa-cilities to best support their mental and physical health.

Justine Larson

As a child and adolescent psychiatrist, I am aware that puberty is a chal-lenging experience for many adolescents and parents. As a parent of a transgender adolescent, I have seen the ways in which the experience of puberty is similar to and different from that of cisgender adolescents. In this article, I describe my thought process behind going forward with several medical interventions for my transgender child and relate this to broader observations about parents and puberty.

CHILD AND ADOLESCENT PSYCHIATRIC CLINICS

SERIES OF RELATED INTEREST
Psychiatric Clinics
https://www.psych.theclinics.com/
Pediatric Clinics
https://www.pediatric.theclinics.com/

AACAP Members: Please go to www.jaacap.org for information on access to the Child and
Adolescent Psychiatric Clinics. *Resident* Members of AACAP: Special access information is
available at www.childpsych.theclinics.com.

THE CLINICS ARE AVAILABLE ONLINE!
Access your subscription at:
www.theclinics.com

Preface

Navigating the Storm: Meeting the Needs of Transgender and Gender-Diverse Youth and Their Families in a Time of Sociopolitical Upheaval

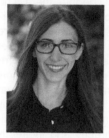 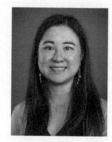 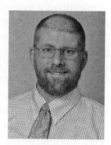

Natalia Ramos, MD, MPH   Serena Chang, MD   Scott Leibowitz, MD
Editors

"The way I see it, if you want the rainbow, you gotta put up with the rain."
–Dolly Parton

We were approached to organize this issue of *Child and Adolescent Psychiatric Clinics of North America* in mid-2021 amidst an epidemic of discrimination against lesbian, gay, bisexual, transgender, and queer (LGBTQ) people in the United States (US) catalyzed by the Trump Administration, including its unrelenting rollback of federal anti-LGBTQ discrimination measures in health care, education, public spaces, and housing; its targeted appointment of judges with anti-LGBTQ records to the Supreme Court; and its refusal to use the US Department of Justice to protect the rights of LGBTQ Americans. Once the Biden Administration took office in January 2021, it began to roll back some of these changes, while also appointing the first openly transgender federal official requiring Senate confirmation, Assistant Secretary of Health Dr Rachel Levine.[1] At that point, anti-LGBTQ efforts pivoted to state leaders and legislatures in conservative states and proliferated.

Currently, over 450 bills across the United States target LGBTQ Americans across all social settings, including in health care, school, workplace, and public settings.[2] The Arkansas state legislature imposed the first ban on gender-affirming care for minors in 2021, followed by an additional ten states. An estimated 77,900 transgender and

Child Adolesc Psychiatric Clin N Am 32 (2023) xiii–xix
https://doi.org/10.1016/j.chc.2023.05.010
1056-4993/23/© 2023 Published by Elsevier Inc.

gender-diverse (TGD) youth reside in states that have enacted bans or limitations on gender-affirming care, and another 68,400 face pending legislation in 19 states.[3] In some states, health care providers face legislation that categorically restricts, forbids, and/or criminalizes gender-affirming services for transgender youth and their families. The resulting backlash on clinicians, universities, and health systems has led to multiple closures of well-regarded programs across the country, many of which served families with no other access to care. It is notable that these politically motivated attacks on services for gender-diverse youth are occurring during a calamitous post-shutdown national shortage of youth mental health services *and* during an era of increasing evidence that gender-affirming care improves health outcomes and overall well-being among TGD youth.

The widespread pathologization and marginalization of TGD youth and their families will likely have vast long-term impacts on mental health that we are yet to fully comprehend. We are in the middle of a traumatic period in history for TGD people; there is no telling when things will shift. Pervasive anti-transgender rhetoric creates unsafe circumstances for TGD youth across social settings, and transgender Americans are already *four* times more likely to be the victims of violent crimes than their cisgender peers.[4] As providers who work with youth and families, we witness firsthand the impacts of these toxic stressors on self-esteem, self-worth, and mental and physical health symptoms. TGD children and adolescents internalize messages they hear from the individuals and media around them, particularly in a world in which they are greatly connected to online spaces.[5,6] Over two decades of rigorous scientific inquiry has shown that mental health among LGBTQ youth is directly and indirectly affected by laws pertaining to LGBTQ civil rights. For example, in states that legalized same-sex marriage before the US Supreme Court required it, the rate of suicide attempts among LGBTQ high school students—and high school students overall—subsequently declined.[7]

Amidst this political backdrop and resulting mental health challenges lies an ever-evolving population of young people seeking care. As the conceptualization of gender becomes more expansive with each successive generation,[8] the clinical care needs of TGD youth have also become increasingly complex. Twenty-five years have passed since the World Professional Association of Transgender Health (WPATH) first recommended that minors as young as 16 who met specific, carefully selected criteria were appropriate to begin hormone treatments (in the fifth version of its Standards of Care).[9] This guideline was released 19 years after the very first guidelines on transgender health (for adults) were published, in 1979.

Between the late 1990s and the early 2010s, the first protocols to delay pubertal onset—with gonadotropin-releasing hormone agonists (GnRHa)—for carefully assessed youth with gender dysphoria (GD) were introduced thanks to the research of Dutch clinicians and researchers at the VU Center of Expertise on Gender Dysphoria in Amsterdam, the Netherlands.[10] This protocol created a safe medical opportunity for transgender youth, whose gender had been very clear and consistent from a young age, to experience *one correctly-gender-aligned* puberty in a similar developmental time frame as their cisgender peers. Prior to this development, transgender adults would have to navigate the experience of *two* puberties: the undesired one first, and then the second, more desired, puberty later on.

By the late 2010s, with promising early data (and clinical experience) coming out of the Dutch clinic,[11] a handful of gender-affirming care clinics for minors opened in the United States. Boston Children's Hospital led the way as the first multidisciplinary service and offered pubertal suppression and gender-affirming hormones to youth utilizing an assessment approach adapted from the Dutch team.[12] Shortly thereafter, in 2011, the long-awaited seventh edition of the Standards of Care (SOC7) was published.[13] SOC7 included treatment recommendations and criteria for treatments based on the preliminary research that demonstrated the benefits of gender-affirming treatments, such as social transition in prepubertal children and puberty suppression, cross-gender hormones, and chest masculinization surgery in adolescents when indicated. Of note, during this time, the *Child and Adolescent Psychiatric Clinics of North America* published its first special issue on TGD youth, including an article that described the development of Boston Children's gender identity clinic.[14]

Following the release of SOC7, gender-affirming clinical services in the United States expanded rapidly.[15] The shift toward greater public recognition and visibility of transgender people was also palpable during this era, with the emergence of mainstream role models like Janet Mock, Jazz Jennings, and Laverne Cox. The appreciation of gender as a dimensional (rather than dichotomous or binary) construct was also evident among both youth and adults, who continued to progress and evolve in their expression of gender along more expansive lines.[8] The contemporaneous *Diagnostic and Statistical Manual of Mental Disorders (Fifth Edition; DSM-5)* even included language that affirmed gender as a spectrum, rather than a binary construct.[16] The Dutch team continued to demonstrate the benefits of gender-affirming medical treatment and, in 2014, published a hallmark longitudinal study in *Pediatrics* that demonstrated the longitudinal benefits of puberty suppression for 55 adolescents who subsequently received gender-affirming hormones and surgery.[11]

Coincidentally, the January 2017 *National Geographic* cover story "Gender Revolution" highlighted the shifting landscape of gender in the same month that Donald Trump became US President. By the late 2010s, more than fifty gender identity clinics in pediatric settings had opened as waitlists surged and clinical complexity increased. With the increase in the number of clinical programs around the country came a marked increase in research being done to better understand TGD patient populations and their clinical care needs.[17-21] Many of the complex, nuanced clinical questions that providers still contemplate emerged during this time, including (1) how long puberty can be suppressed before it is necessary to introduce a sex hormone; (2) the relevance (if any) of the sex ratio of TGD youth presenting for clinical care (e.g., shift from designated-males-at-birth to more designated-females-at-birth); (3) the significance of the length of time during which an adolescent experiences GD when it comes to medical decision making; and (4) how detailed an assessment should be, considering ever-present barriers in accessing care and the ongoing importance of de-pathologizing transgender identities. These questions, among others, continue to dominate the conversations of providers working with young TGD patients.

The September 2022 release of Standards of Care version 8 (SOC8)—the first standards of care document on transgender health that incorporated a Delphi Consensus method[22]—could not have come at a more salient time.[23] Recognizing an evolving evidence base, this process strengthened the integrity of the recommendations by ensuring 75% agreement among an international group of approximately 120 multidisciplinary experts in the field of transgender care. The evidence base now reflects a combination of longitudinal research, short-term research, cross-sectional retrospective surveys, and comparative studies. The evidence base is certainly not "insufficient," as anti-transgender advocates often claim. The evidence base is also not "settled," considering the evolving needs of a patient population that is continuously redefining how we think about gender and bodily autonomy. The SOC8 recommendations for children and adolescents help preserve the integrity of the decision-making process by employing both an affirming and cautious approach simultaneously. So, while some governors and legislatures perseverate on *whether* to do the care, the academics, scientists, and clinicians are figuring out *how* to do the care. SOC8 serves as a vital, yet flexible, guidepost for health care professionals seeking to provide compassionate, affirming, and ethical care.

Given the history described herein, it remains difficult to believe where we find ourselves today. We, as child and adolescent clinician-researchers, did not anticipate the fragility of science-driven progress, the massive resurgence of anti-transgender discrimination, or the related politically-motivated interference. Unfortunately, health care for TGD youth is also being sensationalized in the mainstream media through unsophisticated reporting that oversimplifies the complex experiences of TGD youth and misses the nuances of gender-affirming care.

As many providers are well aware, longitudinal US health data sets on mental and physical health outcomes among TGD youth do remain relatively limited, in large part due to the exclusion of gender identity data from major federally-funded initiatives. Data presented on TGD youth and their families come largely from community-based surveys and university-affiliated research teams. Many of these studies, cited in subsequent articles, exhibit scientifically rigorous and well-designed protocols, especially in light of the methodologic challenges associated with studying marginalized populations often excluded from research and health settings. Existing research data indeed fail to capture the experiences of some of the most isolated and vulnerable TGD youth in the United States, often TGD youth of color and those living in more rural and underserved locations. All youth-serving providers would benefit from increased investment in research on how best to support TGD youth and help them thrive. We offer this issue as a resource for reviewing up-to-date research on TGD youth mental health outcomes and the current care protocols driven by scientific data and expertise. In today's polarizing sociopolitical climate, deciphering study-derived data and examining study design itself are especially useful.

Fortunately, data on TGD youth mental health outcomes are nevertheless more robust than often portrayed in mainstream media. This issue presents a collection of articles written by expert colleagues who are clinicians, educators, parents, and/ or researchers. We aim to support providers navigating the ever-evolving landscape of mental health services for TGD youth and their families through this series of review articles that focus on clinical practice and advocacy within health systems. We aim to highlight the *individualized* nature of mental health presentations among TGD youth across social settings and stages of development.

The issue opens with a primer from Chang, Erickson-Schroth, and Kamceva that provides foundational knowledge pertaining to serving TGD youth, including an overview of common terminology, the nuances of sexual orientation, gender identity, and gender expression, and the interface between these topics, the field of psychiatry, and the *DSM*. Ramos and Marr explore the underlying mechanisms and impacts of traumatic stressors facing TGD youth in today's world, as well as family, community, and school-based resilience factors providers can target. Zhou, Huang, and Howard provide a nuanced examination of intersectional identities, examining some of the unique cultural experiences of black, Latinx, and Asian American and Pacific Islander youth. Importantly, they also examine the challenges facing intersex youth who are pushed to conform to the societal sex binary.

The following three articles summarize important considerations in the assessment of TGD youth, factoring in the varying, and often complex, needs of diverse youth. Leibowitz provides an overview of the recommendations of the *Adolescent* chapter of the WPATH SOC8 and provides a primer on the history and importance of the Standards of Care and the key challenges facing TGD adolescents. Then, Tishelman and Rider provide a parallel overview on the *Childhood* chapter of SOC8 (note that the SOC8 marks the first time that there are two distinct chapters dedicated to children and adolescents). Curtis, Janssen, and Swaringen describe the relationship between complex mental health presentations and gender-diverse identities, providing an affirming framework within which child and adolescent psychiatrists can decipher and prioritize individualized care needs with families and youth. Strang and Van der Miesen, two leading international authorities on the cooccurrence of autism spectrum disorder and gender diversity, provide an overview of its relevance and considerations for treatment.

The next set of articles focuses on gender-affirming treatments and outcomes. Belfort and Brown provide readers with a rich overview of social and psychological interventions designed to help TGD youth navigate the world, highlighting strategies for promoting resilience, supporting healthy exploration of identity, and coping with the adverse effects of minority stress. Ryan, Barba, and Cohen explore the critical role of family support in youth mental health, focusing specifically on provider-parent alignment, parental/caregiver rejecting and supportive behaviors, and the integrated Family Acceptance Project–Trauma-Focused Cognitive Behavioral Therapy model for youth who have experienced trauma. Pediatric endocrinologists Singh and Lopez provide a comprehensive overview of biomedical gender-affirming treatments and the evidence that exists to support their use. Their article is a user-friendly guide for the child and adolescent psychiatrist, as knowledge of these treatments is crucial when working with patients and families seeking them. Finally, Daniolos and Dolotina summarize the existing literature on diverse gender trajectories, specifically those that are nonlinear and may include detransition and/or regret, while integrating real-world clinical presentations.

The last set of articles focuses on the experiences of TGD youth across social systems, including school, faith, welfare, legal, and residential settings. Johnson and Szilagyi explore the vital roles that schools, community organizations, religious groups, and rural communities play in supporting and affirming TGD youth and improving their mental well-being. Balsamo, Wanta, Nguy, and Gianakakos address the needs of TGD youth involved in legal, welfare, and foster care settings. Stevens provides an extensive guide to best practices for TGD youth in inpatient, residential, and other long-term care settings, including recommendations for discharge planning.

Finally, we close with personal reflections from Larson, a child and adolescent psychiatrist whose son came out as transgender at 11 years old. She courageously shares her family's ongoing journey in accessing and exploring gender-affirming care options.

The timeliness of this publication cannot be understated. We present this issue within a climate of intense ongoing anti-transgender rhetoric across the United States—and the fear and chaos it has created for transgender youth and their families, educators, and providers, including us. Many youth and families across the US are directly impacted by discriminatory state bills and laws. Even those youth not directly or practically impacted by legislation are hurt by the pervasive harmful messaging and rampant discrimination they promote. We remain optimistic that science, compassion, morality, and ethics will ultimately prevail, and that we will be able to look back at this moment in history having developed a greater sense of humility and awareness not to take anything for granted. We are grateful to have collaborated with so many inspiring, brave youth and families and our indefatigable colleagues in this work. We appreciate the opportunity to share this important content with you and hope this issue serves as a useful resource for science-driven data and clinical best practices.

Natalia Ramos, MD, MPH
Department of Psychiatry and Biobehavioral Sciences
University of California, Los Angeles
David Geffen School of Medicine
Los Angeles, CA, USA

Serena Chang, MD
Callen-Lorde Community Health Center
New York, NY, USA

Scott Leibowitz, MD
Department of Psychiatry
Nationwide Children's Hospital
Columbus, OH, USA

E-mail addresses:
nramos@mednet.ucla.edu (N. Ramos)
schang@callen-lorde.org (S. Chang)
scottleibowitzmd@gmail.com (S. Leibowitz)

REFERENCES

1. Diamond D. & Schmidt S. Rachel Levine, historic transgender nominee, confirmed as assistant health secretary. Washington Post, 2021. Available at: https://www.washingtonpost.com/health/2021/03/24/rachel-levine-confirmed/. Accessed July 12, 2022.
2. American Civil Liberties Union. Mapping attacks on LGBTQ rights in the U.S. state legislatures. 2023. Available at: https://www.aclu.org/legislative-attacks-on-lgbtq-rights. Accessed April 25, 2023.
3. Redfield E, Conron KJ, Tentindo W, et al. Prohibiting gender affirming medical care for youth. UCLA: The Williams Institute; 2023. Available at: https://williamsinstitute.law.ucla.edu/publications/bans-trans-youth-health-care/. Accessed April 25, 2023.
4. Flores AR, Meyer IH, Langton L, et al. Gender identity disparities in criminal victimization: national crime victimization survey, 2017–2018. Am J Public Health 2021;111(4):726–9.
5. Gay, Lesbian & Straight Education Network (GLSEN), Center for Innovative Public Health Research (CiPHR), Crimes Against Children Research Center (CACRC). Out online: the experiences of lesbian, gay, bisexual and transgender youth on the Internet. 2013. Available at: https://www.glsen.org/sites/default/files/2020-01/Out_Online_Full_Report_2013.pdf. Accessed May 1, 2023.
6. Pew Research Center. Teens, social media and technology 2022. August 2022. Available at: https://www.pewresearch.org/internet/wp-content/uploads/sites/9/2022/08/PI_2022.08.10_Teens-and-Tech_FINAL.pdf. Accessed May 1, 2023.
7. Raifman J, Moscoe E, Austin SB, et al. Difference-in-differences analysis of the association between state same-sex marriage policies and adolescent suicide attempts. JAMA Pediatr 2017;171(4):350–6.
8. Twist J, de Graaf NM. Gender diversity and non-binary presentations in young people attending the United Kingdom's National Gender Identity Development Service. Clin Child Psychol Psychiatry 2019;24(2):277–90.

9. Levine SB, Brown G, Coleman E, et al. The standards of care for gender identity disorders, Fifth Edition. Int J Transgend 1998;2(2). Available at: https://www.brandnewdaycounseling.com/soc9.pdf.

10. De Vries AL, Cohen-Kettenis PT. Clinical management of gender dysphoria in children and adolescents: the Dutch approach. J Homosex 2012;59:301–20.

11. de Vries AL, McGuire JK, Steensma TD, et al. Young adult psychological outcome after puberty suppression and gender reassignment. Pediatrics 2014;134(4): 696–704.

12. Edwards-Leeper L, Spack NP. Psychological evaluation and medical treatment of transgender youth in an interdisciplinary "Gender Management Service" (GeMS) in a major pediatric center. J Homosex 2012;59(3):321–36.

13. Coleman E, Bockting W, Botzer M, et al. Standards of care for the health of trans-sexual, transgender, and gender- nonconforming people, version 7. Int J Trans-gend 2012;13(4):165–232.

14. Leibowitz SF, Spack NP. The development of a gender identity psychosocial clinic: treatment issues, logistical considerations, interdisciplinary cooperation, and future initiatives. Child Adolesc Psychiatr Clin N Am 2011;20(4):701–24.

15. Hsieh S, Leininger J. Resource list: clinical care programs for gender-noncon-forming children and adolescents. Pediatr Ann 2014;43(6):238–44.

16. American Psychiatric Association. Diagnostic and statistical manual of mental disorders. fifth edition. American Psychiatric Publishing; 2013.

17. Arnoldussen M, van der Miesen AIR, Elzinga WS, et al. Self-perception of trans-gender adolescents after gender-affirming treatment: a follow-up study into young adulthood. LGBT Health 2022;9(4):238–46.

18. Olsavsky AL, Grannis C, Bricker J, et al. Associations between gender-affirming hormonal interventions & social support with transgender adolescents' mental health. J Adolescent Health 2023;72(6):860–8.

19. Kuper LE, Stewart S, Preston S, et al. Body dissatisfaction and mental health out-comes of youth on gender-affirming hormone therapy. Pediatrics 2020;145(4): e20193006.

20. Grannis C, Leibowitz SF, Gahn S, et al. Testosterone treatment, internalizing symptoms, and body image dissatisfaction in transgender boys. Psychoneuroen-docrinology 2021;132:105358.

21. Chen D, Berona J, Chan YM, et al. Psychosocial functioning in transgender youth after 2 years of hormones. N Engl J Med 2023;388(3):240–50.

22. Linstone HA, Turoff M. The Delphi method: techniques and applications. Boston: Addison-Wesley; 1975.

23. Coleman E, Radix AE, Bouman WP, et al. Standards of care for the health of trans-gender and gender diverse people, version 8. Int J Transgend Health 2022; 23(Suppl 1):S1–259.

Gender Literacy Across Childhood and Adolescence

Serena M. Chang, MD[a,b,c],*, Laura Erickson-Schroth, MD, MA[d,e],
Marija Kamceva, MD[f]

KEYWORDS

- Sex • Gender • Sexual orientation • Gender expression • Gender identity
- Gender roles • Gender diversity

KEY POINTS

- Children, adolescents, and adults alike have become increasingly comfortable exploring their gender identities and expression.
- This has led to an increase in inquiries regarding gender-affirming care, along with an accompanying sociopolitical backlash resulting in an increasing number of states attempting to enact restrictions and bans, effectively turning health care for transgender and gender diverse youth into a political battlefield.
- Evidence shows that gender-affirming care results in better physical, emotional, social, and psychological health outcomes and well-being for transgender and gender diverse youth and adults.
- This section will define and provide an overview of common gender- and sexual orientation-related terminology and basic topics in order to establish an understanding for the remainder of the chapters in this edition.

Masculine and feminine roles are not biologically fixed but socially constructed.

Gender is not something that one is, it is something one does, an act... a doing rather than a being.

We act as if that being of a man or that being of a woman is actually an internal reality or something that is simply true about us, a fact about us, but actually

[a] Callen-Lorde Community Health Center, 356 West 18th Street, New York, NY 10011, USA;
[b] Department of Psychiatry, New York University, One Park Avenue, New York, NY 10016, USA;
[c] Department of Child and Adolescent Psychiatry, New York University, One Park Avenue, New York, NY 10016, USA; [d] The Jed Foundation, Hetrick Martin Institute for LGBTQ Youth, 530 7th Aveue, Suite 801, New York, NY 10018, USA; [e] Columbia University Medical Center, 530 Seventh Avenue, Suite 801, New York, NY 10018, USA; [f] Department of Psychiatry, Massachusetts General Hospital/McLean Hospital, 1 Fitchburg Street, Apartment F192, Somerville, MA 02143, USA
* Corresponding author.
E-mail address: schang@callen-lorde.org

Child Adolesc Psychiatric Clin N Am 32 (2023) 655–666
https://doi.org/10.1016/j.chc.2023.05.001
1056-4993/23/© 2023 Elsevier Inc. All rights reserved.

it's a phenomenon that is being produced all the time and reproduced all the time, so to say gender is performative is to say that nobody really is a gender from the start.
—Judith Butler, Gender Trouble[1]

INTRODUCTION

A colleague expresses excitement at a group gathering about being 5 months pregnant. After expressing congratulations, what is the inevitable next question?

The "genderization" of children begins long before their birth. From baby outfits to nursery decorations to gender reveal parties, the answer to "is it a boy or a girl?" plays an outsized role in the rituals surrounding anyone caught in the orbit of an impending newborn.

Now think back to your own childhood. What were you taught about "how babies are made"? Did you receive sexual health education in school? How about lessons on sex and gender? How about what it means to "be" a boy or a girl?

Gender—once an afterthought despite its significant yet unspoken role in the average American's daily life (public restrooms, clothes shopping, grooming, sports teams)—has become a fraught sociopolitical issue. The concept of gender as a construct, once relegated to the realm of Women's and Gender Studies courses, went mainstream while concurrently, gender reveal parties have experienced a surge in popularity. Meanwhile, youth (and adults) have become increasingly comfortable exploring their gender identities and expression, which has led to an increase in inquiries regarding gender-affirming care–along with an accompanying backlash resulting in an increasing number of states attempting to enact restrictions and bans, effectively turning health care for transgender youth into the latest political battlefield.

This section will define and provide an overview of common gender- and sexual orientation-related terminology and basic topics in order to establish an understanding for the remainder of the chapters in this edition.

SEXUAL ORIENTATION

The commonly-utilized acronym "LGBTQIA+" is comprised of letters referring to both identities of sexual orientation (lesbian, gay, bisexual, asexual) as well as gender (transgender). It also includes terminology that does not neatly fit into either category: queer and intersex.

Sexual orientation is a term that describes the attraction—romantic and/or sexual—that a person feels toward a certain gender. For instance, heterosexual ("straight") generally implies a binary; of a man exclusively attracted to women, or a woman exclusively attracted to men. The term gay generally refers to men who are attracted to men (although it has also been used colloquially by a spectrum of identities to indicate that one is under the LGB+ umbrella). Lesbian identifies women who are attracted to women, and bisexual indicates one who is attracted to multiple genders, within and beyond the binary. Others use pansexual as a term that similarly indicates an attraction to all genders.

The terms asexual and aromantic refer to a spectrum of identities that generally denote a lack of attraction (sexual and/or romantic) toward others. This is in contrast to those who are allosexual, or who have the capacity to be sexually attracted to others. Queer is also a term used to indicate one is under the "LGBTQIA+" umbrella but is defined less explicitly or specifically. For many members of the community, "queer" has a political connotation, for one who exists beyond the boundaries of a heteronormative, gender-normative nuclear family model. In the mid-twentieth century, "queer" was used as a pejorative term. It has since been "reclaimed" by the younger generation who use the word casually to describe themselves; however, there are many LGBTQIA+ people who avoid the term completely.

It should be noted that there is an under-studied tension between identity and behavior. As these terms are self-defined identities, they do not always reflect *behavior*. Straight and not-straight individuals alike may experiment with or pursue sexual or romantic relationships that do not "align" with their self-reported sexual orientation identity. This does not negate those identities but speaks to the inadequacy of simple identifiers and labels to capture the spectrum, richness, and nuance of human sexuality and experience.

SEX/GENDER

Sexual orientation is partly defined by, but does not otherwise indicate, gender identity. Gender identity is the gender (ie, woman, man, agender, non-binary, and so forth) that a person regards themselves as, or identifies for themself; as in, how one understands their own gender. This may or may not be in contrast to sex, which is typically assigned by a medical professional based on the external genitalia an infant has at birth—"female" for a vagina and "male" for penis/testes.

Hence, a more accurate descriptor for sex is "assigned female at birth" (AFAB) or "assigned male at birth" (AMAB). If someone's gender identity—their internal sense of their gender—aligns with the sex they were assigned at birth, they are cisgender. A cisgender woman would have been assigned "female" at birth and still experiences her own sense of gender as aligned with "girl/woman" as she develops. Transgender individuals are those whose internal sense of their gender is different from the sex they were assigned at birth. This can fall within a binary of gender (ie, boys/men and girls/women) but may not. For instance, a person who was assigned male at birth but who identifies as a woman, may identify as a transwoman. Transgender can also include identities beyond the male/female binary such as non-binary, genderqueer, genderfluid, bigender, or agender. These terms refer to one who does not identify as exclusively as a man or woman, but their specific definition is otherwise not universal. Further, some who identify as non-binary, genderqueer, or agender may not necessarily identify themselves as transgender. Various non-binary, genderqueer, or agender individuals might experience their gender in various ways—as a mix of male and female, as without any gender, as beyond gender, or as a "third" gender.

Additionally, it is essential to note that gender identity does not dictate one's sexual orientation in any way: just like a cisgender woman may identify as heterosexual (attracted only to men), bisexual (attracted to "both" men and women), or lesbian (attracted only to women), a transwoman may identify as heterosexual (attracted only to men), bisexual (attracted to "both" men and women), or lesbian (attracted only to women) as well; she may also use the term "queer" for her sexual orientation if she feels that none of these descriptors are accurate.

As such, gender is frequently understood as a spectrum or gradient, rather than as a binary – the "Gender Unicorn" (**Fig. 1**) is one way of visualizing this concept.[2] Experiences of gender may be difficult to characterize with terminology as well, and individuals may also shift their understanding of their gender over time. New terminology for sexual orientation and gender identity, has and will continue to emerge as culture and society shift. Some of these terms/definitions are limited to the United States, and different countries and cultures may conceptualize orientation and gender in different ways.

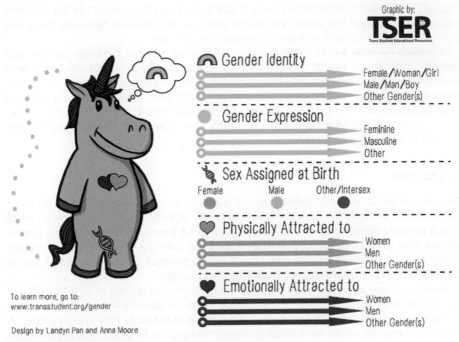

Fig. 1. The gender unicorn.

GENDER EXPRESSION AND GENDER ROLES

Gender identity is related to, but not always in obvious concordance with, gender expression or gender roles. Gender expression is how one presents themselves, in terms of clothing, hairstyle, makeup, or mannerisms. A gender role is an often loosely defined set of social expectations ascribed to a gender. Gender roles themselves are social phenomena, continuously defined and re-defined by society. Many conceptualizations of what it means to be a *man* or *woman* have shifted across time and cultures. These gender "social norms" are frequently transgressed by cisgender individuals, and as such, any number of individuals, cisgender and transgender alike, may not *look* or *act like* their self-defined gender identity. Someone's gender expression—in terms of clothing, hairstyle, mannerisms—may not obviously relate to their gender identity in the dominant social interpretation of that gender expression. A cisgender man may choose to wear their hair long and apply makeup, and still self-identify as a cisgender man, despite not behaving in concordance with the current predominant social role or gender expression of a *man*. Thus, gender role or gender expression is often but not always related to gender identity.

TERMINOLOGY

For a summary of commonly used gender terms, please see **Table 1**, later in discussion. For a summary of commonly used sexual orientation terms, please see **Table 2**, later in discussion.

PRONOUNS

Pronouns are words that can be used to refer to a person or people without using their names. Many transgender people use what are traditionally understood to be male

Table 1
Gender terminology

Term	Definition
Gender identity	The gender (ie, woman, man, agender, non-binary, and so forth) that a person regards themselves as, or identifies for themself; how one understands their own gender
Cisgender ("cis")	Refers to those whose *gender identity* aligns with the sex they were assigned at birth
Sex assigned at birth	Refers to the sex one is assigned at birth based on their external genitalia—includes "assigned female at birth" (AFAB) and "assigned male at birth" (AMAB)
Transgender ("trans")	Refers to those whose internal sense of their gender is different from the sex they were assigned at birth
Gender binary	A distinction of gender into two separate, "opposite" categories: male and female. This is in contrast to an understanding of gender as a spectrum or gradient
Non-binary Genderqueer Genderfluid Bigender	These terms refer to one who does not identify as exclusively male or female, but their specific definition is otherwise not universal; different *non-binary* or *genderqueer* individuals might experience their gender in different ways — as a mix of man and woman, as without any gender, as beyond gender, or as a third gender
Agender	One who does not identify as exclusively male or female, but their specific definition is otherwise not universal. Generally, thought of as a person who does not identify with any gender
Gender expression	How one presents themselves, and specifically their gender identity, in terms of clothing, hairstyle, makeup, mannerisms, or behavior
Gender role	An often loosely defined set of social expectations ascribed to, or generally associated with, a certain gender; the norms a culture associates with a certain gender
Transition	The process of changing legal paperwork, self-expression, social behavior, physiology, or anatomy, amongst others, to align with one's gender identity
Social transition	Involves the changes a person makes to live as their gender in society; these can include choosing a new name or pronouns, or wearing different clothing or hairstyles
Legal transition	The process by which a person's name and gender are recognized legally, that is, by name changes or through changing gender marker on identification documents
Medical transition	Refers to gender-affirming medical interventions, namely medications such as puberty blockers or hormones, that are taken to effect changes to one's body that affirm one's gender identity
Surgical transition	Refers to surgical interventions that are pursued to affect changes in one's body that affirm one's gender identity; these can include chest ("top") surgery or genital ("bottom") surgery

(he/him/his) or female (she/her/hers) pronouns. There are a growing number of non-binary people, as well as others, who use gender neutral pronouns, the most common of which is they/them/theirs. Some people feel comfortable using more than one set of pronouns and may introduce themselves as she/they, he/they, or another combination of pronouns, signaling that others can choose which to use. It can be helpful, especially for children and teens, to try out pronouns to see which fits them best.

Table 2
Sexual orientation terminology

Term	Definition
LGBT LGBTQ LGBTQIA+	Variations of a commonly utilized acronym comprised of letters referring to both identities of sexual orientation (lesbian, gay, bisexual, asexual) and of gender (transgender); it also occasionally includes terminology that does not neatly fit into either category such as "queer" and "intersex"
Sexual orientation	The attraction—romantic and/or sexual—that a person feels toward a certain gender
Heterosexual ("straight")	A term for sexual orientation that generally implies a binary: of a man exclusively attracted to women, or a woman exclusively attracted to men
Gay	A term referring to men who are exclusively attracted to men (although it has also been used colloquially by a spectrum of identities to indicate that one is under the LGB + umbrella)
Lesbian	A term identifying women who are attracted to women
Bisexual	Refers to one who is attracted to multiple genders, both within and beyond the binary
Pansexual	A term that indicates an attraction to all genders
Allosexual	Refers to those who have the capacity to be sexually attracted to others
Asexual Aromantic	Refers to a spectrum of identities that generally denote a lack of attraction (sexual and/or romantic) toward others
Queer	A term used to indicate that one is under the "LGBTQIA+" umbrella, but is defined less explicitly or specifically. For some, "queer" has a political connotation, meaning one who exists beyond the boundaries of a heteronormative, gender-normative, nuclear family model

Referring to someone with their correct pronouns is an essential part of treating them with respect. Bullying and harassment often include the purposeful use of incorrect pronouns to demean someone. The best way to find out someone's pronouns is to ask. The majority of those you ask will be glad that you did so rather than making an incorrect assumption. If you make a mistake, offer a quick apology and move on–it can do more harm than good to focus too much attention on the issue, and over-apologizing puts an emotional burden on the other person.

INTERSEX

Intersex people are those whose bodies or biology do not neatly align with traditional expectations of a "female" or "male" body, with regards to anatomy, hormonal pathways, or chromosomes. Some intersex conditions include androgen insensitivity, congenital adrenal hyperplasia, Klinefelter's, and 5-alpha reductase deficiency. Being intersex is a common, natural variation in biology–between 1% and 2% of people fall into this category.[3] Some people know from birth that they are intersex, while others do not find out until later in life. Despite most intersex people not requiring any gender-specific medical treatment, the standard of care in the past included assigning a gender identity or conducting surgical intervention on intersex infants to ensure external genitalia *looked* "normal" rather than for any medical necessity. Advocacy groups have worked hard to decrease stigma and discourage medical or surgical interventions, especially before a person is able to consent.[4] Some intersex people consider themselves part of transgender communities and others do not.

ETIOLOGY OF GENDER DIVERSITY

Given the increase of interest in gender diversity by medical establishments and media, researchers have attempted to understand its causes. A recent critical review investigated approximately 102 articles studying the etiology of transgender identities, most of which pursued the discovery of a biological feature that might differentiate transgender individuals from their cisgender peers.[5] Results of these studies, which include postmortem tissue, neuroimaging, genetic, digit ratio, and cognitive function studies, frequently contradict one another, and have not been replicable. Further, as the review notes, major methodological gaps exist in article seeking to medicalize and categorize gender identity–much like other social identities, including sexual orientation, race, and ethnicity, gender identity is shaped significantly by cultural and psychosocial factors that are insufficiently explored in biologically oriented studies.

Per WPATH reports, it is not currently "possible to distinguish between those for whom gender identity may seem fixed from birth and those for whom gender identity development appears to be a developmental process"—nor may it matter.[6] Gender diversity itself is not pathological, and as such investigation into etiology may not be necessary, particularly if the purpose is to legitimize identity. The diversity of human experience includes "normal" variations in social identity—gender included—without easily-identifiable "causes."

LGBTQ IDENTITIES AND THE DSM: GENDER DYSPHORIA

Gender diverse youth often interact with mental health or behavioral health institutions in the process of seeking gender-affirming care. When patients experience distress due to an incongruence between their gender identity and sex assigned at birth, this is often referred to as *gender dysphoria*. In the most recent edition of the Diagnostic and Statistical Manual of Mental Disorders (DSM-5), gender dysphoria in children is operationalized as distress due to "a marked incongruence between one's experienced/expressed gender and assigned gender, of at least 6 months' duration," manifested by six additional criteria including dressing as a different gender, preference for toys and activities stereotypically used by a different gender, and a strong dislike of one's sexual anatomy, among others.[7] Notably, not all gender minority youth experience gender dysphoria, and simply identifying as a gender minority is not a pathology.

Prior to this edition, the DSM categorized the experience of being transgender as "gender identity disorder." As observed by changing language in sequential editions of the DSM, psychiatry has a history of pathologizing identities under the LGBTQ+ umbrella. For instance, the first edition of the DSM (1952) classified homosexuality as a "sociopathic personality disturbance" while the subsequent DSM-II (1968) used the categorization of "sexual deviation." Five years later, in 1973, the American Psychiatric Association finally removed homosexuality from DSM-II.[8]

The shift in culture that has begun to understand different sexual orientations and gender identities as normal variations in human experience, has been followed by a shift in language in the DSM, from "transsexuals" (terminology used in the 1950s onward) who were understood to be mentally ill or sexually deviant and categorized under psychosexual disorders and personality disorders, to "gender dysphoria" in the most recent 2013 edition of the DSM.[8]

Even so, patients seeking gender-affirming care often need to obtain a diagnosis of "gender dysphoria" – whether or not they feel it accurately describes their experience – for that care to be covered by medical insurance companies. Without a corresponding medical code that implies pathology, some are concerned that gender-affirming surgical or medical care would then cease to be offered as part of a standard health plan.

Given this history of pathologizing their existence and identities, LGBTQ people often have a complicated relationship with behavioral health care. Psychiatric assessments have been historically required by endocrinologists and surgeons in order for patients to access hormone therapy or gender-affirming surgeries, as recommended by the WPATH's Standards of Care. However, given this pressure, TGNB patients have long felt that they needed to present a certain way to secure such recommendation letters, even if they could also benefit from longer-term engagement in behavioral health support. This is particularly compounded by the context of cost and limited access to psychiatry providers.

PSYCHIATRIC IMPLICATIONS AND PROTECTIVE FACTORS

Numerous studies show that LGBTQ youth (and adults) experience increased rates of violence, trauma, bullying, disproportionate punishment, and other forms of abuse and harassment, social stigmatization, familial rejection, and homelessness when compared to their cisgender heterosexual peers.[8]

Such marginalization and stress can take place across multiple settings including but not limited to: interpersonal, familial, educational, occupational, social, and political, and hence has resulted in chronically increased rates of depression, anxiety, trauma, substance abuse, self-harm, and suicidality.[9,10] More than half of LGBTQ youth endorse symptoms of major depressive disorder and almost two-thirds report symptoms of generalized anxiety disorder.[10] Additionally, symptomology in LGBTQ youth tends to appear sooner in life and with increased duration.[9] It should be noted that there is no evidence of increased risk for psychosis or related conditions such as schizophrenia, schizoaffective disorder, or bipolar disorder.

This is significant because as noted in the landmark Adverse Childhood Experiences (ACE) study, young people exposed to long-term social stressors such as unsafe or rejecting home environments have an especially elevated risk of future chronic health risks including increased rates of multiple causes of adult morbidity and mortality such as substance use, cancers, ischemic events, and other cardiovascular, pulmonary, and hepatic diseases.[11]

Another way to explain the systemic challenges facing LGBTQ populations resulting in disparate behavioral and physical health outcomes is through an intersectional lens. As per Oxford Dictionary, intersectionality is defined as "the interconnected nature of social categorizations such as race, class, and gender as they apply to a given individual or group, regarded as creating overlapping and interdependent systems of discrimination or disadvantage."[12]

In other words, being marginalized in more than one social category (such as race/ethnicity, class, religion, gender, sexuality, ability) makes it harder for minority populations to survive on a daily basis, much less achieve their goals in life. Studies in health disparities show that minority stress and intersectional approaches offer contextualization for how social inequities such as anti-LGBTQ political legislature, homelessness, and education disparities result in increased psychiatric diagnoses such as anxiety, depression, and somatization, as well as external symptomology such as substance use and impulsivity.[13,14]

Unfortunately, compared to their cisgender heterosexual peers, in addition to experiencing increased trauma and stressors, it follows that LGBTQ youth are also less likely to have access to mitigating protective factors, such as supportive families, safe and secure housing, and social support networks.[15,16] Beyond their immediate implications, such context can be concerning for adults concerned about the wellbeing of LGBTQ youth in their lives. Hence, it can be beneficial for clinicians to instead emphasize family, school, and community-based protective factors such as.

- Familial and social support
- Being engaged in one's community, such as serving as a role model for others
- Engagement in social activism, being aware of oppressive social structures
- Receiving gender-affirming care, which may include hormones and/or surgery

Encouraging and building parental/guardian and family support around youth gender identity and sexual orientation is potentially one of the strongest protective factors for LGBTQ youth wellbeing and has been shown to reduce depressive and anxious symptoms as well as reduce risk behaviors in this population.[15] It is particularly notable that transgender pre-pubescent youth who have parental support in their social transitions have rates of depression and anxiety comparable to their cisgender peers.[17]

Similarly, although most LGBTQ youth report experiencing discrimination and harassment in educational settings, it has also been shown that school support, safety, and connectedness result in not only decreased risk behaviors but also increased psychological wellbeing.[18–20]

GENDER TRANSITION

Transition can be divided into several areas, including social transition, legal transition, medical transition, and surgical transition. A person may choose to go through some or all of these, and there is no set order or steps to transitioning.

Social transition involves the changes a person makes to live as their gender in society. These can include choosing a new name or pronoun or wearing different clothing or hairstyles. For children and teens prior to puberty, social transition is the main way that they live authentically in their genders. Young people who are given space to explore their gender identities through social transition have higher life satisfaction and decreased rates of depression.[21] Schools can be supportive of young people's social transition by ensuring they can use the bathrooms and locker rooms consistent with their gender identities as well as participate in sports alongside others of their gender.

Legal transition is the process by which a person's name and gender are recognized legally. Name changes are made on a state level and differ from state to state but generally involve obtaining a court order. Changing gender markers on identification documents is dependent on the document and whether it is state or federally issued. Starting in 2021, passport gender marker changes no longer require a physician's letter and can be made by individuals by filing an application.[22] The same is true of gender on Social Security cards.[23] The steps for changing gender marker on state driver's licenses and non-driver IDs differ by state. Some states allow individuals to file a form on their own behalf, while others make it much more difficult, requiring a physician letter, court order, proof of surgery, or amended birth certificate. The process for amending birth certificates is also state-dependent, with some states continuing to require proof of surgery and a few not allowing amendments at all.[24]

Some transgender people choose to transition medically by taking hormones that affect changes in their bodies. These medications are not used in children or teens before they enter puberty. Once a young person enters puberty, there is the option of taking a gonadotropin-releasing hormone (GnRH) agonist to block further puberty in order to provide time for decisions to be made with their guardians about proceeding with adult hormones. For transmen, testosterone is the primary medication used for transition. Transwomen are often prescribed estrogen along with an androgen blocker such as spironolactone. Hormone treatment has been linked to improvements in mental health and quality of life in both youth and adults.[25,26]

While public perception is that surgery is a major part of transgender experiences, the majority of transgender people do not undergo surgical transition.[27] Some are not interested in this type of transition, while others lack access because of insurance or other financial constraints. Surgical transition generally takes place over the age of 18 in the United States, though certain procedures – most commonly chest surgery – may be available to a small number of those over age 16 with permission from guardians. Chest ("top") surgery is more common than genital ("bottom") surgery. Some transgender people prioritize procedures, such as facial feminization surgeries, that are likely to help them be recognized or "read" as their gender in public, especially those who are vulnerable to harassment and violence.

TREATMENT AND CARE

As seeking gender-affirming care often necessitates interactions with medical establishments, including psychiatry, a number of societies have published best practice guidelines for doing so, most notably including the World Professional Association for Transgender Health (WPATH). The WPATH releases the *Standards of Care for the Health of Transgender and Gender Diverse People* every several years, with the most recent iteration in its eighth edition.[6]

For both children and adolescents, the guidelines recommend an individualized approach to clinical care that integrates patients' families, health care teams, and social environment. The focus of WPATH recommendations for children and adolescents is first on promoting a safe environment for identity exploration, within the medical office and also in other social contexts, including home and school. This exploration can involve a mental health professional, such as a psychiatrist, psychologist, or therapist, whose role is to create an open and non-judgmental environment for youth to process and explore their gender identity. When gender identity seems marked and sustained, various avenues of legal, social, medical, or surgical transition may be pursued.

SUMMARY

Gender identity is a personal understanding of oneself along a vast gradient of possibility, one which is distinct from sexual orientation, and may come with an additional spectrum of gender expressiveness. Pronouns are one of the many ways to respect and affirm someone's gender identity. Transgender and non-binary individuals may seek medical and surgical care, along with other forms of social and legal transition, in order to affirm their identity, which numerous studies have shown to be notably beneficial for their physical, emotional, social, and psychological health and well-being. As the medical field has evolved its understanding of gender diversity, psychiatrists have shifted from pathologizing to affirming gender identity; however, psychiatric and medical evaluation of patients' "gender dysphoria" is still necessary in order to access gender-affirming care, which positions the field both as a source of support and gatekeeping for gender diverse youth.

CLINICS CARE POINTS

- Human beings contain multitudes—don't make assumptions.
- Self-defined identity does not necessary correlate with behavior.

- Using a patient's pronouns are one of the many ways to respect and affirm their gender identity.

- Transgender and non-binary individuals may seek medical and surgical care, along with other forms of social and legal transition, in order to affirm their identity.

- Gender-affirming care results in better physical, social, and psychological health outcomes and well-being for transgender and gender diverse youth and adults.

- As the medical field has evolved its understanding of gender diversity, psychiatrists have shifted from pathologizing to affirming gender identity.

- However, psychiatric and medical evaluation of patients' "gender dysphoria" is still necessary in order to access gender-affirming care, which positions the field both as a source of support and gatekeeping for gender diverse youth.

REFERENCES

1. Butler J. Gender Trouble: Feminism and the subversion of identity. Routledge; 1989.
2. Trans Student Educational Resources. The Gender Unicorn. Published 2015 Available at: https://transstudent.org/gender/. Accessed January 11, 2023.
3. Fausto-Sterling A. *Sexing the body: gender politics and the construction of sexuality.* Basic Books; 2000.
4. InterACT. What is intersex? Available at: https://interactadvocates.org Accessed January 11, 2023.
5. Levin RN, Erickson-Schroth L, Mak K, et al. Biological studies of transgender identity: A critical review. J Gay Lesbian Ment Health 2022;1–30. https://doi.org/10.1080/19359705.2022.2127042.
6. Coleman E, Radix AE, Bouman WP, et al. Standards of care for the health of transgender and gender diverse people, version 8. Int J Transgender Health 2022;23(sup1):S1–259.
7. Diagnostic and Statistical Manual of Mental Disorders: DSM-5TM. 5th edition. American Psychiatric Publishing, a division of American Psychiatric Association; 2013.
8. Drescher J. Out of DSM: Depathologizing homosexuality. Behav Sci 2015;5(4):565–75. https://doi.org/10.3390/bs5040565.
9. Lothwell LE, Libby N, Adelson SL. Mental health care for LGBT youths. FOCUS 2020;18(3):268–76. https://doi.org/10.1176/appi.focus.20200018.
10. The Trevor Project 2021 national survey on LGBTQ youth mental health. The Trevor Project; 2021. Available at: https://www.thetrevorproject.org/survey-2021/. Available at:.
11. Felitti VJ, Anda RF, Nordenberg D, et al. Relationship of childhood abuse and household dysfunction to many of the leading causes of death in adults: the Adverse Childhood Experiences (ACE) Study. Am J Prev Med 1998;14:245–58. https://doi.org/10.1016/S0749-3797(98)00017-8.
12. OED Online. intersectionality, n. Oxford University Press; 2022. Available at: https://www.oed.com/view/Entry/429843. Accessed January 11, 2023.
13. Rhoades H, Rusow JA, Bond D, et al. Homelessness, mental health and suicidality among LGBTQ youth accessing crisis services. Child Psychiatry Hum Dev 2018;49(4):643–51.

14. McInroy LB, Beaujolais B, Leung VWY, et al. Comparing asexual and non-asexual sexual minority adolescents and young adults: stressors, suicidality and mental and behavioural health risk outcomes. Psychol Sex 2022;13(2):387–403.

15. Ryan C, Russell ST, Huebner D, et al. Family acceptance in adolescence and the health of LGBT young adults. J Child Adolesc Psychiatr Nurs 2010;23(4):205–13.

16. Romero Adam P, Goldberg Shoshana K, Vasquez Luis A. LGBT people and housing affordability, discrimination, and homelessness. UCLA. The Williams Institute; 2020. Available at: https://williamsinstitute.law.ucla.edu/publications/lgbt-housing-instability/.

17. Olson KR, Durwood L, DeMeules M, et al. Mental health of transgender children who are supported in their identities. Pediatrics 2016;137(3):e20153223.

18. Eisenberg ME, Resnick MD. Suicidality among gay, lesbian and bisexual youth: the role of protective factors. J Adolesc Health 2006;39(5):662–8.

19. Kosciw Joseph G, Clark Caitlin M, Truong Nhan L, et al. The 2019 National School Climate Survey: The experiences of lesbian, gay, bisexual, transgender, and queer youth in our nation's schools. GLSEN; 2020.

20. Harper C, Dittus P, Steiner R, et al. School connectedness enhances the protective effects of parental monitoring on adolescent sexual risk behavior. J Adolesc Health 2017;60(2):S103–4.

21. Simons L, Schrager SM, Clark LF, et al. Parental support and mental health among transgender adolescents. J Adolesc Health 2013;53(6):791–3.

22. National Center for Transgender Equality. Know Your Rights—Passports. Published 2021 Available at: https://transequality.org/know-your-rights/passports. Accessed January 11, 2023.

23. Social Security Administration. How do I change the sex identification on my Social Security record? Frequenty Asked Questions Available at: https://faq.ssa.gov/en-us/Topic/article/KA-01453. Accessed January 11, 2023.

24. Movement Advancement Project. Equality Maps: Identity Document Laws and Policies. Identity Document Laws and Policies Available at: https://www.lgbtmap.org/equality-maps/identity_document_laws. Accessed January 11, 2023.

25. Mahfouda S, Moore JK, Siafarikas A, et al. Gender-affirming hormones and surgery in transgender children and adolescents. Lancet Diabetes Endocrinol 2019;7(6):484–98.

26. Dhejne C, Van Vlerken R, Heylens G, et al. Mental health and gender dysphoria: a review of the literature. Int Rev Psychiatry 2016;28(1):44–57.

27. Nolan IT, Kuhner CJ, Dy GW. Demographic and temporal trends in transgender identities and gender confirming surgery. Transl Androl Urol Vol 8 No 3 June 27 2019 Transl Androl Urol Urol Manag Transgender Patient. Published online 2019 Available at: https://tau.amegroups.com/article/view/25593. Accessed January 1, 2019.

Traumatic Stress and Resilience Among Transgender and Gender Diverse Youth

Natalia Ramos, MD, MPH[a],*, Mollie C. Marr, PhD[b]

KEYWORDS

- Social stress • Discrimination • Transphobia • Adverse childhood experience
- Resilience • Coping • Transgender • Gender diverse youth • Toxic stress

KEY POINTS

- Traumatic stress during childhood elicits neurobiologic, behavioral, and psychosocial impacts across the lifespan.
- Transgender and gender diverse (TGD) youth face higher rates of abuse and traumatic stress as compared with their cisgender peers.
- Traumatic stressors facing TGD youth include discrete experiences of abuse and recurrent socially-embedded forms of stigma, discrimination, and marginalization.
- TGD youth encounter traumatic stressors across multiple social settings, including at school, at home, and in community settings.
- Clinicians can help TGD youth build resilience by bolstering existing strengths; helping youth heal from trauma; and facilitating connections to supportive activities, peers, and role models.

INTRODUCTION

Childhood trauma is a significant public health problem with lasting consequences. Traumatic stress increases the risk for virtually all mental health conditions and adversely impacts health, academic performance, and coping.[1] The Substance Abuse and Mental Health Services Administration (SAMHSA) defines trauma as an experience of physical, emotional, or life-threatening harm with lasting effects on health and well-being.[2] The terms "toxic stress" and "traumatic stress" refer to stress that overwhelms an individual's support systems, buffering relationships, and coping strategies.[3]

[a] University of California, Los Angeles David Geffen School of Medicine, Jane & Terry Semel Institute for Neuroscience, Los Angeles, CA 90095, USA; [b] Medical Scientist Training Program, Oregon Health & Science University, Portland, OR 97239-3098, USA
* Corresponding author.
E-mail address: nramos@mednet.ucla.edu

Child Adolesc Psychiatric Clin N Am 32 (2023) 667–682
https://doi.org/10.1016/j.chc.2023.04.001
1056-4993/23/© 2023 Elsevier Inc. All rights reserved.

childpsych.theclinics.com

A traumatic experience may present as a single event, such as a physical assault, or a chronic exposure, such as maltreatment in a school setting or family rejection. Transgender and gender diverse (TGD) youth often experience acute and chronic traumatic stressors related to identity-based marginalization and discrimination. Ongoing interpersonal trauma is more likely to cause posttraumatic stress disorder (PTSD)—and is associated with more severe forms of PTSD—than noninterpersonal trauma.[4]

TGD youth face the gamut of common childhood stressors and additionally face higher rates of interpersonal and community-embedded trauma as compared to their cisgender peers. Neurobiologic models of chronic stress and social stress theory provide useful frameworks for conceptualizing how experiences of discrimination, stigma, and rejection across social settings affect mental health. Despite the higher rates of interpersonal traumas facing TGD youth, TGD youth are often quite resilient, particularly when able to access social supports, skill building, and affirming trauma-informed services. Clinicians who identify and address traumatic stress affecting TGD youth patients, while also providing guidance for improving social relationships and accessing supportive activities, can have a profoundly positive impact on mental health.

NEUROBIOLOGICAL UNDERPINNINGS OF TOXIC STRESS

In youth who experience chronic social stress, including family rejection, discrimination, stigma, and/or rejection, physiologic stress response mechanisms become dysregulated. During an acute stress response, changes in neurotransmitters, hormones, and immune mediators promote adaptation and stability, a process known as "allostasis." These time-limited responses are generally protective and helpful to an individual under duress. Chronic activation of stress response systems, however, leads to lasting mental and physical changes that may damage organ systems. Underlying neuroendocrine systems are unable to achieve allostasis when stressors do not remit. As stress builds, an individual exceeds their innate capacity to cope, leading to allostatic overload.[5] Multiple neuroendocrine systems are implicated in the "wear and tear" in the body and brain associated with chronic childhood stress.[6] This model of allostasis (achievement of stability via stress activation) versus allostatic overload (pathophysiologic changes resulting from overuse) helps explain clinical presentations among youth with trauma histories.

Two key neurobiologic systems are known to be affected by toxic stress: the hypothalamic-pituitary-adrenal (HPA) system, which involves glucocorticoids; and the sympathetic adrenomedullary system, which centers on adrenaline (epinephrine and norepinephrine). Areas of the brain implicated in posttraumatic stress symptoms (specifically the hippocampus, amygdala, and prefrontal cortex) are especially sensitive to stress hormones.[6] The amygdala, a region that encodes emotional memories and informs emotional responses,[7] may become hyperresponsive to threats, leading to hypervigilance and a heightened fear response in the absence of true danger—also referred to as "altered fear conditioning."[8,9] Neuroimaging studies have also demonstrated decreased hippocampal volume and abnormal hippocampus functioning in PTSD.[10] Damage to the hippocampus, which helps encode emotional, episodic, and spatial memories, contributes to memory impairment and mood dysregulation seen in PTSD.[11] Lastly, alterations in the shape and/or volume of multiple regions of the prefrontal cortex—in particular the medial prefrontal cortex—impede the extinction of fear responses and downregulation of amygdala activation.[12,13] Stress-related changes in the prefrontal cortex also impact circadian rhythms and memory more generally.[6]

PSYCHOSOCIAL IMPACTS OF IDENTITY-RELATED TOXIC STRESS

Childhood trauma is associated with lasting health effects across the lifespan. Studies have linked childhood trauma to poor physical health,[14–17] greater psychological stress,[15,18] increased risk for psychopathology,[15,16,19–22] and increased risk of substance use.[15] Early studies on childhood trauma centered on childhood adversity, as characterized by the Adverse Childhood Experience (ACE) study.[15] In the ACE study, investigators retrospectively examined adult health outcomes in association with exposure to childhood maltreatment (physical, emotional, and sexual abuse), physical and emotional neglect, and household challenges. Household dysfunction included parental interpersonal violence, a family member with mental illness or substance use, a family member in prison, or parental separation/divorce. The ACE study found a strong direct correlation between the number of ACEs and poor health outcomes. Experiences of early adversity tended to cluster, and data showed a dose-response relationship between the number of ACEs and negative health outcomes in adulthood. For example, participants reporting four or more ACEs had a 4 to 12 times increased risk for alcoholism, drug abuse, depression, and suicide attempts as compared to those who reported no ACEs.[15]

Subsequent studies have added peer rejection, peer victimization, community violence exposure, and socioeconomic status to the ever-growing list of ACEs[23] and emphasized that ACEs all occur within a social context. Historical definitions of ACEs may fail to capture the nuance and pervasiveness of social stress experienced by TGD youth. This expanded definition better captures the experiences of many TGD youth who are repeatedly exposed to peer and family rejection and victimization at higher rates than their cisgender peers.[24]

Risk factors for the development of PTSD following a traumatic event are divided into factors before, during, and after the event. Risk factors before a traumatic event include younger age (when an individual has limited self-regulatory capacity); female sex; lower education level or intelligence; family history of depression, anxiety, or PTSD; history of mental health disorder, temperament, genetic, and/or neurobiologic factors, such as stress reactivity; and a prior individual history of trauma.[25] Risk factors during the event include the level of exposure, intensity of the experience, perception of the event, and whether the trauma is interpersonal and/or intentional. Risk factors after the event include limited social support, limited access to resources/services, ongoing stress, and limited coping skills. Critically, almost none of the risk factors for developing PTSD are within the individual's control. TGD youth often face numerous risk factors for PTSD while experiencing limited social support and reduced access to resources and services. They are also more likely to have experienced prior traumatic events and to face ongoing stressors and instability than cisgender youth.

TGD youth face discrete episodes of maltreatment and abuse and socially embedded discrimination, stigma, and marginalization across community settings. Minority social stress theory explains that both the direct negative consequences of social stressors and the internal experience of anti-transgender discrimination and messaging influence psychological processes.[26] Social stress impacts youths' perception of the external world, fosters concealment of identity, and worsens self-image.[26] Recurrent exposures to traumatic experiences and marginalization compound over time to lower self-image, impede self-efficacy, and decrease health-promoting behaviors. Data clearly show an increased risk for substance use, depression, stress, shame, and loneliness among TGD youth.[27,28] For TGD youth of color, gender minority status intersects with racial-ethnic identity to potentiate social stress. Intersectional framework explains that TGD youth of color experience profound inequities across community, school, legal, and social welfare settings because of compounding marginalization based on race/ethnicity and gender identity and expression.

Clinically, providers often observe internalizing symptoms related to anxiety, depression, and/or PTSD, and, in some youth, externalizing symptoms, such as irritability or reactivity. TGD youth experience disproportionate rates of depression and anxiety disorders as compared to cisgender heterosexual youth.[29-31] LGBTQ individuals also carry a risk of PTSD 1.6 to 3.9 times higher than their cisgender heterosexual peers.[24] Relatedly, the rates of nonsuicidal self-injury, suicidal ideation, planning, and suicide attempts are higher among TGD compared to their cisgender peers.[31] Depression and victimization are significantly associated with higher odds of suicidal ideation among transgender youth[32] and transgender adults.[33] A staggering 45% of LGBTQ youth in the national 2021 Youth Risk Behavior Survey reported seriously considering attempting suicide within the last year, whereas 22% reported an actual attempt in the past year.[34]

Rates of disordered eating are also higher among LGBTQ individuals,[35] with disordered eating behaviors often beginning in childhood or adolescence (as with the general population in the United States [US]).[36] LGBTQ children aged 9 to 10 years old in the Adolescent Brain Cognitive Development Study were more likely to have full or subthreshold binge eating disorder than their cisgender heterosexual peers.[37] Although limited, data on TGD youth and young adults show elevated rates of self-reported eating disorders and, specifically, elevated rates of compensatory behaviors, such as fasting, vomiting, and laxative pill use.[36,38] Increased rates of disordered eating behaviors among TGD youth stem from traumatic experiences, discrimination, gender dysphoria, and body dissatisfaction.[35,36,38,39] Eating disorders are associated with more severe psychiatric symptoms and risk behaviors in early adulthood,[39] presenting additional complex challenges for TGD youth with trauma.

As with cisgender youth, TGD youth with trauma histories are more likely to engage in substance use than peers who have not experienced childhood trauma.[40,41] Among a large national sample, TGD adolescents had higher odds of alcohol use, marijuana use, and illicit drug use over the last year than cisgender adolescents. Experiences of bullying and harassment were associated with increased risk of substance use.[42] Another large cross-sectional analysis conducted among diverse California middle and high school students similarly found elevated rates of heavy alcohol, cigarette, marijuana, illicit drug, and polysubstance use when comparing TGD and cisgender youth (2.4–5 times the odds, depending on the substance). Both recent use (in the last 30 days) and lifetime use were elevated. Not surprisingly, TGD youth were at greater risk for substance use at an earlier age than cisgender peers. Victimization partially mediated the relationship between TGD identity and substance use.[40] Both adolescent PTSD[41] and depression[43,44] have bidirectional, reciprocal effects with substance use, wherein the presence of one increases risk for the other. Adolescents may use substances to mitigate PTSD or depression symptoms, while simultaneously exacerbating underlying symptoms in the long-term. Furthermore, substance use also increases the risk of victimization[45,46] and decreases response to PTSD[45] and depression treatments.[43,44]

PHYSICAL HEALTH IMPACTS OF IDENTITY-RELATED TOXIC STRESS

Minority stress, discrimination, trauma, victimization, and stigma all influence the general health and well-being of LGBTQ people. LGBTQ people experience worse health and more disabilities than their cisgender heterosexual peers, with TGD individuals experiencing the greatest differences in overall health.[47] In addition to minority stress associated with their LGBTQ identities, Black, Native American, and other people of color experience racism and intergenerational and historical racial trauma, which further compounds poor health outcomes.[47] People who experience multiple traumatic events, especially during childhood, are more likely to have a greater burden of persistent somatic symptoms, such as fatigue, dizziness, headaches, gastrointestinal symptoms, and pain.[48–50]

Dysregulation of the HPA axis is one of the lasting effects of childhood adversity, maltreatment, and LGBTQ-related structural stigma.[51–56] HPA axis dysregulation and stress-related disorders are associated with increased inflammatory factors, decreased anti-inflammatory factors, and altered immune responsiveness affecting overall physical health.[57,58] PTSD is also associated with metabolic and autoimmune disorders and increased risk for cardiovascular disease.[59] The autonomic nervous system is undermodulated or overmodulated in PTSD, contributing to a range of gastrointestinal, cardiac, and pulmonary complaints.[49] Neurologic symptoms like gait disturbances, psychogenic nonepileptic seizures, and visual symptoms may also be present. In children and adolescents, traumatic stress has also been associated with catatonia, pseudoneurologic symptoms, and altered arousal states.[49]

The increased vulnerability to somatic symptoms is potentially related to altered physiologic responses and perception of bodily sensations following traumatic events.[48,60] Individuals experiencing interpersonal trauma or multiple traumatic events are more likely to report more severe somatic symptoms.[48] A sense of threat, a common experience for LGBTQ youth, is associated with somatic symptoms.[50] Treatment of PTSD has been shown to improve somatic symptoms.[49]

DISTINCT STRESSORS FACING TGD YOUTH

The true prevalence of traumatic stress among TGD youth is difficult to accurately estimate, because childhood trauma is often underreported as a result of stigma and shame.[61] Exposure to trauma is common in the general US population, with 58% of youth reporting exposure to assault or bullying, sexual victimization, maltreatment by caretaker, property victimization, or witnessed victimization in the past year.[23] The prevalence of childhood trauma is even higher among LGBTQ youth.[62] In a recent cross-sectional study of lifetime exposure to ACEs in LGBTQ youth, 58% reported emotional neglect, 56% reported abuse, and 41% reported living with a family member with mental illness.[63] As with the foundational ACE study,[15] ACEs tended to cluster, with 43% of LGBTQ youth reporting four or more ACEs by age 18.[63] TGD youth report higher rates of maltreatment and ACE scores than cisgender LGBTQ youth.[63] Numerous studies have shown an association between childhood gender nonconformity and an increased risk of childhood abuse.[64,65] In one study, greater gender nonconformity before 11 years of age was associated with greater exposure to childhood abuse and higher rates of PTSD.[24]

Family rejection represents a common form of childhood trauma facing TGD youth.[66] Parental rejection behaviors increase risk for substance use, depression, and suicidality among TGD youth.[66–68] In addition to the direct mental health impacts, family rejection contributes to disproportionate rates of child welfare contact and out-of-home placements for TGD youth.[69] TGD youth additionally face disproportionate rates of homelessness, with family rejection and maltreatment being the leading causes.[70–72] Family conflict, adversarial relationships, and a lack of parent-child closeness are also linked to drug use.[73–76]

LGBTQ youth are also more likely than cisgender heterosexual youth to face bullying and victimization from peers.[77] In a recent national assessment conducted by the Centers for Disease Control and Prevention, almost 25% of LGBTQ students reported bullying at school within the last year, and 30% reported online bullying.[34] One in five LGBTQ students reported ever being forced to have sex, with female students experiencing disproportionate risk compared to male students.[34] In the 2021 National School Climate Survey, 76% of LGBTQ students reported verbal harassment based on identity in the past year.[78] Bullying continues through college and is associated with increased stress, anxiety, and depression, and lower self-esteem.[79,80] Unsurprisingly, LGBTQ youth who experience bullying and victimization in school settings report lower self-esteem and higher levels of depression.[78]

In addition to experiences of bullying and harassment by peers, LGBTQ students experience many other forms of school-based discrimination, including exclusion from school spaces and activities, hearing homophobic and transphobic comments from teachers or staff, and being encouraged to ignore perpetrators and/or to change their own behavior to avoid victimization. More than two-thirds of LGBTQ students report feeling unsafe in school because of factors related to gender or sexual orientation, with 32% missing at least one day of school in the past month as a result. Victimization is itself also associated with an increased risk of school discipline directed toward the LGBTQ student.[78] Bullying and harsher discipline in school settings increase rates of school dropout among LGBTQ youth.[81] These experiences of discrimination are associated with symptoms of PTSD in TGD individuals, even when adjusting for previous traumatic experiences.[82]

The rise of anti-transgender bills around the United States further marginalizes TGD youth, who already face high rates of victimization and discrimination in home and school settings. Public restriction or loss of civil rights among the LGBTQ community contributes to feelings of stigma, hopelessness, internalized homophobia/transphobia, and poor self-image.[83,84] Overall, young LGBTQ Americans experience more profound impacts of discrimination on their psychological well-being than previous generations.[85] TGD youth frequently follow news about transgender rights, with 85% reporting they follow the news closely. More than 85% of TGD youth surveyed nationally reported worsened mental well-being as a result of exposure to debate about anti-transgender state laws.[86] These data align with prior analyses of the effects of political climate on LGBTQ youths' mental health. In the late 2000s, LGB youth living in states that banned same-sex marriage had higher rates of suicide attempts than LGB counterparts in states that legalized same-sex marriage.[87] Data among LGB adults similarly showed higher rates of psychiatric disorders and psychological distress among those living in states that banned same-sex marriage before it was federally recognized[88] and those living in states that do not protect LGBTQ people from employment discrimination or hate crimes.[89]

High rates of abuse and maltreatment, family rejection, and pervasive sociopolitical stress compound to increase psychiatric symptoms, risk behaviors, and maladaptive coping (including substance use and self-harm) among TGD youth. Homelessness, bullying, social stigma, and family rejection are specifically associated with an elevated risk of suicide.[66,90] Additional articles in this special issue detail the roles of school and family environments in the mental well-being of TGD youth.

RESILIENCE AND PROTECTIVE FACTORS FOR TGD YOUTH

Providers can support the mental well-being of TGD youth by recognizing and promoting recovery from trauma and by helping youth build resilience. According to the American Psychological Association, resilience commonly refers to "the process by which people adapt well in the face of trauma, stressors, and adversity."[91] Multiple factors contribute to resilience among TGD youth, including individual coping strategies, interpersonal communication and support, access to resources, and school and community connectedness. Resilience factors can exist at the individual level (eg, self-efficacy skills, strategies for managing stress in helpful ways, social skills, ability to define one's identity), at the relationship level (eg, receiving encouragement and support from others, positive parent-child attachment, family cohesion), and at the community level (eg, reliable support from social networks, engagement in positive extracurricular and community-based activities). Some resilience factors center internal characteristics and skills, whereas others focus on the social support systems around the youth.

The literature on PTSD delineates a set of protective factors that helps prevent the development of clinical PTSD following a traumatic event. Protective factors include: supportive relationships, networks of support, and access to support groups, services, and resources; the response of others to the traumatic event (especially important for children and adolescents); adaptive coping strategies; a strong system of meaning or faith; and opportunities for expression and mastery, stability, hope, or optimism.[25,92] As with PTSD risk factors, many of these protective factors are outside of the individual's control. . Yet, providers who work with TGD youth can often impact the youth's social environment through direct family education and communication; connections to other supportive spaces or resources (e.g., online or in-person youth groups or activities); and safety, interpersonal, and communication skill building.

For many TGD youth, mental health challenges emerge in childhood or adolescence, as gender expression and roles play a larger role in peer socialization. Caregiver attachment and security are foundational to trust and interpersonal relationships throughout the lifespan and highly protective for transgender youth. TGD youth with strong early attachments are often better equipped to buffer socially-embedded discrimination and adversity. Importantly, prepubescent TGD children supported in their gender identity by parents exhibit comparable rates of depression as matched cisgender peers and only slightly higher anxiety scores.[93]

Regardless of age, parental support and engagement are highly impactful. . Studies have consistently shown that parental support and engagement lower the risk of alcohol and drug use in general adolescent populations[94–96] and for LGB adolescents.[97–99] In particular, parental trust, warmth, and involvement decrease tobacco, alcohol, and marijuana use.[100] Research conducted over two decades by the Family Acceptance Project has demonstrated that LGBTQ youth who experience more acceptance and support from their parents display lower rates of depression and suicidality and higher self-esteem.[66,101] Parental behaviors impact youths' social support, self-worth, and overall health. Specific supportive family behaviors associated with improved youth mental well-being include advocating for the youth when mistreated by others, seeking supportive community spaces for the youth, and supporting the youth's gender expression.[66] The Family Acceptance Project provides helpful culturally-tailored guides and handouts for use with families of TGD youth.[101,102]

Peer, community, and school connectedness present additional key targets for bolstering resilience among TGD youth. Positive social support or sense of belonging improves self-esteem; lowers rates of psychological symptoms; and decreases unhealthy adolescent behaviors, such as substance use and high numbers of sexual partners. LGBTQ youth who report acceptance from peers regarding their identity also tend to use substances less than peers who do not experience identity acceptance from peers.[103] Meanwhile, positive relationships with teachers and school staff improve feelings of safety at school,[104] ease the burden of navigating structural barriers at school,[104] and reduce absenteeism among TGD youth.[105] Participation in Gay-Straight Alliance student groups, which offer interpersonal support and educational, advocacy, and/or recreational activities to LGBTQ students and their allies, is associated with better psychological well-being and more social connectedness among LGBTQ students.[106] In fact, the presence of a Gay-Straight Alliance group on a school campus is associated with better overall student well-being[107] and lower rates of risk behaviors among students, including substance use and high numbers of sexual partners.[108]

IMPLICATIONS FOR CLINICAL CARE

Trauma-informed care (TIC), as defined by SAMHSA, is a systems-based approach designed to create safe environments that are responsive to the signs and symptoms of trauma. A trauma-informed approach does the following: "(1) realizes the widespread impact of trauma and understands potential paths for recovery; (2) recognizes the signs and symptoms of trauma in clients, families, staff, and others involved with the system; (3) responds by fully integrating knowledge about trauma into policies, procedures, and practices; and (4) resists re-traumatization."[2] Within health care settings, trauma-informed principles and practices support patients, families, and professionals through trust, collaboration, safety, and empowerment.[2] TIC is of particular relevance to TGD youth, who have often experienced a multitude of traumatic stressors and barriers when presenting to care settings.

In addition to TIC, the gender affirmative framework is another key guiding set of principles for providing high-quality care to TGD youth and their families. TIC and gender-affirming care guide systems of care and individual providers in creating safe, supportive environments for TGD youth.[109] At its core, gender-affirmative framework contends that gender presentations are diverse, vary across cultures, and vary over time and that no gender identity or expression is pathologic. Gender is informed by biology, development, socialization, culture, and context. For some youth, gender is evolving and/or fluid, and for some youth gender is nonbinary. As discussed herein, clinical symptoms and risk-taking behaviors result from TGD youth's experiences in society and by cultural reactions to their gender identities and presentations.[110–113] Providers who adopt gender-affirmative framework engage in the following best practices: (1) approaching LGBTQ identities as natural, normal variations of human sexuality and gender; (2) acquiring and using accurate knowledge to effectively provide mental health care to LGBTQ clients; (3) addressing and counteracting anti-LGBTQ attitudes, stigma, and minority stress; and (4) providing support and promoting resilience and pride.[114–116] SAMHSA further encourages providers to consistently use affirming language (including names and pronouns), support LGBTQ peer support, and ensure that services are responsive to the needs of TGD individuals.[117]

Gender-affirming care is associated with reduced symptoms of depression, suicidal ideation, and suicide attempts.[118–120] The specific act of using pronouns and chosen names has also been shown to reduce depressive symptoms and suicidal behaviors.[119] Importantly, greater symptom reduction was directly associated with the use of pronouns and chosen name in a greater number of contexts.[119] When providers assist families in adopting accepting behaviors, TGD youths' self-esteem, social support, and health are all likely to improve.[66] The improvements in depression and suicidal ideation observed with gender-affirming care are lasting and significant. Over a 1-year follow-up period, gender-affirming care was associated with a 60% lower odds of moderate or severe depression and a 73% lower odds of suicidality.[120] Beyond improvements in depressive symptoms and suicidality, studies demonstrate that gender-affirming care is also associated with improvements in psychosocial functioning, physical health, quality of life, and general well-being.[121–123]

SUMMARY

TGD youth experience higher rates of abuse, assault, and maltreatment than their cisgender peers. Some TGD youth further experience toxic stress associated with identity rejection by family, peers, communities, and societal attitudes and messages.[109] Toxic stress often presents as pervasive interpersonal and community-based discrimination, rejection, and marginalization. Providers working with TGD youth and their families can improve mental well-being by addressing underlying trauma symptoms while bolstering individual skills, family and peer supports, and school and community connectedness.

CLINIC CARE POINTS

- Providers should screen for childhood trauma and toxic stress symptoms among their TGD patients.
- TGD youth benefit from interventions that target individual coping strategies, healthy relationships, and community/school connectedness.
- Trauma-informed care and gender-affirming care principles guide high-quality care for TGD youth.

ACKNOWLEDGMENTS AND SUPPORT

Dr N. Ramos receives funding from the National Institute on Drug Abuse, United States of the National Institutes of Health, United States under the AACAP NIDA K12 program (K12 DA000357). Dr M.C. Marr receives funding from the National Institute of Mental Health, United States (F30 MH118762). The authors report no biomedical financial interests or potential conflicts of interest. Contents are solely the responsibility of the authors and do not necessarily represent the official view of NIH or their institutions.

REFERENCES

1. Bethell CD, Newacheck P, Hawes E, Halfon N. Adverse childhood experiences: assessing the impact on health and school engagement and the mitigating role of resilience. Health Aff (Millwood) 2014;33(12):2106–15. https://doi.org/10.1377/hlthaff.2014.0914.
2. SAMHSA. SAMHSA's Concept of Trauma and Guidance for a Trauma-Informed Approach. 2014.
3. McEwen BS. Neurobiological and systemic effects of chronic stress. Chronic Stress (Thousand Oaks, Calif) 2017;1.
4. Yoo Y, Park HJ, Park S, et al. Interpersonal trauma moderates the relationship between personality factors and suicidality of individuals with posttraumatic stress disorder. PLoS One 2018;13(1):e0191198.
5. Guidi J, Lucente M, Sonino N, et al. Allostatic load and its impact on health: a systematic review. Psychother Psychosom 2021;90(1):11–27.
6. McEwen BS, Morrison JH. The brain on stress: vulnerability and plasticity of the prefrontal cortex over the life course. Neuron 2013;79(1):16–29.
7. Davis M, Whalen PJ. The amygdala: vigilance and emotion. Mol Psychiatry 2001;6(1):13–34.

8. Orr SP, Metzger LJ, Lasko NB, et al. De novo conditioning in trauma-exposed individuals with and without posttraumatic stress disorder. J Abnorm Psychol 2000;109(2):290–8.

9. Peri T, Ben-Shakhar G, Orr SP, Shalev AY. Psychophysiologic assessment of aversive conditioning in posttraumatic stress disorder. Biol Psychiatry 2000; 47(6):512–9.

10. Shin LM, Rauch SL, Pitman RK. Amygdala, medial prefrontal cortex, and hippocampal function in PTSD. Ann N Y Acad Sci 2006;1071:67–79.

11. Yehuda R. Linking the neuroendocrinology of post-traumatic stress disorder with recent neuroanatomic findings. Semin Clin Neuropsychiatry 1999;4(4):256–65.

12. Morgan MA, Romanski LM, LeDoux JE. Extinction of emotional learning: contribution of medial prefrontal cortex. Neurosci Lett 1993;163(1):109–13.

13. Quirk GJ, Russo GK, Barron JL, Lebron K. The role of ventromedial prefrontal cortex in the recovery of extinguished fear. J Neurosci 2000;20(16):6225–31.

14. Anda RF, Felitti VJ, Bremner JD, et al. The enduring effects of abuse and related adverse experiences in childhood. A convergence of evidence from neurobiology and epidemiology. Eur Arch Psychiatry Clin Neurosci 2006;256(3):174–86.

15. Felitti VJ, Anda RF, Nordenberg D, et al. Relationship of childhood abuse and household dysfunction to many of the leading causes of death in adults. The Adverse Childhood Experiences (ACE) Study. Am J Prev Med 1998;14(4): 245–58. http://www.ncbi.nlm.nih.gov/pubmed/9635069. Accessed April 2, 2018.

16. Min MO, Minnes S, Kim H, Singer LT. Pathways linking childhood maltreatment and adult physical health. Child Abuse Negl 2013;37(6):361–73.

17. Springer KW, Sheridan J, Kuo D, Carnes M. The long-term health outcomes of childhood abuse: an overview and a call to action. J Gen Intern Med 2003; 18(10):864–70.

18. D'Andrea W, Ford J, Stolbach B, et al. Understanding interpersonal trauma in children: why we need a developmentally appropriate trauma diagnosis. Am J Orthopsychiatry 2012;82(2):187–200. https://doi.org/10.1111/j.1939-0025. 2012.01154.x.

19. Afifi TO, Boman J, Fleisher W, et al. The relationship between child abuse, parental divorce, and lifetime mental disorders and suicidality in a nationally representative adult sample. Child Abuse Negl 2009;33(3):139–47.

20. Duncan RD, Saunders BE, Kilpatrick DG, Hanson RF, Resnick HS. Childhood physical assault as a risk factor for PTSD, depression, and substance abuse: findings from a national survey. Am J Orthopsychiatry. 1996;66(3):437–448. http://www.ncbi.nlm.nih.gov/pubmed/8827267. Accessed April 2, 2018.

21. Edwards VJ, Holden GW, Felitti VJ, et al. Relationship between multiple forms of childhood maltreatment and adult mental health in community respondents: results from the adverse childhood experiences study. Am J Psychiatry 2003; 160(8):1453–60.

22. Heim C, Newport DJ, Mletzko T, et al. The link between childhood trauma and depression: insights from HPA axis studies in humans. Psychoneuroendocrinology 2008;33(6):693–710.

23. Finkelhor D, Turner HA, Shattuck A, et al. Violence, crime, and abuse exposure in a national sample of children and youth: an update. JAMA Pediatr 2013; 167(7):614–21.

24. Roberts AL, Rosario M, Corliss HL, et al. Elevated risk of posttraumatic stress in sexual minority youths: mediation by childhood abuse and gender nonconformity. Am J Public Health 2012;102(8):1587–93.

25. Sayed S, Iacoviello BM, Charney DS. Risk factors for the development of psychopathology following trauma. Curr Psychiatry Rep 2015;17(8):1–7.

26. Meyer IH. Minority stress and mental health in gay men. J Health Soc Behav 1995;36(1):38–56.

27. Scheer JR, Edwards KM, Helminen EC, Watson RJ. Victimization Typologies Among a Large National Sample of Sexual and Gender Minority Adolescents. https://home.liebertpub.com/lgbt. 2021;8(8):507–518. doi:10.1089/LGBT.2021.0024.

28. Scheer JR, Antebi-Gruszka N. A psychosocial risk model of potentially traumatic events and sexual risk behavior among LGBTQ individuals. J Trauma Dissociation 2019;20(5):603–18.

29. Wallien MSC, Van Goozen SHM, Cohen-Kettenis PT. Physiological correlates of anxiety in children with gender identity disorder. Eur Child Adolesc Psychiatry 2007;16(5):309–15.

30. Cohen-Kettenis PT, Owen A, Kaijser VG, et al. Demographic characteristics, social competence, and behavior problems in children with gender identity disorder: a cross-national, cross-clinic comparative analysis. J Abnorm Child Psychol 2003;31(1):41–53.

31. Atteberry-Ash B, Kattari SK, Harner V, et al. Differential experiences of mental health among transgender and gender-diverse youth in Colorado. Behav Sci (Basel) 2021;11(4). https://doi.org/10.3390/BS11040048.

32. Perez-Brumer A, Day JK, Russell ST, et al. Prevalence and correlates of suicidal ideation among transgender youth in California: findings from a representative, population-based sample of high school students. J Am Acad Child Adolesc Psychiatry 2017;56(9):739.

33. Sutter M, Perrin PB. Discrimination, mental health, and suicidal ideation among LGBTQ people of color. J Couns Psychol 2016;63(1):98–105.

34. Centers for Disease Control and Prevention (CDC). The Youth Risk Behavior Survey Data Summary & Trends Report: 2011–2021. https://www.cdc.gov/healthyyouth/data/yrbs/yrbs_data_summary_and_trends.htm. Published 2023.

35. Nagata JM, Ganson KT, Austin SB. Emerging trends in eating disorders among sexual and gender minorities. Curr Opin Psychiatry 2020;33(6):562.

36. McClain Z, Peebles R. Body image and eating disorders among lesbian, gay, bisexual, and transgender youth. Pediatr Clin North Am 2016;63(6):1079.

37. Schvey NA, Pearlman AT, Klein DA, et al. Obesity and eating disorder disparities among sexual and gender minority youth. JAMA Pediatr 2021;175(4):412–5.

38. Guss CE, Williams DN, Reisner SL, et al. Disordered weight management behaviors, nonprescription steroid use, and weight perception in transgender youth. J Adolesc Health 2017;60(1):17–22.

39. Micali N, Solmi F, Horton NJ, et al. Adolescent eating disorders predict psychiatric, high-risk behaviors and weight outcomes in young adulthood. J Am Acad Child Adolesc Psychiatry 2015;54(8):652–9, e1.

40. Day JK, Fish JN, Perez-Brumer A, et al. Transgender youth substance use disparities: results from a population-based sample. J Adolesc Health 2017;61(6):729–35.

41. Simmons S, Suárez L. Substance abuse and trauma. Child Adolesc Psychiatr Clin N Am 2016;25(4):723–34.

42. Reisner SL, Greytak EA, Parsons JT, Ybarra ML. Gender minority social stress in adolescence: disparities in adolescent bullying and substance use by gender identity. J Sex Res 2015;52(3):243–56.

43. Goldstein BI, Shamseddeen W, Spirito A, et al. Substance use and the treatment of resistant depression in adolescents. J Am Acad Child Adolesc Psychiatry 2009;48(12):1182–92.

44. SAMHSA. Key Substance Use and Mental Health Indicators in the United States: Results from the 2018 National Survey on Drug Use and Health. HHS Public. Rockville: Center for Behavioral Health Statistics and Quality, Substance Abuse and Mental Health Services Administration; 2019. https://www.samhsa.gov/data/.

45. NCTSN. Making the connection: trauma and substance abuse. www.nctsn.org/sites/default/files/assets/pdfs/SAToolkit_1.pdf. Published 2008.

46. Kingston S, Raghavan C. The relationship of sexual abuse, early initiation of substance use, and adolescent trauma to PTSD. J Trauma Stress 2009;22(1):65–8.

47. NASEM. Understanding the Well-Being of LGBTQI+ Populations. Washington, DC: The National Academies Press; 2020.

48. Barends H, van der Wouden JC. Claassen-van Dessel N, Twisk JWR, van der Horst HE, Dekker J. Potentially traumatic events, social support and burden of persistent somatic symptoms: a longitudinal study. J Psychosom Res 2022;159.

49. Gupta MA. Review of somatic symptoms in post-traumatic stress disorder. Int Rev Psych. 2013;25(1):86–99.

50. Jowett S, Shevlin M, Hyland P, et al. Posttraumatic stress disorder and persistent somatic symptoms during the COVID-19 pandemic: the role of sense of threat. Psychosom Med 2021;83(4):338–44.

51. Gerritsen L, Milaneschi Y, Vinkers CH, et al. HPA axis genes, and their interaction with childhood maltreatment, are related to cortisol levels and stress-related phenotypes. Neuropsychopharmacology 2017;42(12):2446–55.

52. Hatzenbuehler ML, McLaughlin KA. Structural stigma and hypothalamic-pituitary-adrenocortical axis reactivity in lesbian, gay, and bisexual young adults. Ann Behav Med 2014;47(1):39.

53. Heim C, Shugart M, Craighead WE, Nemeroff CB. Neurobiological and psychiatric consequences of child abuse and neglect. Dev Psychobiol 2010;52(7):671–90.

54. Mijas M, Blukacz M, Koziara K, et al. Dysregulated by stigma: cortisol responses to repeated psychosocial stress in gay and heterosexual men. Psychoneuroendocrinology 2021;(131):105325.

55. Tarullo AR, Gunnar MR. Child maltreatment and the developing HPA axis. Horm Behav 2006;50(4):632–9.

56. Van Voorhees E, Scarpa A. Effects of child maltreatment on the hypothalamic-pituitary-adrenal axis. Trauma, Violence, Abus 2004;5(4):333–52.

57. Silverman MN, Sternberg EM. Glucocorticoid regulation of inflammation and its functional correlates: from HPA axis to glucocorticoid receptor dysfunction. Ann N Y Acad Sci 2012;1261(1):55–63.

58. Sun Y, Qu Y, Zhu J. The relationship between inflammation and post-traumatic stress disorder. Front Psychiatry 2021;(12):1385.

59. Katrinli S, Oliveira NCS, Felger JC, Michopoulos V, Smith AK. The role of the immune system in posttraumatic stress disorder. Transl Psychiatry 2022;12(1):1–14.

60. Atanasova K, Lotter T, Reindl W, Lis S. Multidimensional assessment of interoceptive abilities, emotion processing and the role of early life stress in inflammatory bowel diseases. Front psychiatry 2021;12.

61. Giovannoni J. Definitional issues in child maltreatment. In: Cicchetti D, Carlson V, editors. Child Maltreatment: Theory and Research on the Causes and Consequences of Child Abuse and Neglect. New York: Cambridge University Press; 1989. p. 3–37.

62. Elze DE. The lives of lesbian, gay, bisexual, and transgender people: a trauma-informed and human rights perspective. Trauma Hum Rights 2019;179–206.

63. Craig SL, Austin A, Levenson J, Leung VWY, Eaton AD, D'Souza SA. Frequencies and patterns of adverse childhood events in LGBTQ+ youth. Child Abuse Negl 2020;107.

64. Warren AS, Goldsmith KA, Rimes KA. Childhood gender-typed behaviour, sexual orientation, childhood abuse and post-traumatic stress disorder: a prospective birth-cohort study. Int Rev Psychiatry 2022;34(3-4):360–75.

65. Bos H, de Haas S, Kuyper L. Lesbian, gay, and bisexual adults: childhood gender nonconformity, childhood trauma, and sexual victimization. J Intepers Violance 2016;34(3):496–515.

66. Ryan C, Russell ST, Huebner D, Diaz R, Sanchez J. Family acceptance in adolescence and the health of LGBT young adults. J Child Adolesc Psychiatr Nurs 2010;23(4):205–13.

67. Grossman AH, D'Augelli AR. Transgender youth: invisible and vulnerable. J Homosex 2006;51(1):111–28.

68. Main M, Goldwyn R. Predicting rejection of her infant from mother's representation of her own experience: implications for the abused-abusing intergenerational cycle. Child Abuse Negl 1984;8(2):203–17.

69. Irvine A, Canfield A. The Overrepresentation of Lesbian, Gay, Bisexual, Questioning, Gender Nonconforming and Transgender Youth Within the Child Welfare to Juvenile Justice Crossover Population. Soc Policy Law. 2016;24(2):243–261. http://digitalcommons.wcl.american.edu/jgsplhttp://digitalcommons.wcl.american.edu/jgspl/vol24/iss2/2. Accessed April 16, 2023.

70. Whitbeck LB, Chen X, Hoyt DR, Tyler KA, Johnson KD. Mental disorder, subsistence strategies, and victimization among gay, lesbian, and bisexual homeless and runaway adolescents. J Sex Res 2004;41(4):329–42.

71. Rew L, Whittaker TA, Taylor-Seehafer MA, Smith LR. Sexual health risks and protective resources in gay, lesbian, bisexual, and heterosexual homeless youth. J Spec Pediatr Nurs 2005;10(1):11–9.

72. Durso LE, Gates GJ. Serving Our Youth: Findings from a National Survey of Services Providers Working with Lesbian, Gay, Bisexual and Transgender Youth Who Are Homeless or At Risk of Becoming Homeless. Los Angeles, CA: The Williams Institute with True Colors Fund and The Palette Fund; 2012.

73. Norem-Hebeisen A, Johnson DW, Anderson D, Johnson R. Predictors and concomitants of changes in drug use patterns among teenagers. J Soc Psychol 1984;124(1ST Half):43–50.

74. Brook JS, Lukoff IF, Whiteman M. Initiation into adolescent marijuana use. J Genet Psychol 1980;137(1st Half):133–42.

75. Kandel DB, Kessler RC, Margulies RZ. Antecedents of adolescent initiation into stages of drug use: a developmental analysis. J Youth Adolesc 1978;7(1):13–40.

76. Guo J, Hill KG, Hawkins JD, Catalano RF, Abbott RD. A developmental analysis of sociodemographic, family, and peer effects on adolescent illicit drug initiation. J Am Acad Child Adolesc Psychiatry 2002;41(7):838–45.

77. Moyano N. Sánchez-Fuentes M del M. Homophobic bullying at schools: a systematic review of research, prevalence, school-related predictors and consequences. Aggress Violent Behav 2020;(53):101441.

78. Kosciw JG, Clark CM, Menard L. The 2021 National School Climate Survey: The Experiences of LGBTQ+ Youth in Our Nation's Schools. New York: GLSEN; 2022.

79. Seelman KL, Woodford MR, Nicolazzo Z. Victimization and Microaggressions Targeting LGBTQ College Students: Gender Identity As a Moderator of Psychological Distress. J Ethnic Cult Div Soc. 2016;26(1-2):112–125.

80. Moran TE, Chen CYC, Tryon GS. Bully victimization, depression, and the role of protective factors among college LGBTQ students. J Community Psychol 2018; 46(7):871–84.

81. Kosciw J.G., Greytak E.A., Giga N.M., et al., The 2015 National School Climate Survey: The Experiences of Lesbian, Gay, Bisexual, Transgender, and Queer Youth in Our Nation's Schools. New York: GLSEN; 2015.

82. Reisner SL, Hughto JMW, Gamarel KE, Keuroghlian AS, Mizock L, Pachankis JE. Discriminatory experiences associated with posttraumatic stress disorder symptoms among transgender adults. J Couns Psychol 2016;63(5): 509–19.

83. Woodford MR, Paceley MS, Kulick A, Hong JS. The LGBQ social climate matters: policies, protests, and placards and psychological well-being among LGBQ emerging adults. J Gay Lesbian Soc Serv 2015;27(1):116–41.

84. Bauermeister JA. How statewide LGB policies go from "under our skin" to "into our hearts": fatherhood aspirations and psychological well-being among emerging adult sexual minority men. J Youth Adolesc 2014;43(8):1295.

85. Gruberg S, Mahowald L, Halpin J. The State of the LGBTQ Community in 2020- Center for American Progress. https://www.americanprogress.org/issues/lgbtq-rights/reports/2020/10/06/491052/state-lgbtq-community-2020/. Published 2020. Accessed May 30, 2021.

86. The Trevor Project. Issues Impacting LGBTQ Youth.; 2022. https://www.thetrevorproject.org/wp-content/uploads/2022/01/TrevorProject_Public1.pdf.

87. Raifman J, Moscoe E, Austin SB, McConnell M. Difference-in-differences analysis of the association between state same-sex marriage policies and adolescent suicide attempts. JAMA Pediatr 2017;171(4):350–6.

88. Scales Rostosky S, Riggle BED, Horne SG, Miller AD. Marriage amendments and psychological distress in lesbian, gay, and bisexual (LGB) adults. J Counsel Phy 2009. https://doi.org/10.1037/a0013609.

89. Hatzenbuehler ML, Keyes KM, Hasin DS. State-level policies and psychiatric morbidity in lesbian, gay, and bisexual populations. Am J Public Health 2009; 99(12):2275.

90. Ream G, Peters A. Working with suicidal and homeless LGBTQ+ youth in the context of family rejection. J Heal Serv Psychol 2021;47(1):41–50.

91. APA Dictionary of Psychology. https://dictionary.apa.org/. Published 2023. Accessed April 15, 2023.

92. Campodonico C, Berry K, Haddock G, Varese F. Protective factors associated with post-traumatic outcomes in individuals with experiences of psychosis. Front Psychiatry 2021;(12):2164.

93. Olson KR, Durwood L, Demeules M, McLaughlin KA. Mental health of transgender children who are supported in their identities. Pediatrics 2016;137(3): 20153223.

94. Resnick MD, Bearman PS, Blum RW, et al. Protecting adolescents from harm. Findings from the National Longitudinal Study on Adolescent Health. JAMA 1997;278(10):823–32.

95. Bukstein OG, Bernet W, Arnold V, et al. Practice parameter for the assessment and treatment of children and adolescents with substance use disorders. J Am Acad Child Adolesc Psychiatry 2005;44(6):609–21.

96. Hawkins JD, Catalano RF, Miller JY. Risk and protective factors for alcohol and other drug problems in adolescence and early adulthood: implications for substance abuse prevention. Psychol Bull 1992;112(1):64–105.

97. Eisenberg ME, Resnick MD. Suicidality among gay, lesbian and bisexual youth: the role of protective factors. J Adolesc Health 2006;39(5):662–8.

98. Needham BL, Austin EL. Sexual orientation, parental support, and health during the transition to young adulthood. J Youth Adolesc 2010;39(10):1189–98.

99. Ryan C, Huebner D, Diaz RM, Sanchez J. Family rejection as a predictor of negative health outcomes in white and Latino lesbian, gay, and bisexual young adults. Pediatrics 2009;123(1):346–52.

100. Hundleby JD, Mercer GW. Family and friends as social environments and their relationship to young adolescents' use of alcohol, tobacco, and marijuana. J Marriage Fam 1987;49(1):151.

101. Ryan C. Helping Families Support Their Lesbian, Gay, Bisexual,and Transgender (LGBT) Children. Washington, DC: National Center for Cultural Competence, Georgetown University Center for Child and Human Development; 2009.

102. Ryan C. Supportive Families, Healthy Children: Helping Families with Lesbian, Gay, Bisexual & Transgender Children. San Francisco: Family Acceptance Project, San Francisco State University; 2009.

103. Rosario M, Schrimshaw EW, Hunter J. Disclosure of sexual orientation and subsequent substance use and abuse among lesbian, gay, and bisexual youths: critical role of disclosure reactions. Psychol Addict Behav 2009;23(1):175.

104. McGuire JK, Anderson CR, Toomey RB, Russell ST. School climate for transgender youth: a mixed method investigation of student experiences and school responses. J Youth Adolesc 2010;39(10):1175–88.

105. Greytak EA, Kosciw JG, Boesen MJ. Putting the "T" in "Resource": The Benefits of LGBT-Related School Resources for Transgender Youth. J LGBT Youth 2013; 10(1–2):45–63. https://doi.org/10.1080/19361653.2012.718522.

106. Herdt G, Russell ST, Sweat J, Marzullo M. Sexual inequality, youth empowerment, and the GSA: a community study in California. Sex Inequalities Soc Justice 2006;233–51.

107. Ioverno S, Baiocco R, Belser AB, Grossman AH, Russell ST. The protective role of gay-straight alliances for lesbian, gay, bisexua and questioning students: a prospective analysis. Psychol Sex Orientat Gend Divers 2016;3(4):397–406.

108. Poteat VP, Sinclair KO, Digiovanni CD, Koenig BW, Russell ST. Gay–straight alliances are associated with student health: a multischool comparison of LGBTQ and heterosexual youth. J Res Adolesc 2013;23(2):319–30.

109. Clarke M, Farnan A, Barba A, et al. Gender-Affirming Care Is Trauma-Informed Care. Los Angeles, CA, and Durham, NC: National Center for Child Traumatic Stress; 2022.

110. Hidalgo MA, Ehrensaft D, Tishelman AC, et al. The gender affirmative model: what we know and what we aim to learn. Hum Dev 2013;56(5):285–90.

111. Hendricks ML, Testa RJ. A conceptual framework for clinical work with transgender and gender nonconforming clients: an adaptation of the minority stress model. Prof Psychol Res Pract 2012;43(5):460–7.

112. Ehrensaft D. The Gender Creative Child : Pathways for Nurturing and Supporting Children Who Live Outside Gender Boxes. New York: The Experiment

Publishing; 2016. https://theexperimentpublishing.com/catalogs/spring-2016/gender-creative-child/. Accessed April 15, 2023.

113. Keo-Meier C, Ehrensaft D. The Gender Affirmative Model: An Interdisciplinary Approach to Supporting Transgender and Gender Expansive Children. Washington, DC: American Psychological Association (APA); 2018.

114. Moradi B, Budge SL. Engaging in LGBQ+ affirmative psychotherapies with all clients: defining themes and practices. J Clin Psychol 2018;74(11):2028–42.

115. Pepping CA, Lyons A, Morris EMJ. Affirmative LGBT psychotherapy: outcomes of a therapist training protocol. Psychotherapy (Chic) 2018;55(1):52–62.

116. Pachankis JE. The scientific pursuit of sexual and gender minority mental health treatments: toward evidence-based affirmative practice. Am Psychol 2018; 73(9):1207.

117. Levenson JS, Craig SL, Austin A. Trauma-informed and affirmative mental health practices with LGBTQ+ clients. Psychol Serv 2023;20(Suppl 1).

118. van Bergen DD, Dumon E, Parra LA, et al. "I don't feel at home in this world" sexual and gender minority emerging adults' self-perceived links between their suicidal thoughts and sexual orientation or gender identity. Can J Psychiatry 2023. https://doi.org/10.1177/07067437221147420/ASSET/IMAGES/LARGE/10.1177.

119. Russell ST, Pollitt AM, Li G, Grossman AH. Chosen name use is linked to reduced depressive symptoms, suicidal ideation, and suicidal behavior among transgender youth. J Adolesc Health 2018;63(4):503–5.

120. Tordoff DM, Wanta JW, Collin A, Stepney C, Inwards-Breland DJ, Ahrens K. Mental health outcomes in transgender and nonbinary youths receiving gender-affirming care. JAMA Netw Open 2022;5(2):e220978.

121. Allen LR, Watson LB, Egan AM, Moser CN. Well-being and suicidality among transgender youth after gender-affirming hormones. Clin Pract Pediatr Psychol 2019;7(3):302–11.

122. Achille C, Taggart T, Eaton NR, et al. Longitudinal impact of gender-affirming endocrine intervention on the mental health and well-being of transgender youths: preliminary results. Int J Pediatr Endocrinol 2020;(1):2020. https://doi.org/10.1186/S13633-020-00078-2.

123. White Hughto JM, Reisner SL. A systematic review of the effects of hormone therapy on psychological functioning and quality of life in transgender individuals. Transgender Heal 2016;1(1):21–31.

Beyond Race, Sex, and Gender

Mental Health Considerations of Transgender Youth of Color, Intersex Youth, and Nonbinary Youth

A. Ning Zhou, MD[a,b,*], Kai J. Huang, MD Candidate[c],
Terence L. Howard, MD, MS[b]

KEYWORDS

- Intersectionality • Black • Latinx • Asian American Pacific Islander (AAPI)
- Transgender youth of color • Intersex • Differences of sex development
- Nonbinary gender identity

KEY POINTS

- Race, sex, and gender, which have traditionally been depicted in binary categories, are better understood as a continuum of identities and experiences.
- Black, Latinx, and Asian American Pacific Islander (AAPI) transgender and nonbinary youth experience unique challenges and stressors relating to their cultural context and values, racism and discrimination in the LGBTQ community and in the larger society, as well as transphobia within their racial communities, which can lead to adverse mental health consequences such as elevated rates of depression and suicidality.
- Variations in sexual development can lead to a variety of intersex traits that are outside of binary views of sex; intersex youth face a number of challenges and barriers as they are often coerced to conform to society's sex binary.
- Nonbinary youth have a gender identity that differs from traditional binary categories of boy/man and girl/woman; affirming their gender requires individually-tailored interventions.
- Despite experiencing many challenges and stressors, transgender, nonbinary, and intersex youth find ways to express their authentic identities and are resilient.

[a] San Francisco Department of Public Health Behavioral Health Services and Primary Care Behavioral Health, 3850 17th Street, San Francisco, CA 94114, USA; [b] University of California, San Francisco Department of Psychiatry and Behavioral Sciences, Box 3134, 675 18th Street, San Francisco, CA 94107, USA; [c] University of California, San Francisco School of Medicine, Program in Medical Education - Urban Underserved, 513 Parnassus Avenue, Suite S221, San Francisco, CA 94143, USA
* Corresponding author. 3850 17th Street, San Francisco, CA 94114.
E-mail address: a.ning.zhou@ucsf.edu

Child Adolesc Psychiatric Clin N Am 32 (2023) 683–705
https://doi.org/10.1016/j.chc.2023.04.002
1056-4993/23/© 2023 Elsevier Inc. All rights reserved.

childpsych.theclinics.com

Abbreviations	
LGBTQ	Lesbian, Gay, Bisexual, Transgender, and/or Queer
TNBY	Transgender and Nonbinary Youth
TNBYOC	Transgender and Nonbinary Youth of Color
ERI	Ethnic-Racial Identity
E-R	Ethnic-Racial
AAPI	Asian American Pacific Islander

INTRODUCTION

Our society deals with many binaries: male versus female, boy versus girl, black versus white. However, the human experience is complex and does not easily fit into binary categories; instead, it is helpful to view our identities in a continuum and take a dimensional perspective. This article will be divided into three sections to explore care for specific marginalized youth communities that do not neatly fit into defined categories and benefit from a more expansive approach: transgender youth of color, intersex youth, and nonbinary youth. The first section will provide an overview of the concept of intersectionality with a focus on ethnic-racial identity, highlighting the challenges and disparities that transgender and nonbinary youth of color experience, as well as their strengths and resilience. A framework for thinking about intersectionality and ethnic-racial identity will be provided. There will be subsections to highlight specific ethnic-racial groups, including Black, Latinx, and Asian American Pacific Islander (AAPI) transgender and nonbinary youth, and relevant cultural considerations. Next, this article will explore intersex traits and variations in sex development, including definitions, terminology, and psychosocial implications, such as intersex stigma. Finally, this article will discuss nonbinary gender identities, how gender shows up in social interactions, disparities and barriers to care, and considerations for gender affirmation. In all sections, we highlight the strengths and resilience of these diverse youth and provide practical clinical recommendations for child and adolescent mental health providers.

INTERSECTIONAL CARE FOR TRANSGENDER AND NONBINARY YOUTH OF COLOR
Overview

Audre Lorde famously said: "There is no such thing as a single-issue struggle because we do not live single-issue lives."[1] Intersectionality refers to the way systems of power and oppression based on axes of social identities, such as race, ethnicity, class, gender identity, sexual orientation, religion, ability, age, body size, nationality, and additional identities intersect in complex ways that allow for privilege or marginalization; these intersections produce an impact that is greater than the sum of privilege or marginalization for each individual identity.[2–5]

Challenges and disparities

For transgender and nonbinary youth of color (TNBYOC), their various identities intersect in different dimensions that often lead to compounding marginalization. For example, TNBYOC may experience transphobia within their racial communities, as well as racism within lesbian, gay, bisexual, transgender, and/or queer (LGBTQ) communities. The resulting stress and mental health challenges can be understood through minority stress theory,[6] which was originally developed for sexual minority people[7] and adapted for transgender and nonbinary individuals.[8,9] Minority stress theory describes distal stress processes (ie, discrimination, violence) and proximal stress processes (ie, expectations of rejection, concealment, internalized stigma).[6] These stressors lead to adverse mental and physical health outcomes. For example, 57% of transgender youth from unsupportive families had a past year suicide attempt, compared to 4% of transgender youth from supportive families.[10] TNBYOC have elevated rates of depression, anxiety, suicidal ideation, and suicide attempts.[11–14] In a study of transgender youth and life-threatening behaviors, half of whom were youth of color, 45% reported seriously thinking about suicide, and 26% reported attempting suicide.[15] In addition, TNBYOC are at risk of experiencing homelessness, police and community harassment, sexualization, commodification, and have higher rates of HIV infection.[16,17]

Strengths and resilience

A greater sense of school belonging was found to be protective for TNBYOC and decreased negative outcomes like substance use.[18] A study with transgender people of color who have survived traumatic events found that creating social networks, finding pride in one's racial/ethnic and gender identity, navigating family, accessing financial resources and healthcare, and other coping mechanisms were important aspects of the participants' resilience.[19] Additional resilience strategies used by TNBYOC include using their own words to describe their racial/ethnic and gender identities, developing self-advocacy skills, finding one's place in the LGBTQ youth community, and using social media to affirm one's identity.[20]

Later in discussion are several core principles from intersectionality as they apply to TNBYOC:[21]

1. Individuals have multiple simultaneous social identities that interact (eg, a Latina trans woman who is upper middle class will have a different experience from an Asian American, nonbinary, lower socioeconomic class individual).
2. These identities are not static and can evolve with the youth depending on their setting and circumstances (eg, an individual may have greater clarity of gender identity after pubertal changes and the development of secondary sex characteristics).
3. Holding a particular social identity does not equate to having the same experience; there is large intragroup variation (eg, people who identify as nonbinary can have very different experiences and embodiment goals—some pursue medical/surgical interventions, some do not).
4. Various social identities offer privilege or oppression dependent on the context (eg, TNBYOC at home may receive more support for their ethnic/racial identity than their gender identity, whereas at school they may receive more support for their gender identity than their ethnic/racial identity).

Intersectionality is particularly relevant for TNBYOC as they may change social identities or be perceived differently during and after their transitions. These new social identities may confer additional privilege or oppression.[4,5] For example, a Black transgender man after affirming his male gender may have more negative encounters with the law enforcement system. Facial feature changes with gender affirmation may push an individual to appear either more racialized or more white-passing, which further influences their social position.[4,5]

Ethnic-racial identity

While TNBYOC have a myriad of social identities (eg, gender, race) that become relevant in certain contexts, ethnic-racial identity (ERI) is especially salient in ethnically-conscious societies such as the United States.[22] ERI is a multidimensional construct that reflects the content, or beliefs and attitudes individuals have about their ethnic-racial (E-R) group, as well as the processes by which these beliefs and attitudes develop over time.[23] Content components include affirmation (ie, positive affect individuals have toward their E-R group), centrality (ie, how important ethnicity and race are to an individual's self-concept), and public regard (ie, how much individuals feel that others positively view their E-R group). Process components include exploration (ie, learning about traditions or history of one's E-R group) and resolution (ie, achieving a clear sense of the meaning of ethnicity in an individual's life).[24] Higher levels of ethnic affirmation were predictive of less anxiety and fewer depressive symptoms among African American, Latinx, and Asian American college students, and these associations were stronger for students who reported higher levels of ethnic centrality.[25] Ethnic minority high school students who had high levels of exploration also had high levels of resolution and affirmation.[22] Per socio-ecological theory, individuals are embedded in many social contexts, both proximal (eg, family, peer, community) and distal (eg, local, national, global).[as cited in 23(p30),26] For ethnic minority youth attending predominantly white schools, ethnic identity affirmation increase significantly, a finding that does not happen when youth are in majority ethnic minority settings.[23] Thus, ERI centrality is dependent on social context. There are limited studies that examine identity centrality in LGBTQ individuals who are also ethnic-racial minorities; however, those studies that do exist find the primacy of ERI and also find that sexual and gender identities have high centrality and intersect with ERI.[27,28]

In the coming sections, we have highlighted three ethnic-racial groups to demonstrate how intersectionality may apply to these specific groups: Black, Latinx, and Asian American Pacific Islander transgender and nonbinary youth.

Black Transgender and Nonbinary Youth

Background
Despite widespread awareness of social justice principles in modern American culture, there have been purposeful efforts to diminish the constitutional rights of traditionally marginalized citizens. Spanning voting rights to healthcare, Black communities, as well as LGBTQ communities, have been prime targets, with Black transgender and nonbinary persons being particularly vulnerable. Historically dehumanized in media,[29] Black transgender and nonbinary Americans encounter oppression from a multitude of structural systems including racism, sexism, classism, and transphobia that maintain white supremacy.[29–31] Even though more authentic representations of these identities have been recently highlighted, Black transgender and nonbinary individuals still disproportionately live under the poverty line, experience violence, engage with the U.S. industrial carceral system, and experience various physical and mental health issues from the compounding effects of stress from discrimination.[31–34] As transgender adults often report knowing their identity during childhood,[32] these risks likely develop from progressive exposure as Black transgender and nonbinary youth (TNBY).

Hardships for Black transgender and nonbinary youth
Black TNBY exist at the intersection of multiple marginalized identities. Just like Black and LGBTQ communities are not monoliths, it is imperative to note the diversity of experience amongst Black TNBY. However, Black TNBY often find themselves at odds with loved ones and others who may believe their gender identity conflicts with traditional Black cultural norms. A national survey of LGBTQ youth found that for Black transgender youth, 67% had relatives shame them for their gender identity, 57% felt unsafe in school bathrooms, and only 29% were comfortable wearing clothing which accurately reflected their gender identity.[29] It should be noted that

Black Americans are not inherently more homophobic than other races.[35,36] The structural violence found within American society unsurprisingly causes real violence for Black TNBY. The same survey indicated that 82% experienced verbal insults, 41% were physically assaulted, and 27% survived unwanted sexual acts.[29] In fact, 2021 had the highest number of tracked fatal violence against transgender and nonbinary Americans, with 33 of the 57 victims identified as Black.[37] Even more worrisome is how Black transgender youth are 1.6 times more likely than other queer youth to endorse suicidal ideation and attempt suicide.[38] Since rejection from parents and peers is a critical predictive factor for suicidality,[39] the alienation that Black TNBY may encounter due to the heteronormativity often prevalent in Black communities and racism pervasive in mainstream queer culture can exacerbate already dire circumstances.[40]

Uniquely Black spaces
A prominent cultural and political pillar since the time of slavery, the Black Church has acted as a safe haven and source of identity for many Black Americans especially in the Southern United States.[34,35] Although not more homophobic than other religious bodies,[35,36] some postulate that the queerphobia within Black communities stem from the tenets preached and atmosphere cultivated amongst certain church denominations.[40] Queer individuals have always discreetly existed in the church; however, this must be more challenging for Black TNBY whose expression may be more apparent and thus creates conflict that may force them to abandon their faith or suppress parts of themselves to avoid ostracization. Of course, there are Black TNBY who find solace in their faith outside of the Black Church. Many have also survived and found refuge while voguing in the ballroom scene. Immortalized in media such as *Paris is Burning* and *Legendary*, vogue is a style of dance and self-expression involving hand movements, runway walking, and acrobatics that grew to prominence amongst Black and Latinx social networks in the 1980s. "Houses" of unrelated individuals, typically unhoused youth rejected by blood relatives, lived as a family unit and competed against other houses in categories at "balls" for trophies and monetary prizes.[30] Not only providing food and shelter, the ballroom scene encourages creativity and leadership, acts as a positive recreational outlet, cultivates confidence, and offers mentorship from an elder house mother or father.[30] Though observed to have increased numbers of sexually transmitted infections and other pitfalls,[30,41] the ballroom scene unmistakably allows Black TBNY to live authentically and unapologetically.

Approaching care for Black transgender and nonbinary youth
Potentially having to brave one, if not multiple, traumatic events and developmentally appropriate stressors of adolescence, it is no wonder Black TNBY endorse higher rates of mood, anxiety, and substance use disorders in their lifetime.[30,31,33,42] In spite of these elevated risks, Black queer youth engage with mental health providers at decreased rates even when they have suicidal thoughts.[38] Multiple intersecting structural forces limit Black TNBY from getting safe reliable healthcare,[41] but past negative encounters and fear of future intolerance in medical systems are major reasons Black TNBY postpone seeking care.[42] Transgender youth appreciate having providers of similar racial or ethnic backgrounds, as they believe it results in greater empathy and understanding.[42] As Black queer mental health clinicians are scarce in number, it behooves child mental health providers to be more knowledgeable of psychiatric concerns specific to Black TNBY. Transgender youth also reported comfort with providers who were "transgender friendly" and did not need education from the youth.[42] Since Black TNBY can endure a plethora of adversities, utilizing a trauma-informed

approach or dialectical behavior techniques for emotional dysregulation may prove beneficial. A strength-based framework that validates and affirms Black TNBY can be extremely helpful in a society that tends to demonize their existence. The therapeutic alliance remains paramount and can truly be life-saving for Black TNBY.

Latinx Transgender and Nonbinary Youth

Background

Latinx Americans make up about 20% of the US population,[43] and include a heterogenous group of people with Black/African, indigenous, and white/European heritage.[44] Latinx individuals come from various regions of Latin America where Spanish or Portuguese are formally spoken, including Mexico, Central and South America, and the Caribbean.[45] Approximately one-third of Latinx Americans in the US are foreign born.[46] For Latinx youth whose parents are immigrants, their parents' limited English proficiency is an additional challenge that can affect school participation, and may lead some youth to serve as language brokers and interpret for their parents.[47–49] The term *Afro-Latinx* refers to individuals who trace their roots back to Africa and Latin America[50] and/or Spanish-speaking folks of African descent living in the United States.[51] This term has been used to highlight the racial heterogeneity of Latin America and the cultural influence of Africa in Latin America.[52] Latinx children are more likely to live in neighborhoods of concentrated poverty, and about one-third of Latinx youth live below the poverty line.[53] The terms *Latinx* and *Latine* were developed to be gender-inclusive terms, in contrast to the binary gender assumption in Latino/a.[45,54] This article will use the term *Latinx* and recognizes that *Latine* could also be used.

Culture

Family plays a key role in Latinx culture. *Familismo* is a Latinx concept that involves dedication, commitment, and strong loyalty to the family.[46] *La familia* (the family) is a close unit, supporting each other and sticking together through adversity.[55] The concept of *respeto* (respect) explains obedience to one's elders and other authority figures, which can make coming out challenging as it can be viewed as a *falta de respeto* (lack of respect).[55] *Marianismo* is shaped by the religious ideals of the Virgin Mary, where girls and women are socialized to be subservient, self-sacrificing, pure, and nurturing, and have a lot less independence than the men in their families.[56–58] *Machismo* encourages specific male gender role values and behaviors that include aggressiveness, bravado, being controlling, hardworking, providing for one's family, and being more independent.[56,57,59] While traditional *machismo* can be described as aggressive, sexist, chauvinistic, and hypermasculine, *caballerismo* highlights positive aspects of masculinity and can be described as nurturing, family centered, and chilvalrous.[60] Latinx individuals who do not conform to societally-driven gender roles experience increased levels of mental distress and abuse.[61] In addition, religion plays an important role in Latinx culture, with more than 70% of Latinx individuals attending religious services regularly, and 57% identifying as Catholic.[46] Finally, Latinx youth may acculturate more quickly to US culture, which can lead to an acculturation gap with their parents (eg, Latina girls may want more independence such as white American girls, which might cause tensions with parents who have more strict and traditional views) (Frias A. Personal communication regarding Latinx trans youth. Published online July 23, 2022.).

Indigenous heritage

Most indigenous cultures in the Americas have long traditions of third gender or gender-expansive people.[46] For example, the Muxes of the indigenous Zapoteca culture in Juchitán, Mexico, are identified as male at birth but choose to be raised as female at a young age; the Muxes are embraced as part of the community and are viewed as good luck and blessings.[62–64] Unfortunately, during colonization, Christian Europeans condemned gender variance as sinful which led to the marginalization of diverse sexualities and genders and the stripping away of rich traditions of gender diversity.[65,66] As a result, many Latinx trans and nonbinary youth may face accusations from other Latinxs that their gender variance is imported from white European-American culture and that they are losing their native culture (Frias A. Personal communication regarding Latinx trans youth. Published online July 23, 2022.). However, connecting with their indigenous history of gender diversity during traditions of ancestor worship such as Día de los Muertos in Mexico can be a powerful experience (Frias A. Personal communication regarding Latinx trans youth. Published online July 23, 2022.).

Latinx transgender and nonbinary youth
While there is limited literature on Latinx TNBY, the existing literature reveals that Latinx TNBY experience significant challenges. Forty-five percent of Latinx TNBY have been taunted or mocked by family.[13] 93% of gender queer Latinx youth rate stress a 5 or higher on a 10-point scale. Latinx LGBTQ youth experience high rates of depression (79%), anxiety (82%), insomnia (95%), and racial discrimination (80%).[13] Increased bullying leads to more isolation from social supports and increased likelihood to experience depression and suicidal ideation.[67] One study examining Black and Latinx transgender youth found that the prevalence of depressive symptoms was 50% and suicidality was 46%, with higher levels of harassment/victimization and lower levels of school connectedness.[68] In addition, Latinx LGBTQ youth have low levels of parental acceptance, which is a strong predictor for experiencing depression.[69]

Resilience
Youth who fully embraced their Latinx and LGBTQ identities and who were part of communities where they could authentically be themselves had increased resilience and were better able to combat experiences of adversity.[70] Gender & Sexuality Alliances (GSAs) and LGBTQ social justice activities were positively associated with school belonging and grade point average for LGBTQ Latinx youth.[67] Latinx youth may feel more comfortable with family members knowing their sexuality because they believe they won't be abandoned given strong family cultural norms.[55] Having a strong connection to family and an additional minority identity may serve to buffer negative effects such as minority stress.[71] Visibility and representation in the media can also serve to enhance resilience. For example, Vico Ortiz is a nonbinary Puerto Rican actor who plays a nonbinary character on the show "Our Flag Means Death."[72] In addition, the character Luz on the show "The Owl House" is Latinx, bisexual, and gender non-conforming.[73,74]

Asian American and Pacific Islander Transgender and Nonbinary Youth

Background
Asian Americans and Pacific Islanders (AAPIs) represent a heterogenous group of over forty different ethnicities and languages, making up about 7% of the United States (U.S.) population.[75–77] Ancestral homes for AAPIs include East Asia (eg, China, Japan, Korea), Southeast Asia (eg, Vietnam, Thailand, Cambodia, Philippines), South Asia (eg, India, Pakistan, Sri Lanka), and the Pacific Islands (eg, Polynesia, Micronesia, Melanesia). AAPIs are the fasting growing population in the U.S., increasing by 88% in the last two decades, and are projected to become the largest immigrant group in the US by the middle of the century.[75,76] The six largest Asian ethnicities (in descending order:

Chinese, Indian, Filipinx, Vietnamese, Korean, Japanese) make up 85% of all Asian Americans.[75]

Model minority myth

AAPIs are considered the "model minority" as they are perceived to work hard and value education. On average, AAPIs are more likely to be highly educated and earn a high median income. However, the "model minority" label reflects only a subgroup of AAPIs who have found academic success and does not reflect the experience of most AAPIs. Certain Southeast Asian and Pacific Islander groups have high rates of poverty and low educational attainment. The "model minority" label is considered more of a "bane than a blessing" as it masks those AAPIs who are not fairing so well, and the labeling may prevent AAPI individuals from seeking the support they need.[78]

Asian cultural values

Asian cultural values such as collectivism (ie, emphasizing group harmony over individual needs), filial piety (ie, loyalty and obedience to one's parents and elders), adherence to traditional gender roles, family recognition through achievement, emotional self-control, and humility[79,80] can make it more challenging to express a sexual or gender minority identity. In one study, higher adherence to Asian cultural values was associated with decreased likelihood to disclose one's sexual orientation, a relationship that was mediated by internalized heterosexism (ie, internalized stigma against sexual minority identities).[81] While gender identity was not specifically examined in that study, it is likely that the same cultural values would similarly make it challenging to express a transgender or nonbinary identity.

Anti-Asian racism

Since the start of the COVID pandemic and President Trump's use of the term "the Chinese virus," racism against AAPIs has drastically increased in the US, with over 10,000 hate incidents reported between March 2020 and December 2021.[82] Compared to AAPI men and women, AAPI nonbinary people experienced more physical assault, being coughed or spat at, deliberate avoidance or shunning, denial of service, and online harassment compared to AAPI women and men.[82] In addition, 85% of AAPI LGBTQ people report experiencing discrimination and/or harassment based on their race or ethnicity, 78% experienced racism within the predominantly white LGBTQ community, and 69% of AAPI transgender people reported experiencing discrimination due to their gender identity.[83] Moreover, AAPI individuals also experience stigma within the LGBTQ community while attempting to date, either being devalued or fetishized/exoticized.[84,85]

Asian American Pacific Islander transgender and nonbinary youth

Many AAPI cultures have strong traditions of third gender and/or gender-expansive people, such as the Hijra in South Asia, Bakla in the Philippines, Kathoeys in Thailand, Wakashu in Japan, and RaeRae and Mahu in Polynesia.[65,86–89] Limited studies have been conducted on AAPI TNBY. One study found that AAPI TNBY emphasize their gender identity over their ethnicity, and feel less safe expressing their authentic gender in Asian contexts.[90] AAPI TNBY are also less likely to share their gender identity with their parents compared to non-AAPI LGBTQ youth.[14,91] Asian parents are more resistant to prescribing medicine and surgical procedures.[90] Gender is a salient characteristic in how AAPIs view people, with gender nonconformity being a strong source of discomfort about LGBTQ people for some AAPIs.[92] Heterosexism, anti-LGBTQ bias, and adherence to traditional gender roles are perceived to be stronger in Asian

American cultures than in mainstream U.S. culture.[93–95] Moreover, AAPI LGBTQ individuals also have higher levels of internalized oppression than other groups.[96,97]

Health disparities

There are significant mental health disparities among AAPI TNBY: they are three times more likely to report a past year suicide attempt compared to cisgender AAPI LGBQ youth.[91] Many also reported experiencing discrimination, racism, being verbally insulted or physically threatened, and feeling unsafe or unprotected at school.[14] In addition, AAPI LGBTQ youth experience more familial physical abuse compared to LGBTQ youth from other ethnic groups.[98]

Resilience

Despite the significant challenges that AAPI TNBY face, they are incredibly resilient. AAPI TNBY find ways to express themselves authentically in the face of cultural and societal pressures to conform to traditional gender roles; they actively create their own communities, both online and offline, and engage in socio-political activism.[99] One study on AAPI youth suggested that fostering authenticity protected against depression, anxiety, and school isolation.[100] Another study on AAPI LGBQ individuals described building resilience by drawing strength and meaning from one's Asian culture and values.[95] Finally, a study of AAPI TNB adults found that they were able to negotiate their various identities toward integration to find and achieve a sense of authenticity.[101]

Summary

Black TNBY encounter many adversities due to multiple intersecting oppressive societal forces ingrained in American culture and internalized within already marginalized communities. Many find solace in networks of chosen family that allow them to be their truest selves. To help reduce the increased risk for psychiatric distress and suicide, providers should prioritize fostering trust and make good efforts to learn about psychosocial plights that are specific to Black TNBY.

Latinx TNBY experience many challenges and stressors relating to tensions with their cultural values, racial discrimination, immigration concerns, and more. Cultural values such as familismo, marianismo, machismo, and respeto can make it difficult for Latinx TNBY to disclose and express their authentic gender identities. Despite these challenges, Latinx TNBY can find resilience by embracing their Latinx and TNB identities and cultivating authenticity.

AAPI TNBY experience many challenges due to tensions with Asian cultural values, anti-Asian racism in society and within the LGBTQ community, and anti-LGBTQ bias within the AAPI community. Asian cultural values such as collectivism, filial piety, and conformity to traditional gender roles can make it challenging for AAPI TNBY to disclose and express their authentic gender identities, especially to their parents. Despite the many challenges AAPI TNBY face, they are quite resilient.

Intersectional Clinical Care Points

- Transgender and nonbinary youth of color (TNBYOC) encompass individuals with differing national origins, primary languages, levels of religiosity, and socioeconomic status so mental health providers should take the time to learn the individual before making presumptions in their care.
- It is important for mental health providers to have cultural competence and humility regarding racial-ethnic and TNB identities, so that patients do not have to take the role of educating providers.

- The family is often very important to TNBYOC, so cutting off the family to express TNB identities may not be an option.
- It is important to create spaces at schools and community-based organizations that are specifically for Black, Latinx, and AAPI TNBY, encouraging a sense of connection and belonging.
- There is stigma in many racial/ethnic minority communities regarding accessing mental health services, leading to a decreased likelihood of seeking services; partnership with local community groups, such as the Ballroom Scene or nightlife venues, could be another avenue to promote trust and mental health engagement amongst TNBYOC who may be hesitant to seek care.
- Clinicians should utilize medical interpreters when working with parents or guardians of patients who do not speak English and not rely on TNBYOC to interpret for their families.
- Clinicians should find ways to help families accept their TNBYOC and preserve family harmony, emphasizing values of loving their children and wanting their children to thrive.
- Clinicians should help TNBYOC find ways to cultivate authenticity, strengths, and resilience in their daily lives.
- Clinicians should help TNBYOC draw strength and meaning from their culture and values and, if relevant, connect with their indigenous traditions of gender diversity.
- Clinicians should assess for trauma and discrimination, as well as how TNBYOC have coped with this trauma/discrimination, and incorporate trauma-informed, culturally-sensitive interventions.
- When there is a conflict in values related to culture and LGBTQ identities, clinicians should help TNBYOC explore which values they want to prioritize to maximize authenticity while recognizing the importance certain cultural values may have.
- Clinicians should help TNBYOC explore which social identities to prioritize in any given context. Integration of ethnic-racial and TNB identities may be desired by some youth and not desired by other youth. Clinicians should follow the youth's lead in determining priorities and support them in achieving their goals.

INTERSEX YOUTH
Sex and Gender: a Binary System, or a Continuum?

Sex is often portrayed as a binary of male and female, rather than as a (more accurate) bimodal distribution spanning variations in multiple sex characteristics from chromosomes, external genitalia, internal reproductive organs, gonads, hormone secretion, hormone response, and secondary sex characteristics. Typically, a sex marker such as male or female is assigned to an infant at birth based on the appearance of their external genitalia and is then indicated on a birth certificate. Recently, the U.S. Department of State added an X gender marker to recognize intersex and nonbinary individuals.[102] Some infants develop variations in their external or internal genitalia that differ from the expected male or female appearance. These infants typically undergo a diagnostic process of identifying the factors contributing to the variations in sexual differentiation, followed by an "assignment" to a binary sex category so that they fit into the societal expectations within a binary sex and gender system.

Given the many biological factors involved in the sexual differentiation of the reproductive system—including the fetus's genetic and associated endocrine status and the pregnant parent's health, exposure to stress, and intake of medications—there exists a great diversity of intersex traits that vary in etiologic factors and affect sex characteristics to different degrees. In many cases, the etiologic factors cannot be clearly identified.[103] Raising an intersex child in a society that imposes expectations of sex as a binary may bring challenges. Moreover, in some intersex traits, the sexual differentiation variations become apparent only at the time of puberty. While intersex variations constitute part of the continuum of biological sex,[104] differences in the reproductive system, sex hormone regulation, and/or the gonads that are associated with some intersex traits may affect reproductive capability.

Terminology

In 2005, an international conference on the management of intersex traits developed the term "Disorders of Sex Development" (DSD), defined "by congenital conditions, in which the development of chromosomal, gonadal, or anatomic sex is atypical."[105] As many intersex people found the term "disorder" to be stigmatizing and pathologizing, the term "disorder" was replaced with "differences" so that DSD can be read "Differences of Sex Development." The intersex community organization interACT Advocates has put out a statement clarifying that "intersex" and "intersex traits" are preferred terms to be used instead of "intersexual," "intersexed," or "DSD."[106,107]

Psychosocial Implications

Intersex stigma in its various forms (structural, institutional, interpersonal, experienced, anticipated, internalized) may affect an intersex individual at all stages of development and in all spheres of life.[108–112] Presumably as an attempt to minimize stigma (through a cissexist lens), sometimes surgeons perform surgery during early childhood to conform the child's genital appearance to that "typical" of the assigned gender. This is a highly controversial decision, objected to by ethicists and by intersex activists, because early surgery is done without the child's informed consent and, thereby, violates the child's human rights to autonomy, self-determination, and an open future.[113–115] Early surgical intervention may feel especially violating for individuals who later identify with a gender other than the one assigned at birth.

From preschool age on, individuals with somatic intersex traits tend to have higher rates of gender-expansive behavior than non-intersex individuals.[116] At later stages of development, several factors may contribute to questioning of the assigned gender, affect social relations, and/or increase isolation. These factors include: awareness of the incongruence of sex characteristics with the assigned sex, need for sex-hormone treatment from pubertal age on, infertility, and awareness of any previous genital surgery. Increased rates of mental health conditions have been documented in intersex individuals, including high rates of depression and suicidality.[117–119]

Resilience

In light of the many challenges that intersex youth face, they are also resilient. One study found that having positive parental experiences, a confidant in childhood, and a "best friend" correlated with improved adult wellbeing, more body satisfaction, and fewer suicidal thoughts.[120] Access to affirming spaces, either at home, at school, or online, was associated with decreased rates of suicide attempts.[121] Though understudied, peer support groups are another important resource that further bolster the resilience of intersex youth. These organizations aim to provide emotional support, increase social well-being, and facilitate exchanges of information.[122]

Psychosocial Management

Given the number of diverse intersex traits and youths' varied hormonal, surgical, and mental health care needs across stages of development, clinical management for intersex youth is best provided by a multidisciplinary clinical team[105] whose members are well-trained and experienced in intersex-related topics. Given the limited numbers of such teams and their distance from many families, linkages to community practitioners, possibly utilizing telehealth, need to be developed. Providers themselves can also take steps to become better educated and prepared to provide high-quality care to intersex youth and their families. At its core, mental health care for intersex youth needs to focus on the bodily autonomy and mental wellbeing of the individual. For additional guidance and support, we recommend 4intersex, a project of interACT Advocates that provides many helpful resources, including content on what intersex youth wish their doctors, friends, and teachers knew.[107]

Summary

Intersex youth have variations in sex development that may lead to internal or external sex characteristics outside of the male/female binary. Due to pressures to conform to society's sex binary, intersex youth may be forced to undergo early childhood genital surgeries. They frequently experience multiple forms of intersex stigma and, as a result, experience more mental health symptoms. Despite these imposed challenges, intersex youth can thrive when appropriately supported. Providers can further support intersex youth by participating in interdisciplinary care teams, where available, and by building personal awareness, knowledge, and sensitivity.

Intersex Clinical Care Points

Clinicians working with intersex youth should:

- Center intersex youths' bodily autonomy, voices, and mental health.
- Ask intersex youth which terms they use to describe themselves—without making assumptions.
- Connect intersex youth with supportive counseling and mental health services, when needed.
- Link intersex youth (when old enough) and/or their caregivers to appropriate support groups of other youth or caregivers who have shared experiences.
- Assist the intersex youth and their parents in handling disclosure of the selected aspects of medical condition to people outside the family, as indicated.
- Support intersex youth in discovering their authentic gender identity and sexual orientation without trying to influence them toward any particular identity.
- Help parents accept the youth's intersex traits, gender identity, gender expression, and sexual orientation, if needed.
- Help intersex youth and their family access gender-affirming care, if needed.

NONBINARY YOUTH
Background

Nonbinary individuals do not solely identify as women/girls or men/boys.[123] The transgender umbrella encompasses people whose genders differ from their assigned sex at birth, which includes nonbinary people.[123,124] Some nonbinary people, however, do not identify with or use the label transgender, which is a personal choice.[123,124] The label nonbinary itself also serves as an umbrella term for a wide range of identities, including but not limited to genderqueer, genderfluid, agender, and bigender. The number of openly nonbinary youth is increasing as youth find the language and safety to openly identify as nonbinary. In a national Trevor Project survey from 2020, 26% of LGBTQ youth identified as nonbinary and an additional 20% reported questioning if they were nonbinary.[125]

How Gender Shows Up in Social Interactions

The concept of gender, and especially the gender binary, frequently appears in social interactions. People often make assumptions about other people's gender identities based on their perception and interpretation of those people's gender expressions.[126] They may then address or treat people differently based on these gendered assumptions. For example, people may address strangers with gendered terms such as "sir" or "miss," which may be misgendering someone if they do not use that term for themselves. Nonbinary youth may feel invalidated or unsafe when other people misgender them, whether it is due to lack of awareness or overt dismissal of nonbinary gender identities.[126,127] As a result, nonbinary youth may choose not to disclose their gender identities, which may lead to further feelings of invalidation and invisibility.[127]

Medical and Mental Health Care Disparities

Transgender and nonbinary youth who are unable to access gender-affirming care such as puberty blockers or gender-affirming hormone therapy have higher rates of depression as well as self-harm or suicidal thoughts compared to their transgender and nonbinary peers who received puberty blockers or gender-affirming hormone therapy.[128] In a study with 202 transgender and nonbinary youth ages 15 to 24 in the U.S., nonbinary youth had significantly higher stress levels and were less likely to have already accessed gender-affirming medical care, compared to their binary transgender peers.[129] Additionally, nonbinary youth whose pronouns are not respected had a rate of attempting suicide more than 2.5 times that of nonbinary youth who reported that "all or most of the people" in their life used their pronouns.[125] Respecting a nonbinary youth's asserted name and pronouns can reduce negative mental health outcomes,[130] as explained by gender minority stress and resilience model.[8]

Medical transition

For nonbinary youth under the age of 18, legal guardian consent is necessary to access gender-affirming medical care such as puberty blockers, hormones, surgery, and other interventions. While there is no one way to medically transition in a binary or nonbinary way, some nonbinary people may have different goals than other transgender people.[131] For example, some nonbinary people may seek fewer medical interventions than binary transgender people, such as chest surgery without hormone therapy.[131,132] Nonbinary patients seeking gender-affirming surgeries may also ask for more androgynous or non-traditional aesthetic results, such as top surgery removal of chest tissue with larger areola and nipples that are placed more centrally on the chest, no areola or nipples, or preservation of some chest tissue.[133] Hormone therapy regimens may also be adjusted based on individuals' goals, such as to slow down or minimize certain changes.[134] While nonbinary people may have gender expression goals that differ from stereotypical masculine or feminine presentation, some nonbinary people may feel more comfortable with a more traditionally masculine or feminine presentation. Importantly, each person's gender expression goals are deeply personal and unique. Thus, providers should avoid assumptions and work with individuals to tailor their gender-affirming interventions.

Societal and Structural Barriers to Accessing Care

Nonbinary young adults may avoid health care or feel pressure to present themselves as binary transgender people to access care due to gatekeeping or providers' lack of understanding of nonbinary identities.[135] In gatekeeping systems, health care providers such as therapists or physicians may pose additional barriers to access (ie, gender-affirming care that first requires patients to be assessed for gender dysphoria by a mental health provider).[136] Individuals who seek access to care may feel the need to perform their gender in a way that aligns with providers' views on how transgender people should feel or present, in order to gain access.[136] They also may have to navigate medical providers' assumptions about their gender transition goals and/or pushes for them to medically transition even if they did not express interest in doing so.[137] Nonbinary minors and young adults who rely on their parents or guardians may be unable to pursue gender-affirming medical care due to lack of parental or guardian support.[127]

Strengths and Resilience

Protective factors such as online or in-person support, family support, and online resources can mitigate negative mental health outcomes for transgender and nonbinary youth.[138,139] Additional resilience strategies include: ability to self-define and theorize one's gender, proactive agency, access to supportive educational systems, connection to a trans-affirming community, reframing of mental health challenges, and navigation of relationships with family and friends.[140]

Summary

Nonbinary youth face unique challenges in both social and health care settings that may overlap or differ from those faced by binary transgender youth. Both societal and structural barriers to feeling seen and respected in their authentic selves and to accessing care and resources may negatively impact the mental health of nonbinary youth. Community support, family support, and access to other resources and sources of support are protective. It is important for clinicians to create welcoming environments where nonbinary youth feel safe and respected. More research focusing on nonbinary youth is needed given the limited scholarship on this growing population.

Nonbinary Clinical Care Points

- It is important to create an affirming environment through practices such as training all staff who interact with clients, ensuring safe access to gender-inclusive restrooms, and integrating gender-inclusive language and options into intake forms, materials, and electronic records.
- Nonbinary youth should be given the agency to define their gender identity and gender expression, especially if they are seeking letters of support for gender-affirming care.
- Nonbinary genders are diverse and personal. Clinicians should not assume how a patient identifies or their goals for transition (if any).
- Clinicians should allow clients to take the lead on how much they want to focus on their gender in their clinical care, rather than focusing on gender simply because a client is transgender or nonbinary.[8]
- Protective factors may include a variety of support systems such as peer support, community spaces, family support, affirming healthcare, and other resources.

SUMMARY

This article explored how race, sex, and gender exist on a continuum, rather than fitting neatly into binary categories. Transgender and nonbinary youth of color, intersex youth, and nonbinary youth face significant challenges relating to the intersection of their various social identities and also face many societal and structural barriers to receiving high-quality care. Mental health providers should support these youth in cultivating their strengths, authenticity, and resilience.

DISCLOSURE

The authors have no commercial or financial conflicts of interests to disclose.

ACKNOWLEDGMENTS

The authors would like to acknowledge Aza Frias (they/them, elle/le/-e) for their contributions to the Latinx Trans and Nonbinary Youth section. A.N. Zhou uses he/him/his pronouns. K.J. Huang uses they/them/theirs, he/him/his, and ze/zir/zirs pronouns. T.L. Howard uses he/him/his pronouns.

REFERENCES

1. Lorde A. Learning from the 60s. In: Sister outsider: essays & speeches by Audre Lorde. Berkeley: Crossing Press; 2007. p. 138.
2. Crenshaw K. Demarginalizing the intersection of race and sex: a black feminist critique of antidiscrimination Doctrine, feminist theory and antiracist politics. Univ Chic Leg Forum 1989;1989(1):31.
3. Crenshaw K. Mapping the margins: intersectionality, identity politics, and violence against women of color. Stanford Law Rev 1991;43(6):1241.
4. de Vries KM. Intersectional identities and conceptions of the self: the experience of transgender people: intersectional identities. Symb Interact 2012;35(1): 49–67.
5. de Vries KM. Transgender people of color at the center: conceptualizing a new intersectional model. Ethnicities 2015;15(1):3–27.
6. Meyer IH. Prejudice, social stress, and mental health in lesbian, gay, and bisexual populations: conceptual issues and research evidence. Psychol Bull 2003;129(5):674–97.
7. Meyer IH. Minority stress and mental health in gay men. J Health Soc Behav 1995;36(1):38–56.
8. Hendricks ML, Testa RJ. A conceptual framework for clinical work with transgender and gender nonconforming clients: an adaptation of the Minority Stress Model. Prof Psychol Res Pract 2012;43(5):460–7.
9. Meyer IH. Resilience in the study of minority stress and health of sexual and gender minorities. Psychol Sex Orientat Gend Divers 2015;2(3):209–13.
10. Travers R, Bauer G, Pyne J, et al. Impacts of strong parental support for trans youth: a report prepared for Children's. Toronto, ON: Aid Society of Toronto and Delisle Youth Services; 2012.
11. The Trevor Project. 2022 National Survey on LGBTQ Youth Mental Health.; 2022. Available at: https://www.thetrevorproject.org/survey-2022/. Accessed June 22, 2022.
12. Human Rights Campaign. 2019 Black & African American LGBTQ Youth Report.; 2019. Available at: https://www.hrc.org/resources/black-and-african-american-lgbtq-youth-report. Accessed June 22, 2022.

13. Human Rights Campaign. 2018 LGBTQ Latinx Youth Report.; 2018. Available at: https://www.hrc.org/resources/latinx-lgbtq-youth-report. Accessed June 26, 2022.

14. Human Rights Campaign. 2019 LGBTQ Asian and Pacific Islander Youth Report.; 2019. Available at: https://assets2.hrc.org/files/assets/resources/FINAL-API-LGBTQ-YOUTHREPORT.pdf. Accessed April 18, 2022.

15. Grossman AH, D'Augelli AR. Transgender youth and life-threatening behaviors. Suicide Life Threat Behav 2007;37(5):527–37.

16. Reck J. Homeless gay and transgender youth of color in san Francisco: "No one likes Street Kids"—even in the castro. J LGBT Youth 2009;6(2–3):223–42.

17. Garofalo R, Deleon J, Osmer E, et al. Overlooked, misunderstood and at-risk: exploring the lives and HIV risk of ethnic minority male-to-female transgender youth. J Adolesc Health 2006;38(3):230–6.

18. Hatchel T, Marx R. Understanding intersectionality and resiliency among transgender adolescents: exploring pathways among peer victimization, school belonging, and Drug use. Int J Environ Res Public Health 2018;15(6):1289.

19. Singh AA, McKleroy VS. Just getting out of bed is a revolutionary act": the resilience of transgender people of color who have survived traumatic life events. Traumatology 2011;17(2):34–44.

20. Singh AA. Transgender youth of color and resilience: negotiating oppression and finding support. Sex Roles 2013;68(11–12):690–702.

21. Golden RL, Oransky M. An intersectional approach to therapy with transgender adolescents and their families. Arch Sex Behav 2019;48(7):2011–25.

22. Umaña-Taylor AJ, Yazedjian A, Bámaca-Gómez M. Developing the ethnic identity Scale using eriksonian and social identity perspectives. Identity 2004;4(1):9–38.

23. Umaña-Taylor AJ, Quintana SM, Lee RM, et al. Ethnic and racial identity during adolescence and into young adulthood: an integrated conceptualization. Child Dev 2014;85(1):21–39.

24. Sladek MR, Umaña-Taylor AJ, McDermott ER, et al. Testing invariance of ethnic-racial discrimination and identity measures for adolescents across ethnic-racial groups and contexts. Psychol Assess 2020;32(6):509–26.

25. Brittian AS, Umaña-Taylor AJ, Lee RM, et al. The moderating role of centrality on associations between ethnic identity affirmation and ethnic minority college students' mental health. J Am Coll Health 2013;61(3):133–40.

26. Bronfenbrenner U. Ecological systems theory. Ann Child Dev 1989;6:187–249.

27. Moore K, Camacho D, Spencer-Suarez KN. A mixed-methods study of social identities in mental health care among LGBTQ young adults of color. Am J Orthopsychiatry 2021;91(6):724–37.

28. Shramko M, Toomey RB, Anhalt K. Profiles of minority stressors and identity centrality among sexual minority Latinx youth. Am J Orthopsychiatry 2018;88(4):471–82.

29. Human Rights Campaign Foundation. Black & African-American LGBTQ Youth Report. Available at: https://www.hrc.org/resources/black-and-african-american-lgbtq-youth-report. Accessed May 6, 2022.

30. Harper GW, LaBoy R, Castillo M, et al. It's a Kiki!: Developmental benefits of the Kiki scene for Black gay/bisexual/transgender adolescents/emerging adults. J LGBT Youth 2022;19(1):31–52.

31. Lassiter JM, Follins LD, Smallwood SW, et al. Black U.S. sexual and gender minority mental health. In: The Oxford Handbook of sexual and gender minority

mental health. Oxford library of psychology. Oxford University Press; 2020. p. 175–85.

32. Restar A, Jin H, Breslow AS, et al. Developmental milestones in young transgender women in two American cities: results from a racially and ethnically diverse sample. Transgender Health 2019;4(1):162–7.

33. Murphy J, Hardaway R. LGBTQ adolescents of color: considerations for working with youth and their families. J Gay Lesbian Ment Health 2017;21(3):221–7.

34. Follins LD, Garrett-Walker JJ, Lewis MK. Resilience in black lesbian, gay, bisexual, and transgender individuals: a critical review of the literature. J Gay Lesbian Ment Health 2014;18(2):190–212.

35. Hill MJ. Is the black community more homophobic?: reflections on the intersectionality of race, class, gender, culture and religiosity of the perception of homophobia in the black community. J Gay Lesbian Ment Health 2013;17(2):208–14.

36. Walsh CF. It really is not just gay, but african American gay": the impact of community and church on the experiences of black lesbians living in North central Florida. J Homosex 2016;63(9):1236–52.

37. Human Rights Campaign Foundation. Fatal Violence against the Transgender and Gender Non-Conforming Community in 2021. Available at: https://www.hrc.org/resources/fatal-violence-against-the-transgender-and-gender-non-conforming-community-in-2021. Accessed July 29, 2022.

38. The Trevor Project. Black LGBTQ Youth Mental Health.; 2020. Available at: https://www.thetrevorproject.org/research-briefs/black-lgbtq-youth-mental-health. Accessed May 31, 2022.

39. Diamond GM, Shilo G, Jurgensen E, et al. How depressed and suicidal sexual minority adolescents understand the causes of their distress. J Gay Lesbian Ment Health 2011;15(2):130–51.

40. Lewis MW, Ericksen KS. Improving the climate for LGBTQ students at an historically black university. J LGBT Youth 2016;13(3):249–69.

41. Ezell JM, Ferreira MJ, Duncan DT, et al. The social and sexual networks of black transgender women and black men who have sex with men: results from a representative sample. Transgender Health 2018;3(1):201–9.

42. Panchal Z, Piper C, Whitmore C, et al. Providing supportive transgender mental health care: a systemized narrative review of patient experiences, preferences, and outcomes. J Gay Lesbian Ment Health 2022;26(3):228–64.

43. United States Census Bureau. Race and Ethnicity in the United States: 2010 Census and 2020 Census. Available at: https://www.census.gov/library/visualizations/interactive/race-and-ethnicity-in-the-united-state-2010-and-2020-census.html. Published 2021. Accessed June 26, 2022.

44. Noe-Bustamante L, Gonzalez-Barrera A, Edwards K, Mora L, Hugo Lopez M. Measuring the racial identity of Latinos. Pew Research Center. Available at: https://www.pewresearch.org/hispanic/2021/11/04/measuring-the-racial-identity-of-latinos/. Published November 4, 2021. Accessed June 26, 2022.

45. Pastrana A (Jay), Battle J, Harris A. An Examination of Latinx LGBT populations across the United States: intersections of race and sexuality. New York: Palgrave Macmillan US; 2017.

46. Human Rights Campaign. Coming Out: Living Authentically as LGBTQ Latinx Americans. Available at: https://www.hrc.org/resources/coming-out-living-authentically-as-lgbtq-latinx-americans. Accessed June 26, 2022.

47. Turney K, Kao G. Barriers to school Involvement: are immigrant parents Disadvantaged? J Educ Res 2009;102(4):257–71.

48. Anderson M, Cox RB, Giano Z, et al. Latino parent-child English language Fluency: implications for maternal school Involvement. Hisp J Behav Sci 2020; 42(4):547–62.

49. Morales A, Hanson WE. Language brokering: an integrative review of the literature. Hisp J Behav Sci 2005;27(4):471–503.

50. Vargas MP, Kuhl PE. Bridging the communication gap between afro-Latino and african American individuals: an interdisciplinary curriculum Initiative. J Hisp High Educ 2008;7(4):336–45.

51. Higgins S. Afro-Latinos: An annotated guide for collection building. Ref User Serv Q 2007;47(1):10–5.

52. Flores J, Román MJ. Triple-consciousness? Approaches to afro-Latino culture in the United States. Lat Am Caribb Ethn Stud 2009;4(3):319–28.

53. Murphey D, Guzman L, Torres A. America's Hispanic Children: gaining ground, looking forward. Child Trends Hisp Inst; 2014. p. 36.

54. callmelatine.com. Call me Latine. Frequently Asked Questions. Available at: callmelatine.com. https://callmelatine.com/faq/. Accessed July 16, 2022.

55. Rosario M, Schrimshaw EW, Hunter J. Ethnic/racial differences in the coming-out process of lesbian, gay, and bisexual youths: a comparison of sexual identity development over time. Cultur Divers Ethnic Minor Psychol 2004;10(3): 215–28.

56. Miville ML, Mendez N, Louie M. Latina/o gender roles: a content analysis of empirical research from 1982 to 2013. J Lat Psychol 2017;5(3):173–94.

57. Cerezo A, Camarena J, Ramirez A. Latinx sexual and gender minority mental health. In: Rothblum ED, editor. The Oxford Handbook of sexual and gender minority mental health. Oxford: Oxford University Press; 2020. p. 185–98. https://doi.org/10.1093/oxfordhb/9780190067991.013.17.

58. Raffaelli M, Ontai LL. Gender Socialization in Latino/a families: results from two retrospective studies. Sex Roles 2004;50(5/6):287–99.

59. Torres JB, Solberg VSH, Carlstrom AH. The myth of sameness among Latino men and their machismo. Am J Orthopsychiatry 2002;72(2):163–81.

60. Arciniega GM, Anderson TC, Tovar-Blank ZG, et al. Toward a fuller conception of machismo: development of a traditional machismo and caballerismo Scale. J Couns Psychol 2008;55(1):19–33.

61. Sandfort TGM, Melendez RM, Diaz RM. Gender nonconformity, homophobia, and mental distress in Latino gay and bisexual men. J Sex Res 2007;44(2): 181–9.

62. Muxes - Mexico's Third Gender. the Guardian Documentaries; 2017. Available at: https://www.youtube.com/watch?v=iiek6JxYJLs&ab_channel=TheGuardian. Accessed July 22, 2022.

63. Natural History Museum Los Angeles County. Beyond Gender: Indgenous Perspectives, Muxe: A limited series on some of the world's third gender indigenous people. Natural History Museum Los Angeles County Stories. Available at: https://nhm.org/stories/beyond-gender-indigenous-perspectives-muxe. Published 2019. Accessed July 22, 2022.

64. Stephen L. Sexualities and genders in Zapotec Oaxaca. Lat Am Perspect 2002; 29(2):41–59.

65. Human Rights Campaign Staff. Two Spirit and LGBTQ+ Identities: Today and Centuries Ago. Human Rights Campaign News. Available at: https://www.hrc.org/news/two-spirit-and-lgbtq-idenitites-today-and-centuries-ago. Published November 23, 2020. Accessed July 23, 2022.

66. Express Web Desk. Indigenous tribes embraced gender fluidity prior to colonisation, but Europeans enforced specific gender roles. The Indian Express. Available at: https://indianexpress.com/article/world/indigenous-tribes-embraced-gender-fluidity-prior-to-colonisation-but-europeans-enforced-specific-gender-roles/. Published July 27, 2017. Accessed July 23, 2022.

67. Garcia-Perez J. Lesbian, gay, bisexual, transgender, queer + Latinx youth mental health disparities: a systematic review. J Gay Lesbian Soc Serv 2020; 32(4):440–78.

68. Vance SR, Boyer CB, Glidden DV, et al. Mental health and psychosocial risk and protective factors among black and Latinx transgender youth compared with peers. JAMA Netw Open 2021;4(3):e213256.

69. Abreu RL, Lefevor GT, Gonzalez KA, et al. Bullying, depression, and parental acceptance in a sample of Latinx sexual and gender minority youth. J LGBT Youth 2022;1–18. https://doi.org/10.1080/19361653.2022.2071791.

70. Gonzalez M, Reese BM, Connaughton-Espino T. I'm going to live my life Freely": authenticity as an indicator of belonging among urban Latinx LGBTQ+ youth. JHSE 2022;10(2):21.

71. Hatchel T, Ingram KM, Mintz S, et al. Predictors of suicidal ideation and attempts among LGBTQ adolescents: the roles of help-seeking beliefs, peer victimization, depressive symptoms, and Drug use. J Child Fam Stud 2019;28(9): 2443–55.

72. Spielberger D. Vico Ortiz Plays a Pirate Grappling with Gender on Our Flag Means Death. Them. Available at: https://www.them.us/story/vico-ortiz-our-flag-means-death-q-and-a. Published March 3, 2022. Accessed July 25, 2022.

73. Rude M. The Owl House's Luz & Amity Just Had Their Gayest Episode Yet. Out. Available at: https://www.out.com/television/2021/7/12/owl-houses-luz-amity-just-had-their-gayest-episode-yet. Published July 12, 2021. Accessed July 25, 2022.

74. The Negative Space Podcast. Dana Terrace & The Truffles of Discontent (Compromise in Collaborative Work). Available at: https://anchor.fm/negativespacepod/episodes/009–Dana-Terrace–The-truffles-of-discontent-compromise-in-collaborative-work-evb9af. Accessed July 31, 2022.

75. Budinman A, Ruiz NG. Key facts about Asian Americans, a diverse and growing population. Pew Research Center. Available at: www.pewresearch.org/fact-tank/2021/04/29/key-facts-about-asian-americans/. Published April 29, 2021. Accessed February 28, 2022.

76. Jones N, Marks R, Ramirez R, Rios-Vargas M. 2020 Census Illuminates Racial and Ethnic Composition of the Country. United States Census Bureau. Available at: https://www.census.gov/library/stories/2021/08/improved-race-ethnicity-measures-reveal-united-states-population-much-more-multiracial.html#:~:text=Asian%20Population,people%20(4.8%25)%20in%202010. Published August 12, 2021. Accessed April 30, 2022.

77. Sue DW. Counseling the culturally diverse: theory and practice. 8th edition. Hoboken, NJ: John Wiley & Sons, Inc; 2019.

78. Wong F, Halgin R. The "model minority": bane or blessing for asian Americans? J Multicult Couns Dev 2006;34(1):38–49.

79. Kim BSK, Atkinson DR, Yang PH. The asian values Scale: development, factor analysis, validation, and reliability. J Couns Psychol 1999;46(3):342–52.

80. Kim BK, Li LC, Ng GF. The asian American values Scale–multidimensional: development, reliability, and validity. Cultur Divers Ethnic Minor Psychol 2005; 11(3):187–201.

81. Szymanski DM, Sung MR. Asian cultural values, internalized heterosexism, and sexual orientation disclosure among asian American sexual minority persons. J LGBT Issues Couns 2013;7(3):257–73.
82. Jeung R, Horse AY, Popovic T, et al. Stop AAPI hate national report. Ethn Stud Rev 2021;44(2):19–26.
83. Dang AAT, Vianney C. Living in the margins: a national survey of lesbian, gay, bisexual and transgender Asian and Pacific islander Americans. New York: National Gay and Lesbian Task Force Policy Institute; 2007.
84. Wade RM, Harper GW. Racialized sexual discrimination (RSD) in the age of online sexual networking: are young black gay/bisexual men (YBGBM) at elevated risk for adverse psychological health? Am J Community Psychol 2020;65(3–4): 504–23.
85. Callander D, Newman CE, Holt M. Is sexual racism really racism? Distinguishing attitudes toward sexual racism and generic racism among gay and bisexual men. Arch Sex Behav 2015;44(7):1991–2000.
86. Hossain A. The paradox of recognition: hijra, third gender and sexual rights in Bangladesh. Cult Health Sex 2017;19(12):1418–31.
87. Stip E. Les RaeRae et Mahu : troisième sexe polynésien. Santé Ment Au Qué 2016;40(3):193–208.
88. Jackson PA. An explosion of Thai identities: global queering and re-imagining queer theory. Cult Health Sex 2000;2(4):405–24.
89. Bohnke C. The Disappearance of Japan's "Third Gender." JSTOR Daily. Available at: https://daily.jstor.org/the-disappearance-of-japans-third-gender/. Published December 22, 2021. Accessed July 25, 2022.
90. Tan S, Weisbart C. Asian-Canadian trans youth: identity development in a hetero-cis-normative white world. Psychol Sex Orientat Gend Divers 2021. https://doi.org/10.1037/sgd0000512.
91. The Trevor Project. The Trevor Project Research Brief: Asian/Pacific Islander LGBTQ Youth Mental Health.; 2020. Available at: https://www.thetrevorproject. org/wp-content/uploads/2021/08/Understanding-the-Mental-Health-of-API-Youth-May-Research-Brief-1.pdf. Accessed April 17, 2022.
92. Tseng T. Understanding anti-LGBT bias: an analysis of Chinese-speaking Americans' attitudes toward LGBT people in Southern California. LGBTQ Policy J Harv Kennedy Sch 2010;1:11.
93. Chung YB, Szymanski DM. Racial and sexual identities of asian American gay men. J LGBT Issues Couns 2006;1(2):67–93.
94. Kimmel DC, Yi H. Characteristics of gay, lesbian, and bisexual asians, asian Americans, and immigrants from Asia to the USA. J Homosex 2004;47(2): 143–72.
95. Sung MR, Szymanski DM, Henrichs-Beck C. Challenges, coping, and benefits of being an Asian American lesbian or bisexual woman. Psychol Sex Orientat Gend Divers 2015;2(1):52–64.
96. Pyun T, Santos GM, Arreola S, et al. Internalized homophobia and reduced HIV testing among men who have sex with men in China. Asia Pac J Public Health 2014;26(2):118–25.
97. Ratti R, Bakeman R, Peterson JL. Correlates of high-risk sexual behaviour among Canadian men of South Asian and European origin who have sex with men. AIDS Care 2000;12(2):193–202.
98. Balsam KF, Lehavot K, Beadnell B, et al. Childhood abuse and mental health Indicators among ethnically diverse lesbian, gay, and bisexual adults. J Consult Clin Psychol 2010;78(4):459–68.

99. Tan S, Weisbart C. I'm me, and I'm Chinese and also transgender': coming out complexities of Asian-Canadian transgender youth. J LGBT Youth 2022;1–27. https://doi.org/10.1080/19361653.2022.2071789.

100. Luthar SS, Ebbert AM, Kumar NL. Risk and resilience among Asian American youth: ramifications of discrimination and low authenticity in self-presentations. Am Psychol 2021;76(4):643–57.

101. Thai JL, Budge SL, McCubbin LD. Qualitative examination of transgender Asian Americans navigating and negotiating cultural identities and values. Asian Am J Psychol 2021;12(4):301–16.

102. Blinken A. X gender marker available on U.S. Passports starting April 11. U.S. Department of State Press Release. Available at: https://www.state.gov/x-gender-marker-available-on-u-s-passports-starting-april-11/. Published March 31, 2022. Accessed July 24, 2022.

103. Délot EC, Vilain E. Towards improved genetic diagnosis of human differences of sex development. Nat Rev Genet 2021;22(9):588–602.

104. Štrkalj G, Pather N. Beyond the sex binary: toward the inclusive anatomical Sciences education. Anat Sci Educ 2021;14(4):513–8.

105. Hughes IA. Consensus statement on management of intersex disorders. Arch Dis Child 2005;91(7):554–63.

106. interACT. interACT Statement on Intersex Terminology. Available at: https://interactadvocates.org/interact-statement-on-intersex-terminology/#. Accessed July 25, 2022.

107. interACT: Advocates for Intersex Youth. #4intersex.Available at: https://4intersex.org/#yourself. Accessed July 25, 2022.

108. Ediati A, Juniarto AZ, Birnie E, et al. Social stigmatisation in late identified patients with disorders of sex development in Indonesia. BMJ Paediatr Open 2017;1(1):e000130.

109. Joseph AA, Kulshreshtha B, Shabir I, et al. Gender issues and related social stigma affecting patients with a disorder of sex development in India. Arch Sex Behav 2017;46(2):361–7.

110. Meyer-Bahlburg HFL, Khuri J, Reyes-Portillo J, et al. Stigma in medical settings as reported retrospectively by women with congenital adrenal hyperplasia (CAH) for their childhood and adolescence: table I. J Pediatr Psychol 2016;jsw034. https://doi.org/10.1093/jpepsy/jsw034.

111. Meyer-Bahlburg HFL, Khuri J, Reyes-Portillo J, et al. Stigma associated with classical congenital adrenal hyperplasia in Women's sexual lives. Arch Sex Behav 2018;47(4):943–51.

112. Meyer-Bahlburg HFL, Reyes-Portillo JA, Khuri J, et al. Syndrome-related stigma in the general social environment as reported by women with classical congenital adrenal hyperplasia. Arch Sex Behav 2017;46(2):341–51.

113. Carpenter M. Intersex human rights, sexual orientation, gender identity, sex characteristics and the Yogyakarta Principles plus 10. Cult Health Sex 2021;23(4):516–32.

114. Jorge JC, Valerio-Pérez L, Esteban C, et al. Intersex care in the United States and international standards of human rights. Glob Public Health 2021;16(5):679–91.

115. Jürgensen M, Rapp M, Döhnert U, et al. Assessing the health-related management of people with differences of sex development. Endocrine 2021;71(3):675–80.

116. Callens N, Van Kuyk M, van Kuppenveld JH, et al. Recalled and current gender role behavior, gender identity and sexual orientation in adults with Disorders/Differences of Sex Development. Horm Behav 2016;86:8–20.

117. de Vries ALC, Roehle R, Marshall L, et al. Mental health of a large group of adults with disorders of sex development in six European countries. Psychosom Med 2019;81(7):629–40.

118. Godfrey LM. Mental health outcomes among individuals with 46,XY disorders of sex development: a systematic review. J Health Psychol 2021;26(1):40–59.

119. Rosenwohl-Mack A, Tamar-Mattis S, Baratz AB, et al. A national study on the physical and mental health of intersex adults in the U.S. PLoS One 2020; 15(10):e0240088.

120. Schweizer K, Brunner F, Gedrose B, et al. Coping with diverse sex development: treatment experiences and psychosocial support during childhood and adolescence and adult well-being. J Pediatr Psychol 2016;jsw058.

121. Trevor Project. The Mental Health and Well-being of LGBTQ Youth who are Intersex. Published online 2021. Available at: https://www.thetrevorproject.org/wp-content/uploads/2021/12/Intersex-Youth-Mental-Health-Report.pdf. Accessed July 25, 2022.

122. Baratz AB, Sharp MK, Sandberg DE. Disorders of sex development peer support. In: Hiort O, Ahmed SF, editors. Endocrine development, vol. 27. Basel, Switzerland: S. Karger AG; 2014. p. 99–112. https://doi.org/10.1159/000363634.

123. Chew D, Tollit MA, Poulakis Z, et al. Youths with a non-binary gender identity: a review of their sociodemographic and clinical profile. Lancet Child Adolesc Health 2020;4(4):322–30.

124. Diamond LM. Gender Fluidity and nonbinary gender identities among children and adolescents. Child Dev Perspect 2020;14(2):110–5.

125. Diversity of Nonbinary Youth. The Trevor Project; 2021. Available at: https://www.thetrevorproject.org/research-briefs/diversity-of-nonbinary-youth/. Accessed July 25, 2022.

126. Barbee H, Schrock D. Un/gendering social selves: how nonbinary people navigate and experience a binarily gendered world. Sociol Forum 2019;34(3): 572–93.

127. Johnson KC, LeBlanc AJ, Deardorff J, et al. Invalidation experiences among non-binary adolescents. J Sex Res 2020;57(2):222–33.

128. Tordoff DM, Wanta JW, Collin A, et al. Mental health outcomes in transgender and nonbinary youths receiving gender-affirming care. JAMA Netw Open 2022;5(2):e220978.

129. Todd K, Peitzmeier SM, Kattari SK, et al. Demographic and behavioral profiles of nonbinary and binary transgender youth. Transgender Health 2019;4(1): 254–61.

130. Russell ST, Pollitt AM, Li G, et al. Chosen name use is linked to reduced depressive symptoms, suicidal ideation, and suicidal behavior among transgender youth. J Adolesc Health 2018;63(4):503–5.

131. Koehler A, Eyssel J, Nieder TO. Genders and individual treatment progress in (non-) binary trans individuals. J Sex Med 2018;15(1):102–13.

132. Sayyed AA, Haffner ZK, Abu El Hawa AA, et al. Mutual understanding in the field of gender affirmation surgery: a systematic review of techniques and preferences for top surgery in nonbinary patients. Health Sci Rev 2022;3: 100024.

133. McTernan M, Yokoo K, Tong W. A comparison of gender-affirming chest surgery in nonbinary versus transmasculine patients. Ann Plast Surg 2020;84(5S): S323–8.
134. Cocchetti C, Ristori J, Romani A, et al. Hormonal treatment strategies tailored to non-binary transgender individuals. J Clin Med 2020;9(6):1609.
135. Schulz SL. The informed consent model of transgender care: an alternative to the diagnosis of gender dysphoria. J Humanist Psychol 2018;58(1):72–92.
136. Ashley F. Gatekeeping hormone replacement therapy for transgender patients is dehumanising. J Med Ethics 2019;45(7):480–2.
137. Lykens JE, LeBlanc AJ, Bockting WO. Healthcare experiences among young adults who identify as genderqueer or nonbinary. LGBT Health 2018;5(3): 191–6.
138. Evans YN, Gridley SJ, Crouch J, et al. Understanding online resource use by transgender youth and caregivers: a qualitative study. Transgender Health 2017;2(1):129–39.
139. Valente PK, Schrimshaw EW, Dolezal C, et al. Stigmatization, resilience, and mental health among a diverse community sample of transgender and gender nonbinary individuals in the U.S. Arch Sex Behav 2020;49(7):2649–60.
140. Singh AA, Meng SE, Hansen AW. I Am my own gender": resilience strategies of trans youth. J Couns Dev 2014;92(2):208–18.

Assessment of Transgender and Gender-Diverse Adolescents
Incorporating the World Professional Association of Transgender Health Standard of Care 8th Edition

Scott F. Leibowitz, MD, DFAACAP

KEYWORDS

- Transgender and gender-diverse (TGD) adolescents • Gender-affirming care
- Assessment • Decision-making capacity

KEY POINTS

- Standards of Care for transgender health have existed since 1979, however the most recent edition, the 8th version (SOC8), was published in 2022 and its recommendations were approved by a Delphi consensus process of approximately 120 multidisciplinary international transgender health experts.
- TGD adolescents are presenting for gender-affirming care at rates exponentially higher than they did even a decade ago, and with increased complexity.
- Recommendations in the Adolescent chapter of the SOC8 emphasize the importance of doing a comprehensive biopsychosocial assessment of TGD youth seeking gender-affirming medical treatment to assess for maturity, decision-making capacity, and other psychiatric/psychological vulnerabilities that may need prioritizing.
- Supporting gender-diverse expression and identity is important in order to promote positive psychological and emotional development.
- The SOC8 recommends involving parents and caregivers in decision-making process for TGD adolescents.

INTRODUCTION

The leading international authority on transgender health, World Professional Association of Transgender Health (WPATH), published the long-awaited 8th edition of its

Nationwide Children's Hospital, The Ohio State University College of Medicine, 700 Children's Drive, Columbus, OH 43205, USA
E-mail address: scottleibowitzmd@gmail.com

Child Adolesc Psychiatric Clin N Am 32 (2023) 707–718
https://doi.org/10.1016/j.chc.2023.05.009
1056-4993/23/© 2023 Elsevier Inc. All rights reserved.

childpsych.theclinics.com

Standard of Care (SOC8) in September 2022, 10 years after its previous update.[1] The organization formed in 1979 and published its first standard of care in that same year, under the former name Harry Benjamin International Gender Dysphoria Association (HBIGDA). The newly updated guidelines, specifically as they pertain to the care of transgender and gender-diverse (TGD) adolescents, could not have come at a more needed time.

Clinically, TGD adolescents have been presenting to gender-affirming multidisciplinary care clinics at exponentially higher rates than in the past, often seeking gender-affirming medical treatments to help align their body with their experienced gender.[2,3] While there is a growing body of research that points toward treating appropriately assessed youth,[4–12] the population's clinical needs have outpaced the research advancements that provide answers to some of the more complex questions that come up every day in contemporary practice. While longitudinal research is typically needed to demonstrate causation, these studies take time to conduct. Meanwhile, the ways in which adolescents express and assert their gender are constantly evolving and changing. Just as in other evolving areas of medicine, providers need to rely on clinical experience/consensus and biomedical ethical principles *in addition to* the evidence when assisting families with care decisions. Considering adolescents with gender-diverse experiences have become ubiquitous within most child and adolescent psychiatric settings, many child and adolescent psychiatrists are playing catch up to understand the needs of this complex population. Therefore, clinical guidelines such as SOC8 serve as a crucial guidepost for *how* to approach assessment and treatment for this patient population.

Politically, TGD youth, and specifically the gender-affirming care that has increasingly been provided to them over the past decade, have arguably become one of the most contentious culture wars in modern times.[13] Politicians, *not* the care experts or scholars experienced in this area, are legislating clinical practices.[14] They often claim that the existing research is insufficient and convince themselves and their followers that this should justify banning the treatments. Instead of respecting the debates on *how* to do the care among academics, clinicians, and scientists, politicians believe they can legislate *whether* the care occurs at all. In the United States, the political machine has been particularly brutal, with gender-affirming bans for minors passing numerous state legislatures and some even being signed into law. In this polarized environment, *any* Standard of Care document that recommends gender-affirming care treatments for minors, no matter how careful or cautious, would be considered ideologically rooted in nature to those who seek to ban it. So, while the clinical world has desperately needed updated evidence-informed recommendations, many politicians have been quick to leverage the publishing of such recommendations for politically motivated reasons and to delegitimize the guidelines they contain. This anti-science climate is the context in which Chapter 6 on Adolescents in the SOC8 was published.

BACKGROUND

Gender-affirming hormone treatments—testosterone for assigned-female-at-birth (AFAB) transmasculine persons and estrogen for assigned-male-at-birth (AMAB) transfeminine persons—was first recommended for adolescents in the 5th edition of the WPATH SOC in 1998.[15] In this document, the minimum age for hormone therapy was lowered from 18 years to 16 year old, recognizing that some adolescents are sufficiently mature enough to make decisions that have irreversible implications for their body. Waiting until an arbitrary distant point in the future (eg, 18 years of age) to better align one's body with their gender keeps the young person in psychological and physical limbo, forced to navigate the discomforts and challenges of a disharmonious mind-body connection. This experience, clinically described as Gender Dysphoria in the Diagnostic and Statistical Manual of Mental Disorders, Fifth Edition (DSM-5),[16] has been associated with an increased risk for a number of negative mental health experiences,[17–19] often compounded by an immense amount of minority stress from a discriminatory, stigmatizing, and rejecting environment.[20–22] In the International Classification of Diseases (ICD), Gender Incongruence simply refers to the misalignment between gender identity and sex anatomy.[23]

As the years progressed, child and adolescent issues were addressed in one combined section within both the 6th and 7th editions of the SOC.[24,25] In this same timeframe, advances in the field of gender-affirming care had been introduced (eg, puberty suppression in the early 2000's in the Netherlands),[26] and the research for those treatments has been evolving in response. Other complex issues became more commonplace as well, including changing trends in the patient population (eg, a significant shift in the sex ratio of those seeking care[27]; a shift in the conceptualization of gender as a dimensional construct rather than dichotomous[28]; more young people presenting in adolescence without childhood histories of gender diversity[29]), many of which are listed in **Fig. 1**. The prior version, SOC7,[22] had criteria for gender-affirming care in adolescents as depicted in **Fig. 2**, however it became clear that these recommendations would not sufficiently guide health care professionals to address the increasingly more complex issues that have naturally presented over time.

Therefore, when the SOC8 committee was formed in 2017, the task ahead of it was enormous. With so many unanswered questions, how would the authors translate the available evidence into a set of ethical, globally relevant, and practical recommendations on such a complex topic? The committee consisted of 119 international, multidisciplinary experts who were selected to develop 18 chapters relevant to transgender health. For the first time, the child and adolescent chapters were separated, given the degree of attention that each developmental group would require on its own. Seven clinicians and clinician-researchers in the field of adolescent gender-affirming care were selected to author Chapter 6 (Adolescents), representing the disciplines of adolescent medicine, child and adolescent psychiatry, neuropsychology, pediatric endocrinology, and pediatric psychology.

Selected current debates/questions in pediatric gender affirming care addressed by SOC8
• Unexplained shift in sex ratio where AFAB outnumber AMAB patients by almost 2:1.
• Evolving description of identities while conceptualizing gender as a spectrum.
• Increased youth who first experience gender diverse identities in adolescence and not in childhood.
• Puberty suppression clinical factors (length of treatment, when to start, etc.).
• Hormone clinical factors (fertility, long-term medical implications, etc.).
• Decision-making capacity in adolescence (ability to understand irreversible changes; ability to conceptualize regret/evolution of identity; ability to weigh pros/cons of different pathways, etc.).
• Degree of comprehensiveness and relevance of a psychodiagnostic assessment considering access difficulties within pediatric mental health and gender care.
• Who is best trained and positioned to perform such an assessment.
• Impact that autism spectrum disorder and other mental health experiences have on diagnostic clarity and appropriateness for gender care.

Fig. 1. Debates and current complexities in the field of adolescent gender-affirming care addressed in the World Professional Association of Transgender Health, Standard of Care 8th Edition, 2022.

Criteria for Gender Affirming Medical Care ,Standard of Care 7th Edition, 2012
General criteria • Persistent, long (childhood) history of gender non-conformity/dysphoria; worsening at the onset of puberty; • Co-existing problems do not interfere with assessment or treatment, or are addressed; • Adolescent able to provide informed consent, and parents also provide consent when adolescent has not reached the age of medical consent; • Adolescent is supported by parents or other caregivers throughout the treatment process. **Puberty Suppression** • Tanner 2 minimum **Hormones** • 16 y of age **Chest Masculinization Surgery for transmasculine youth** • Could be done younger than 18 for appropriate patients, preferably after one year on testosterone **Other Surgeries, including bottom surgery** • Deferred until 18+ y of age

Fig. 2. Adolescent criteria for gender-affirming medical and surgical care in the 2012 World Professional Association of Transgender Health Standard of Care 7th edition.

The development of the SOC8 marked the first time in its history that a Delphi consensus process determined whether or not a recommendation would be included. Chapter authors drafted the initial recommendations and then 75% of all 119 co-authors for the SOC8 needed to approve the statement in order for it to be included. Utilizing a consensus-based process strengthens the legitimacy of the guidelines by incorporating the collective thousands of hours of experience of all 119 co-authors. Once the statements passed, then the guidelines were drafted and, ultimately, a draft version was presented for public review. The final version of the chapter incorporated feedback from the review process. In the end, 12 statements were published that included criteria for gender-affirming medical/surgical treatments (**Fig. 3**). Chapter authors were instructed to use the word "recommend" when the statements were more evidence-informed and "suggest" when the recommendation relied more on experience-informed consensus.

SUMMARY OF CONTENT

A detailed description of the SOC8 adolescent chapter goes beyond the scope of this chapter, however the guidelines are readily available online at the WPATH website (www.wpath.org), and this chapter can serve as a summary overview of the content. The SOC8 Adolescent Chapter contextualizes the recommendations as the gold standard, appreciating variability in available resources within different cultures, countries, and environments. This is important because the absence of resources should not preclude the provision of important treatments when appropriate.

The chapter begins with an introduction that summarizes adolescent identity development and decision-making capacity in general. This helps distinguish adolescents and their care needs from the developmental groups that precede and succeed them. The chapter acknowledges that the borders between childhood and adolescence and

Recommendations for TGD adolescents, standard of care 8th edition, 2022

6.1 We recommend that health care professionals working with gender diverse adolescents:

- Are licensed by their statutory body and hold a postgraduate degree or its equivalent in a clinical field relevant to this role granted by a nationally accredited statutory institution.
- Receive theoretical and evidenced-based training and develop expertise in general child, adolescent, and family mental health across the developmental spectrum.
- Receive training and have expertise in gender identity development, gender diversity in children and adolescents, have the ability to assess capacity to assent/consent, and possess general knowledge of gender diversity across the life span.
- Receive training and develop expertise in autism spectrum disorders and other neurodevelopmental presentations or collaborate with a developmental disability expert when working with autistic/neurodivergent gender diverse adolescents.
- Continue engaging in professional development in all areas relevant to gender diverse children, adolescents, and families.

6.2 We recommend health care professionals working with gender diverse adolescents facilitate the exploration and expression of gender openly and respectfully so that no one particular identity is favored.

6.3 We recommend health care professionals working with gender diverse adolescents undertake a comprehensive biopsychosocial assessment of adolescents who present with gender identity-related concerns and seek medical/surgical transition-related care, and that this be accomplished in a collaborative and supportive manner.

6.4 We recommend health care professionals work with families, schools, and other relevant settings to promote acceptance of gender diverse expressions of behavior and identities of the adolescent.

6.5 We recommend against offering reparative and conversion therapy aimed at trying to change a person's gender and lived gender expression to become more congruent with sex assigned at birth.

6.6 We suggest that health care professionals provide transgender and gender diverse adolescents with health education on chest binding and genital tucking, including review of benefits and risks.

6.7 We recommend providers consider prescribing menstrual suppression agents for adolescents experiencing gender incongruence who may not desire testosterone therapy, who desire but have not yet begun testosterone therapy, or in conjunction with testosterone therapy for breakthrough bleeding.

6.8 We recommend health care professionals maintain an ongoing relationship with the gender diverse and transgender adolescent and any relevant caregivers to support the adolescent in their decision-making throughout the duration of puberty suppression treatment, hormonal treatment, and gender- related surgery until the transition is made to adult care.

6.9 We recommend health care professionals involve relevant disciplines, including mental health and medical professionals, to reach a decision about whether puberty suppression, hormone initiation, or gender-related surgery for gender diverse and transgender adolescents are appropriate and remain indicated throughout the course of treatment until the transition is made to adult care.

6.10   We recommend health care professionals working with trans and gender diverse adolescents requesting gender-affirming medical or surgical treatments inform them, prior to initiating treatment, of the reproductive effects, including the potential loss of fertility and available options to preserve fertility within the context of the youth's stage of pubertal development.

6.11   We recommend when gender-affirming medical or surgical treatments are indicated for adolescents, health care professionals working with transgender and gender diverse adolescents involve parent(s)/guardian(s) in the assessment and treatment process, unless their involvement is determined to be harmful to the adolescent or unnecessary.

6.12   We recommend health care professionals assessing transgender and gender diverse adolescents only recommend gender-affirming medical or surgical treatments requested by the patient when:

A. The adolescent meets the diagnostic criteria of gender incongruence as per the ICD-11 in situations where a diagnosis is necessary to access health care. In countries that have not implemented the latest ICD, other taxonomies may be used although efforts should be undertaken to utilize the latest ICD as soon as practicable review of benefits and risks.

B. The experience of gender diversity / incongruence is marked and sustained over time.

C. The adolescent demonstrates the emotional and cognitive maturity required to provide informed consent/assent for the treatment.

D. The adolescent's mental health concerns (if any) that may interfere with diagnostic clarity, capacity to consent, and gender-affirming medical treatments have been addressed.

E. The adolescent has been informed of the reproductive effects, including the potential loss of fertility and the available options to preserve fertility, and these have been discussed in the context of the adolescent's stage of pubertal development.

F. The adolescent has reached Tanner stage 2 of puberty for pubertal suppression to be initiated.

Fig. 3. WPATH SOC8 Adolescent recommendations for gender-affirming medical and surgical care, 2022.

between adolescence and adulthood are imprecise and cannot be determined by age alone. Therefore, the adolescent chapter may be more appropriate to use for pubertal children who are approaching their teenage years, while it may also be relevant for transitional-age youth who are no longer minors yet have not individuated from their caregivers nor demonstrated steps toward independence.

The introduction of the chapter continues to describe the state of evidence for what is and is not known about gender identity development and the relevance this has for clinical care decisions. The introduction then concludes with an overview of the state of evidence for gender-affirming care treatments, indicating that reliance on the existing evidence should only be one factor that informs treatment decisions.[30] Taking a human rights perspective within a biomedical ethical framework is also important.

The chapter then lists the approved recommendations, each with a detailed justification written to support it. The main topic areas will be described herein.

Qualifications of the Provider

Statement 1 describes the ideal qualifications for providers working with TGD youth and families. In addition to local licensing requirements, providers assisting TGD youth should have training and/or competence in 3 main areas: (1) Working with adolescent identity development and family dynamics; (2) Understanding what is and is not known about gender identity development and gender dysphoria; and (3) Appreciation of the unique needs of individuals who are neurodiverse and/or have autism spectrum disorder (ASD). When training or experience lacks in any of these areas, providers should do their best to engage in professional development activities that help build competence in those areas.

Support for gender diversity

Statement 2 recommends that providers approach gender openly and without a preconceived notion that any one particular gender identity experience is favorable. This approach is consistent with the conversion therapy policy statement from the American Academy of Child and Adolescent Psychiatry (AACAP), which maintains that "variations in sexual orientation and gender expression represent normal and expectable dimensions of human development."[31] Statement 2 promotes the idea that gender identity and gender expression can be experienced and expressed in many different ways, none of which reflect inherent psychopathology. Appreciating what this means for an individual is important before recommending a particular biomedical treatment that presumes variations in gender identity or expression automatically implies gender dysphoria/incongruence.

Statements 4 and 5 are also important recommendations that promote support for gender diversity. Statement 4 discusses the implications of gender minority stress and the importance of fostering healthy development for adolescents in different settings, including school, their families, and communities. Statement 5 reaffirms the harmful nature of conversion therapy, which are efforts that promote cisgender, heterosexual experiences as favorable and preferred outcomes.

Comprehensive assessment to determine treatment needs

The hallmark recommendation of the chapter, Statement 3, specifies the importance of conducting a comprehensive biopsychosocial assessment for TGD youth presenting for care. One significant reason for this recommendation is that the most robust longitudinal evidence for the benefits of gender-affirming care in minors was obtained in a clinical setting where a prolonged diagnostic period was used to ensure that the youth were appropriate for treatment.[4] Therefore, generalizing the benefits of gender-affirming care to all youth who seek hormones (some of whom may not have decision-making capacity or identity stability) is not evidence-informed.

By obtaining a holistic psychological/psychiatric profile for the young person, providers are better equipped to prioritize and address mental health treatment needs, if they exist. In some clinical scenarios, addressing family dynamics may be an important first priority, whereas in other scenarios in which mental health issues do not interfere with clarity of identity stability, prioritizing the consent process for irreversible gender-affirming medical treatments may be the next step. The assessment helps determine the need for different therapies and psychosocial supports (described in more detail in the chapter on *Psychological and Social Approaches to TGD youth*) that may support young people in a gender exploration process, should that be determined appropriate. By identifying possible co-occurring mental health conditions, providers are better equipped to provide individualized care. Navigating a gender-diverse identity presents different challenges for youth with differing co-occurring mental health conditions or psychological profiles.

Parameters of the treatment frame- multidisciplinary care and family involvement

Statement 9 specifies the importance of multidisciplinary care, specifically involving mental health professionals in addition to medical providers, when assisting with care decisions. Statement 8 addresses the importance of maintaining an ongoing clinical relationship with patients and families throughout their period of transition and gender-affirming medical treatment, given that developmental factors are highly important for different treatments and therefore appreciating decision-making capacity over time is easier when the clinical relationship is maintained.

Statement 11 specifies the importance of involving parents and caregivers in the decision-making process. Considering that, in most countries, parents or caregivers are required to consent for most treatments in minors, understanding the parents' perspective on the young person's desire for treatment is important. Another significant reason why inclusion of parents/caregivers in the process is important is due to the beneficial impact of family acceptance on mental health outcomes.[32-36] The chapter specifies that there may be clinical scenarios where including parents or caregivers may be harmful (eg, abusive parent) or unnecessary (eg, foster care, child abandonment, and so forth), and therefore provides flexibility to account for those outlier situations.

Consideration of Reversible and Supportive Physical Interventions

Statements 6 and 7 provide information to providers regarding use of menstrual suppression, chest binding, and/or penile tucking for young people with gender dysphoria. These actions might be initial steps with less irreversible implications for young people who either:(1) May have their needs met through these treatments alone; and/or (2) Require more time and treatment to improve decision-making capacity for the treatments that are more irreversible. In the chapter, the evidence is reviewed to support the recommendations for these interventions.

Criteria for gender-affirming medical treatments

Statement 12 provides several criteria for puberty suppression, gender-affirming hormones, and surgical treatments for adolescents. The criteria specify that adolescents: (1) Meet criteria for Gender Incongruence in the ICD or Gender Dysphoria in the DSM, if those classifications are used in a particular country; (2) Have experienced gender-diverse identities for a sustained period of time; (3) Are sufficiently mature enough to be able to appreciate the risks/benefits and long term implications of the treatments they seek; (4) Have sufficient treatment for any mental health conditions that impact the clarity of their identity experience; and (5) Have been informed of the reproductive effects of the treatments they seek, with education on fertility preservation should that be desired. Specifically, for puberty suppression, the guidelines specify that adolescents should be in Tanner 2 stage of puberty in order for gonadotropin-releasing hormone (GnRH) agonists to be considered.

Diagnostic Criteria and Maturity
Statements 6.12 A and 6.12 C are criteria for the initiation of pubertal suppression, gender-affirming hormones, and/or gender-affirming surgical treatments. In combination, they provide both a subjective and objective component to the criteria. 12A states that if a particular diagnostic classification system is used in a given country (eg, DSM or ICD), then the adolescent should meet such criteria in order to access treatment. 12C describes the adolescent demonstrating sufficient emotional and cognitive maturity to appropriately and proactively weigh the risks and benefits of an important decision. Adolescents should be able to appreciate the different outcomes that may exist for a given treatment, even for outcomes that the adolescent does not believe will happen for them (eg, concept of regret).

Sustained experience over time
Statement 6.12 B specifies that the adolescent's experience of gender incongruence/dysphoria is sustained and marked over time. This ensures that the adolescent's experience sufficiently informs their capacity to make decisions with irreversible implications. Defining the exact amount of time necessary to inform the decision is arbitrary and, therefore, it is more important that the concept of a prolonged experience is emphasized (typically years, as is discussed in the text of the chapter), rather than specifying an exact timeframe that can vary from individual to individual.

Fertility options
Statement 6.12 E (which is a replication of Statement 6.10) guides providers to review reproductive effects of the different sought treatments. Often parents and adolescents have different views and priorities regarding reproductive capacity, so facilitating a discussion of options is important.[37]

Mental Health Stability and Co-Occurring Mental Health Diagnoses
Statement 6.12D addresses the importance of addressing and prioritizing mental health conditions that may impact diagnostic clarity for gender dysphoria/gender incongruence. This does not imply that all mental health symptoms must be resolved in order to understand an adolescent's identity experience. Some mental health conditions may present additional challenges in appreciating a young person's experience, while other mental health challenges may be the manifestation of untreated gender dysphoria. Therefore, it is incumbent on the provider to understand the relationship between the mental health issues (if they exist) and the person's experience of gender dysphoria. It is also important to support gender diversity psychologically and socially and/or consider less irreversible gender-affirming treatments, while addressing mental health challenges that create complexity in understanding identity stability and decision-making capacity.

One common mental health diagnosis that often co-occurs with gender dysphoria/gender diversity is autism spectrum disorder (ASD).[38] The presence of ASD should not preclude an adolescent from accessing gender-affirming care, but rather should guide the *way* providers navigate the treatment frame. Considering those with ASD often present with inflexibility, difficulties with theory of mind (appreciating others' perspectives), and black-or-white thinking, appreciating the decision-making capacity of the young person often involves working with them through the lens of autism treatment.[39]

Age and stage

Of note, there are no age minimums included in the final version of the Adolescent SOC8 chapter. While a draft of the document that was seen in public review included different age minimums (for each intervention), after the period of public review, it was determined that age minimums were arbitrary and detracted from the more important criteria that emphasize maturity, identity stability, and parent/caregiver involvement. One negative implication to not including agreed-upon age minimums is that outside entities (eg, insurance companies) may develop their own policies, often using arbitrary age minimums without scientific justification. Therefore, in the future, clinicians and clinician-researchers may want to consider the *beneficial* implications with using age minimums (eg, preventing outside entities from creating arbitrary policies) that *they* agree are appropriate for health-related policies, given their extensive experience working with the population.

For pubertal suppression, which is more impactful when provided in the earlier stages of puberty, Tanner staging, not age, is considered more important.[40] Statement 12F states that adolescents should be at least Tanner stage 2 in order to be eligible for pubertal suppression (in addition to the other criteria).

SUMMARY

Given the increasing clinical demand for gender-affirming and evidence-based care for TGD adolescents, updated guidelines are important for child and adolescent psychiatrists around the world. In today's current political climate, approaching the care from a pragmatic and practical standpoint is more crucial than ever, despite legislative efforts to mischaracterize the care as "experimental." The WPATH SOC8, a multidisciplinary, international, consensus-informed, evidence-based document, serves as a guideline for providers across disciplines regarding how to best approach the decision-making process for important gender-affirming treatments. Such treatments help align a young person's body with their experienced gender identity, maximizing their chance to feel the same sense of comfort and harmony that is naturally afforded to their cisgender adolescent peers during the same developmental period. Conducting a comprehensive biopsychosocial assessment to determine identity stability and the priority and sequence of treatment needs, all while supporting gender diversity and promoting parental acceptance, are important steps in the process. Knowledge of the debates in the field, existing evidence, and the steps necessary to preserve the integrity of the decision-making process are crucial to providing ethical care.

CLINICS CARE POINTS

- TGD adolescents are increasingly presenting to child and adolescent psychiatry practices, and they have complex needs which may include the provision of gender-affirming medical treatment.

- Clinical guidelines are important in the provision of care, and the WPATH Standard of Care 8th edition provides evidence-informed, consensus-based recommendations that translate the available evidence into practical care recommendations.

- TGD adolescents vary in the degree of family acceptance they receive, capacity to make appropriate decisions, and degree to which they experience sustained gender dysphoria, which necessitates an individualized approach to care that involves key family members.

- Starting with a comprehensive biopsychosocial assessment helps to determine a psychiatric and psychological profile that helps guide treatment priorities and when young people seek treatments that may have irreversible implications.

- The evidence base supports the crucial importance of family acceptance and gender-affirming care (social, psychological, and sometimes medical/surgical) for TGD youth, and clinicians can support youth through family therapy and individual therapeutic treatment modalities.

DISCLOSURE

SFL: Co-Investigator for research funded by the National Institute of Mental Health (NIMH). The Impact of Pubertal Suppression on Neural and Mental Health Trajectories R01 MH123746-01A1(MPIs: E. Nelson, J.F. Strang, D. Chen).

REFERENCES

1. Coleman E, Radix AE, Bouman WP, et al. Standards of care for the health of transgender and gender diverse people, version 8. Int J Transgend Health 2022; 23(Suppl 1):S1–259.
2. Arnoldussen M, Steensma TD, Popma A, et al. Re-evaluation of the Dutch approach: are recently referred transgender youth different compared to earlier referrals? Eur Child Adolesc Psychiatr 2020;29(6):803–11.
3. Kaltiala R, Bergman H, Carmichael P, et al. Time trends in referrals to child and adolescent gender identity services: a study in four Nordic countries and in the UK. Nord J Psychiatr 2020;74(1):40–4.
4. de Vries ALC, McGuire JK, Steensma TD, et al. Young adult psychological outcome after puberty suppression and gender reassignment. Pediatrics 2014; 134(4):696–704.
5. Costa R, Dunsford M, Skagerberg E, et al. Psychological support, puberty suppression, and psychosocial functioning in adolescents with gender dysphoria. J Sex Med 2015;12(11):2206–14.
6. Arnoldussen M, van der Miesen AIR, Elzinga WS, et al. Self-perception of transgender adolescents after gender-affirming treatment: a follow-up study into young adulthood. LGBT Health 2022;9(4):238–46.
7. Grannis C, Leibowitz SF, Gahn S, et al. Testosterone treatment, internalizing symptoms, and body image dissatisfaction in transgender boys. Psychoneuroendocrinology 2021;132:105358.
8. Kuper LE, Stewart S, Preston S, et al. Body dissatisfaction and mental health outcomes of youth on gender-affirming hormone therapy. Pediatrics 2020;145(4): e20193006.
9. Morningstar M, Thomas P, Anderson AM, et al. Exogenous testosterone administration is associated with differential neural response to unfamiliar peer's and own caregiver's voice in transgender adolescents. Dev Cogn Neurosci 2023;59: 101194.
10. Nieder TO, Mayer TK, Hinz S, et al. Individual treatment progress predicts satisfaction with transition-related care for youth with gender dysphoria: a prospective clinical cohort study. J Sex Med 2021;18(3):632–45.
11. Olsavsky AL, Grannis C, Bricker J, et al. Associations between gender-affirming hormonal interventions & social support with transgender adolescents' mental health. J Adolesc Health 2023;S1054-139X(23):00097.

12. Chen D, Berona J, Chan YM, et al. Psychosocial functioning in transgender youth after 2 years of hormones. N Engl J Med 2023;388(3):240–50.

13. Barbee H, Deal C, Gonzales G. Anti-transgender legislation-a public health concern for transgender youth. JAMA Pediatr 2022;176(2):125–6.

14. Cole, D. GOP Lawmakers Escalate Fight Against Gender Affirming Care with Bills Seeking to Expand the Scope of Bans. CNN website. https://www.cnn.com/2023/02/11/politics/gender-affirming-care-bans-transgender-rights/index.html. Published 2023. Accessed May 8, 2023.

15. Levine SB, Chairperson), Brown G, et al. The standards of care for gender identity disorders Fifth edition. Int J Transgenderism 1998;2(2). Available at. http://www.symposion.com/ijt/ijtc0405.htm.

16. American Psychiatric Association. Diagnostic and statistical manual of mental disorders. In: DSM-5). 5th edition. Arlington, VA: American Psychiatric Association Publishing; 2013.

17. de Graaf NM, Steensma TD, Carmichael P, et al. Suicidality in clinic-referred transgender adolescents. Eur Child Adolesc Psychiatr 2022;31:67–83.

18. Leibowitz S, de Vries AL. Gender dysphoria in adolescence. Int Rev Psychiatr 2016;28(1):21–35.

19. van der Miesen Anna IR, Steensma TD, de Vries ALC, et al. Psychological functioning in transgender adolescents before and after gender-affirmative care compared with cisgender general population peers. J Adolesc Health 2020; 66(6):699–704.

20. Hendricks ML, Testa RJ. A conceptual framework for clinical work with transgender and gender nonconforming clients: an adaptation of the minority stress model. Prof Psychol Res Pract 2012;43(5):460–7.

21. Chavanduka TMD, Gamarel KE, Todd KP, et al. Responses to the gender minority stress and resilience scales among transgender and nonbinary youth. J LGBT Youth 2021;18(2):135–54.

22. Chodzen G, Hidalgo MA, Chen D, et al. Minority stress factors associated with depression and anxiety among transgender and gender-nonconforming youth. J Adolesc Health 2019;64(4):467–71.

23. International statistical classification of Diseases and related health problems. 11th edition. World Health Organization; 2019. https://icd.who.int/browse11/l-m/en#/http://id.who.int/icd/entity/90875286.

24. Meyer W III, Bockting W, et al. The standards of care for gender identity disorders- sixth version. Int J Transgenderism 2001;5(1). Available at: http://www.symposion.com/ijt/soc_2001/index.htm.

25. Coleman E, Bockting W, Botzer M, et al. Standards of care for the health of transsexual, transgender, and gender- nonconforming people, version 7. Int J Transgenderism 2012;13(4):165–232.

26. de Vries ALC, Cohen-Kettenis PT. Clinical management of gender dysphoria in children and adolescents: the Dutch approach. J Homosex 2012;59(3):301–20.

27. Aitken M, Steensma TD, Blanchard R, et al. Evidence for an altered sex ratio in clinic-referred adolescents with gender dysphoria. J Sex Med 2015;12(3): 756–63.

28. Twist J, de Graaf N. Gender diversity and non-binary presentations in young people attending the United Kingdom's National Gender Identity Development Service. Clin Child Psychol Psychiatry 2019;24(2):277–90.

29. Sorbara JC, Ngo HL, Palmert MR. Factors associated with age of presentation to gender-affirming medical care. Pediatrics 2021;147(4). e2020026674.

30. de Vries ALC, Richards C, Tishelman AC, et al. Bell v Tavistock and Portman NHS Foundation Trust [2020] EWHC 3274: weighing current knowledge and uncertainties in decisions about gender-related treatment for transgender adolescents. International Journal of Transgender Health 2021;22(3):217–24.

31. American Academy of Child and Adolescent Psychiatry (AACAP) Sexual Orientation and Gender Identity Issues Committee. Conversion Therapy Policy Statement. Retrieved from: https://www.aacap.org/AACAP/Policy_Statements/2018/Conversion_Therapy.aspx. Published 2018. Accessed May 8, 2023.

32. Gower AL, Rider GN, Brown C, et al. Supporting transgender and gender diverse youth: protection against emotional distress and substance use. Am J Prev Med 2018;55(6):787–94.

33. Grossman AH, Park JY, Frank JA, et al. Parental responses to transgender and gender nonconforming youth: associations with parent support, parental abuse, and youths' psychological adjustment. J Homosex 2021;68(8):1260–77.

34. Lefevor GT, Sprague BM, Boyd-Rogers CC, et al. How well do various types of support buffer psychological distress among transgender and gender nonconforming students? Int J Transgenderism 2019;20(1):39–48.

35. Ryan C, Russell ST, Huebner D, et al. Family acceptance in adolescence and the health of LGBT young adults. J Child Adolesc Psychiatr Nursing 2010;23(4):205–13.

36. Pariseau EM, Chevalier L, Long KA, et al. The relationship between family acceptance-rejection and transgender youth psychosocial functioning. Clinical Practice in Pediatric Psychology 2019;7(3):267–77.

37. Quain KM, Kyweluk MA, Sajwani A, et al. Timing and delivery of fertility preservation information to transgender adolescents, young adults, and their parents. J Adolesc Health 2021;68(3):619–22.

38. de Vries ALC, Noens ILJ, Cohen-Kettenis PT, et al. Autism spectrum disorders in gender dysphoric children and adolescents. J Autism Dev Disord 2010;40(8):930–6.

39. Strang JF, Meagher H, Kenworthy L, et al. Initial clinical guidelines for Co-occurring autism spectrum disorder and gender dysphoria or incongruence in adolescents. J Clin Child Adolesc Psychol 2018;47(1):105–15.

40. Hembree WC, Cohen-Kettenis PT, Gooren L, et al. Endocrine treatment of gender-dysphoric/gender-incongruent persons: an endocrine society clinical practice guideline. J Clin Endocrinol Metab 2017;102(11):3869–903.

Assessment of Gender Diverse Children
Incorporating the Standard of Care 8th Edition

Amy Tishelman, PhD[a],*, G. Nic Rider, PhD[b]

KEYWORDS

- Transgender • Gender diverse • TGD • Childhood • Standards of care
- Assessment

KEY POINTS

- Standards of care for prepubescent children have been developed for the World Professional Association of Transgender Health (WPATH) Standards of Care 8th edition (SOC8) based on research, clinical consensus, and general psychological literature pertaining to child development.
- The prepubescent developmental period for children is an important time to promote well-being, to enhance childhood quality of life, and to set the stage for a positive transition to adolescence and adulthood, and this includes supporting a child's gender development, including for those who are gender diverse.
- Foundational, stipulated, principles of care for TGD youth underlie the Child chapter of SOC8, including a strong repudiation of attempts to compel a child to reject a TGD identity.
- Gender identity can be fluid in children; thus, children and caretakers need to be aware that change over time is possible and a child should be supported if they experience gender fluidity over time.
- Mental health professionals with broad training in general child clinical care and assessment, as well as specifically gender care can be helpful in facilitating positive development in children, healthy coping, and strongly supportive intra-family, peer, and community relationships.

INTRODUCTION

The SOC 8 child chapter was initially written by a European and American group of clinicians, researchers, and stakeholders all with demonstrable expertise in the area

[a] Department of Psychology and Neuroscience, Boston College, 140 Commonwealth Avenue, Chestnut Hill, MA 02467, USA; [b] Department of Family Medicine and Community Health, Institute for Sexual and Gender Health, University of Minnesota Medical School, 1300 South 2nd Street, Suite 180, Minneapolis, MN 55454, USA
* Corresponding author.
E-mail address: amy.tishelman@bc.edu

Child Adolesc Psychiatric Clin N Am 32 (2023) 719–730
https://doi.org/10.1016/j.chc.2023.05.008
1056-4993/23/© 2023 Elsevier Inc. All rights reserved.

childpsych.theclinics.com

of TGD youth, whether through lived experience and advocacy, clinical care, research, or a combination thereof.[1] The authorship was deliberately comprised to represent a diversity of perspectives. Nevertheless, authors overall shared an overarching vision, and consensus upon practice statements and text was less of a challenge than might have been anticipated. At the outset, all authors agreed upon certain working principles, including a stipulation of mutual respect for one another, an understanding that differences of opinion were welcome and would help facilitate a thoughtful approach to serious topics, and that working group members would retain a collegial appreciation for one another, even if emotionally laden disagreements occurred during discussions. The final Child SOC chapter is a document with strong support from each primary author and represents consensus for best practices in support of TGD children.

Child Chapter Considerations

- *Limited Empirical Research*: Although there has long been recognition that TGD children exist and may benefit from care and support, very little empirical study has been devoted to pre-adolescent TGD children. Thus, by necessity, the SOC 8 Child chapter reflects synthesized knowledge gleaned from a combination of areas, including: a) review of extant empirical literature on TGD children; b) review of non-empirical scholarship relevant to TGD children; c) examination of prior WPATH SOC recommendations; d) expert clinical consensus; and e) ethical considerations.
- *Developmental Perspective:* The Child SOC were created with the understanding that children are not just "little adults." Family, peer, community, and cultural factors can play an enormous role in the well-being of children, including their confidence, sense of self, and overall behavioral and mental health.
- *Ecological Framework:* An ecological approach[2–7] to care emphasizes that children influence and are influenced by each environment or setting of importance in their lives (eg, home, school, religious institution, and so forth). Thus, each setting frequented by children should be safe and welcoming of a child to the extent possible. Research consistently shows that TGD youth are at higher risk for significant childhood adversities compared to cisgender peers (eg, maltreatment, bullying)[8–10] and thus the consideration of safety concerns are paramount. Significant childhood adversities have been linked to some lifelong medical and mental health sequelae,[11–13] and ensuring and/or creating safety to the extent possible is a first step in any work with a TGD child. Gender minority stress can be particularly salient and challenging for TGD children and present in many forms, including being oppressed, stigmatized, antagonized, and/or negated and experiencing threat or actual violence in direct response to a gender diverse identity and/or expression.[14] Children may internalize negative messages encountered in their environments, leading to a sense of low self-worth and other self-diminishing characteristics. On the other hand, the literature indicates that acceptance and support for a TGD child can add to a sense of well-being and diminish mental health risks.[15,16]
- *Global Legal Contexts*: The Child SOC is meant to be relevant and used in a global context. Therefore, the development of the SOC required the consideration of resources and realities in diverse legal, cultural, and social environments. Overly proscriptive standards can preclude their applicability across diverse environments, while vague standards can weaken their meaning and importance. Thus, the authors attempted to balance these considerations, with the expectation that whenever possible efforts will be extended

to employ the SOC 8 recommended care approaches with children and their families.

- *Cultural Considerations* are pertinent to all clinical work, including with TGD youth and their families. Culture can broadly refer to myriad facets of identity and experience, including racial, ethnic, religious, geographic, citizen/immigrant status, and so forth. Many cultures can exist within an individual as well as within a family. Clinicians should strive to understand the impact and meaning of culture and experience for a child and family members, while avoiding biases or stereotyping based on preconceived ideas about identities. Intersections of gender identity and other cultural influences are important to comprehend for each child individually, particularly with regard to socio-structural factors (eg, gendered racism and transphobia) that may negatively impact resources available and can materially affect the daily lives of the child and family. Further, it is important to understand cultural strengths to build upon or draw from, which can be important for resilience building.
- **Box 1** refers to consensus-driven principles that underlie the SOC practice statements and which must be understood while working with TGD children, family members, and others.

SUMMARY OF CHILD STANDARD OF CARE 8 CONTENT

The Child chapter begins with an Introduction summarizing the foundational principles delineated above, the importance of cultural considerations, and the ecological and developmental perspectives helping to shape practice standards. The fifteen consensus-driven practice recommendations are then presented, as depicted in **Box 2**, followed by text elaboration.

Given that the guidelines and accompanying text are available to the public, a full explanation of the entire SOC 8 Child chapter is unnecessary and beyond the scope of this article. Instead, the following discussion will focus on the assessment of TGD children (recommendations 7.5, 7.6, and 7.7)

Assessments with Transgender and Gender Diverse Children

The American Psychological Association defines assessment partially as "the gathering and integration of data to evaluate a person's behavior, abilities, and other characteristics."[17] Thus, a primary assessment function includes synthesizing information to derive a full understanding of the child and their needs to address assessment goals and inform next steps, including a psychotherapeutic process as appropriate. Medical/surgical gender-affirming interventions are not used with prepubescent children; thus, effective treatments occur within psychosocial realms alone, which can include psychiatric/pharmacological assessment and intervention if necessary.

Child assessment in general is a complex endeavor, and can itself act as an intervention, in the sense that any interaction with a child may be replete with messages and sometimes unacknowledged or unintended communications. For instance, psychological literature has examined the effects that interviewers may have on child beliefs about their potential experiences of child sexual abuse, and developmental literature has examined child suggestibility (ie, inadvertent influence of children's beliefs and reports).[18] Therefore, it is critical that any provider is aware of their own biases and approaches assessment with an open and neutral stance. In other words, preconceived ideas about a child or family can lead to confirmation bias, thus skewing assessment findings and recommendations. Importantly, *TGD children do not always need to have a mental health and/or gender assessment*. Assessment will typically only

> **Box 1**
> **Stipulated principles and beliefs serving as foundations for the child standard of care practice statements for transgender and gender diverse children**
>
> - Gender diversity is an expected aspect of general human development.
> - Gender diversity is not a pathology or mental health disorder.
> - Each child should be accepted and respected in their individual gender identities and expressions.
> - Diverse gender expressions cannot be assumed to reflect a transgender identity or gender incongruence.
> - Gender identity may not be static and may change in ways that we cannot predict.
> - TGD children, or their family members, do not always need input from mental health providers.
> - Guidance from mental health providers with expertise in child gender care can be helpful in supporting a child's well-being, positive quality of life, strong relationships in and outside of the family and a comprehension of gender-related needs over time.
> - Gender-affirming medical treatments are not used in prepubescent children.
> - Attempts to "convert" a child's gender identity or expressions to accord with a sex assigned at birth are never acceptable.
> - Parents, caregivers, providers, and others should never overtly or covertly privilege any gender identity for a child, including a cisgender identity.

take place at the discretion of parents/guardians, sometimes upon the request of a child, or after encouragement from another health care provider, such as a pediatrician.

Many types of psychological assessments are possible.[19] Providers needs to be clear about what type of assessment is being requested, and the ultimate goal of the assessment. For instance, some assessments can be crisis or risk assessments, and others may be screening assessments to ensure that a child/family is appropriate for a particular service. In the Child SOC 8 chapter, the authors focused on comprehensive assessments, appropriate when a family is seeking to understand their TGD child's needs from a holistic or whole child perspective. This type of assessment is often used as a first step to developing therapeutic or psycho-educational recommendations for a child, parents/guardians, and/or family, if any, which can be discussed collaboratively with a child and other significant family members.[20–22]

Comprehensive assessments with transgender and gender diverse children should access and integrate information from multiple sources, domains, and methods as part of the assessment

Sources of Information: Almost all assessments of TGD youth will involve parents/guardians, unless they are unavailable, such as when a TGD child is residing in a therapeutic residential facility and parents or legal caregivers are inaccessible or otherwise inappropriate to include (maltreating, non-custodial parents, for example) We recommend the consideration of including cisgender siblings in an assessment process if they have a significant impact on the TGD child, as is suggested by some research,[23,24] or if they may have unexplored needs related to their relationship with their TGD sibling. Other extended family members can also participate in a child assessment, at the discretion of the child, parents/guardians, and the provider performing the assessment.

Box 2
Standard of care 8 child recommendations

7.1. We recommend that health care professionals working with gender diverse children receive training and have expertise in gender development and gender diversity in children, and general knowledge of gender diversity across the life span.

7.2. We recommend that health care professionals working with gender diverse children receive theoretical and evidenced-based training and develop expertise in general child and family mental health across the developmental spectrum.

7.3. We recommend that health care professionals working with gender diverse children receive training and develop expertise in autism spectrum disorders and other neurodiversity or collaborate with an expert with relevant expertise when working with autistic/neurodivergent, gender diverse children.

7.4. We recommend that health care professionals working with gender diverse children engage in continuing education related to gender diverse children and families.

7.5. We recommend that health care professionals conducting an assessment with gender diverse children access and integrate information from multiple sources as part of the assessment.

7.6. We recommend that health care professionals conducting an assessment with gender diverse children consider relevant developmental factors, neurocognitive functioning and language skills.

7.7. We recommend that health care professionals conducting an assessment with gender diverse children consider factors that may constrain accurate reporting of gender identity/gender expression by the child and/or family/caregiver(s).

7.8. We recommend that health care professionals consider consultation and/or psychotherapy for a gender diverse child and family/caregivers when families and health care professional believe this would benefit the well-being and development of a child and/or family.

7.9. We recommend that health care professionals offering consultation and/or psychotherapy to gender diverse children and families/caregivers work with other settings and individuals important to the child in order to promote the child's resilience and emotional well-being.

7.10. We recommend that health care professionals offering consultation and/or psychotherapy to gender diverse children and families/caregivers provide both with age-appropriate psychoeducation about gender development.

7.11. We recommend that health care professionals provide information to gender diverse children and their families/caregivers as the child approaches puberty about potential gender-affirming medical interventions, the effects of these treatments on future fertility, and options for fertility preservation.

7.12. We recommend that parents/caregivers and health care professionals respond supportively to children who desire to be acknowledged as the gender that matches their internal sense of gender identity.

7.13. We recommend that health care professionals and parents/caregivers support children to continue to explore their gender throughout the pre-pubescent years, regardless of social transition.

7.14. We recommend that health care professionals discuss the potential benefits and risks of a social transition with families who are considering it.

7.15. We suggest that health care professionals consider working collaboratively with other professionals and organizations to promote well-being of gender diverse children and minimize adversities they may face.

As noted earlier, as recommended by the SOC 8 Child chapter, a comprehensive assessment will be informed by a developmental and ecological framework. Thus, with family/guardian permission (when appropriate and safe) such an assessment will often include outreach to schools, or individuals in other settings of importance to a child.

The specific reasons for accessing multiple informants for a comprehensive assessment are multifold and can include the following:

- To understand a child's needs across contexts and settings.
- To understand the perspectives, observations, and interactions of a child with multiple influential people in their life.
- To identify child strengths and supports so these can be recognized and buoyed.
- To identify areas of risk or safety concerns, so these can be rectified.
- To understand who the child and family considers to be part of their support network

Domains of Inquiry Areas of inquiry for comprehensive assessments enable the provider to understand and integrate factors, currently and historically, that may impact a child's well-being and needs, both with regard to gender and in other areas of life as well. Thus, assessment domains include gender-related domains as well as those not related to gender. In addition, assessment should more broadly focus on the well-being of all family members, and family dynamics; children are impacted by all family members, and thus parents/guardian, grandparents and sibling stability and support are crucial to understand and integrate into recommendations. The SOC 8 Child chapter lists domains of inquiry for an assessment, summarized here in **Box 3** (gender-related domains) and **Box 4** (non–gender-related domains).

METHODS OF INFORMATION GATHERING

Typically, comprehensive psychological assessments of youth employ a number of means of data collection, which are then synthesized to develop recommendations based on the thorough picture that emerges. Information can be gathered to note if there are inconsistencies in reports or contradictions, and to understand the child's needs to the extent possible in the larger context of their life and development. The evaluation may also pinpoint areas of family need (conflict resolution between guardians, parental stress due to hostilities they may endure for supporting their TGD child, for example), and/or areas for advocacy (eg, working with a school to bolster safety,

---

Box 3
Gender-related domains to assess

- Child's asserted gender identity, currently and historically
- Child's gender-related expressions, currently and historically
- Evidence of gender dysphoria, gender incongruence or both
- Child and family members' experiences of gender minority stress, hostility, rejection, and so forth due to the child's gender diversity
- Level of support for gender diversity in social contexts (schools, camps, faith communities, extended family, preferred activities such as sports or drama, and so forth)
- Evaluation of conflict or concerning behaviors, within or outside the family, related to the child's gender diversity.

Box 4
Non-gender-related domains to assess

• Child mental health status, strengths, and concerns, currently and historically.

• Child communication skills and/or cognitive strengths, neurodivergencies, and/or areas of challenge.

• Behavioral challenges in one or more settings causing significant functional difficulties.

• Relevant medical and developmental history.

• Areas that may cause risk, family stressors.

• Family strengths and protective factors

• Parent/guardian and sibling mental health and behavioral strengths and challenges

• Areas of TGD child talents, abilities, and sources of joy.

---

reduce bullying, and so forth). Importantly, and as noted in the recommended assessment domains, a child and family's strengths and talents can be employed as part of the final assessment recommendations, as areas to build upon and preserve. As an example, if a child reports deriving joy from a hobby, that can be highlighted as an important factor to ensure is valued when recommending ways to support their positive sense of self and quality of life.

Several complexities sometimes intersect with gender-related assessment of TGD children. First, many paper and pencil gender measures have been criticized for any number of reasons, including for not being adequately validated, collapsing the constructs of gender identity and gender expression, and for assuming a binary gender identity, thus foreclosing the option of reporting a non-binary gender identity. Additionally, many measures are not attuned to the communication needs of youth who are on the autism spectrum.[25] More recently, a new tool for gender assessment, accounting for these critiques, has been published, the Gender Self-Report (GSR), attuned for use with TGD and cisgender youth, as well as for autistic and non-autistic young people, and for children as young as age 10 through adulthood.[25] However, standardized gender characterization remains complex, especially for the youngest children who at times may be most challenged when attempting to verbally express the nuances of their inner experiences.

A second concern with some standardized psychological measures is that they are normed by gender. However, these measures do not report norms for youth with a non-binary gender identity, nor do they give guidance for whether to score them based on a gender assumed at birth or a more current asserted gender identity. Some research has suggested that it makes little difference which normative scores are used,[26] while other studies suggest that some caution in the interpretation of gender norms for transgender youth is warranted.[27]

Some potential methods of data collection for a comprehensive assessment are listed in **Box 5**.

Comprehensive assessment with TGD children should consider factors that may constrain accurate reporting of gender identity/gender expression by the child and/or family/caregiver(s).

Many factors shape a child's development, and thus potentially influence what a child may be thinking, perceiving about their internal experiences of gender, or be willing to report to a provider during an initial assessment. Providers should avoid asking leading questions of children or adult family members –that is, questions that embed the expected response in the query itself (eg, you don't feel like a boy, do

---

Box 5
Possible methods of information-gathering

- Interviews, structured and/or unstructured, of child and family members
- Interviews, structured and/or unstructured, of collateral sources (eg, teachers, principals, coaches, clergy, current psychotherapists, and so forth)
- Parent/guardian, child and other (eg, teacher) completed paper and pencil standardized measures related to gender, child well-being, family functioning, acceptance and support, child development, cognitive and communications skills, and/or other areas as warranted based on clinical judgment.
- Structured assessment techniques, often visually supported, such as child worksheets, self-portraits, and family drawings.

---

you?). Leading questions reveal a provider's biases and may be most likely to result in invalid responses, especially with children or parents who may be eager to please or responsive to social expectations.[28]

Children who have experienced negative consequences for making certain statements about their gender identity or expressing themselves in ways considered by others to be non-conforming to gender expectations, may be reluctant to convey some aspects of their experience, fearing rejection and/or other adverse reactions. At times, it is possible that children may need more support to understand the meaning of gender for themselves. Thus, assessment may be a steppingstone in an unfolding process of self-understanding and self-advocacy, which can be acknowledged and continue following assessment, often in a therapeutic process. Parents/guardians and others in a family's life may be reluctant to share aspects of the family dynamic or history, including interactions with their child that may cause embarrassment or shame, or other areas of family unrest or conflict (including relatively common family challenges such as substance abuse, domestic violence, and so forth). Again, a comprehensive assessment may raise hypotheses about hidden family issues that may be affecting a child, but more information may emerge in a follow-up to the assessment.

General Clinical Guidance: Child Assessment

In general, when working with children, comfort and safety should be prioritized. This sometimes means, clinically, that a child may be reluctant to engage with questions or areas of inquiry. A provider needs to be able to follow the lead of a child if they demonstrate hesitancies or resist a provider's agenda when gathering specific information. This may mean that delaying the gathering of information in favor of developing rapport with a child can be important in certain situations. It can actually be a protective inclination for a child to be slow to convey sensitive or emotionally laden information to a provider who is a relative stranger. On the other hand, it is also important to recognize when a child may be *overly* trusting from the outset, demonstrating the possibility for other potential dynamics that may or may not be worth addressing clinically. Similar interpersonal dynamics may prevail with parents/guardians as well.

Box 6 summarizes some basic tenets of child assessment best practices.

Pre-pubescent social gender transition

As noted, medical/surgical interventions are not used with pre-pubescent children. Instead, interventions are relegated to the psychosocial arena. One of these

---

Box 6
Child assessment clinical guidance

- Assessment should be child-centered and child sensitive.
- Assessment should occur in a safe space.
- Assessment should be attuned to a child's developmental, and communicative abilities and preferences.
- All providers conducting assessments should maintain neutrality and avoid biased interactions.
- Assessment should not include coercive or leading questions.
- Assessments should follow a child's needs, especially if a child signals that they need to feel in control.
- Assessors should be aware that certain sensitive information may not be shared initially, or at all, including family "secrets."
- A child or others may have multiple factors influencing what they communicate.
- Prioritize child safety in all settings.

---

interventions may include a gender social transition process, referring to actions taken by child to live in some or all situations in a way that feels consistent with the gender identity they affirm and the gender-related expressions they prefer.[29] Gender social transition is an individualized process and can include gradual or abrupt modifications a child makes to their overt presentations and other behaviors. These can include changes in pronouns, names, hairstyle, clothing, participation in gender-segregated activities, and so forth. This is best viewed as a child-driven decision and can occur gradually or all at once. Children may choose to only share their gender social transition with certain people or in certain settings and may, as well, choose to change only certain aspects of their gender-related expressions. Although social gender transition may include a transition to a non-binary presentation, much of the research on child social transition thus far has included children who initiated a full binary transition. In a series of studies, Kristina Olson and colleagues examined the well-being and functioning of self-selected prepubescent children following social transition, and compared them to cisgender siblings and colleagues. They found, overall, that TGD youth who had socially transitioned were generally well-adjusted and indistinguishable from their cisgender siblings and peers aside from some non-clinically meaningful elevations in anxiety.[16,30] Although, this research has some limitations (self-selected, non-representative participants, for example), it does indicate that TGD youth are not inevitably beset by mental health struggles and can enjoy a generally positive quality of life. The SOC 8 recognizes these positive research findings, as well as the need for continued research, and advises an individualized and thoughtful decision-making process with TGD children and their parents/guardians in order to foster both acceptance and safety. The SOC 8 also recommends that children be supported in continued reflection regarding gender as needed, with an understanding that gender may be fluid (see recommendation 7.13). When considering a social gender transition, the following considerations may be helpful.

- Recognize the nuances of a social gender transition to assist children and families with decision-making, weighing individualized priorities.

- Ensure that children understand that they have the freedom to evolve in gender identity/expression over time, as best suits them and their needs, leaving all pathways open.
- Ensure continuing safety, emotional and physical, in all settings in which a social gender transition process takes place. Dynamic processing of challenges can be ongoing during a social transition process.

SUMMARY

Childhood is a distinct and critical developmental period in the life of any individual. During this time, children acquire massive amounts of information, including important foundational academic, social, and life skills. Psychological literature demonstrates that children can develop risks and resiliencies during this time period that can persist as trajectories of development through adolescence and adulthood. Childhood is also an opportunity to shape experience in way that diminishes distress, promotes self-worth, confidence, and positive coping skills, and sets up a child to be able to traverse the stressors of life adaptively, and while drawing on strong and trusting established relationships. This is, thus, a critical time period for TGD youth, who are more likely than cisgender peers and siblings to encounter significant life stressors, and to be burdened with adversities not experienced by others such as gender minority stressors. The SOC 8 Child chapter is the first to illuminate best practices during these important years in a TGD young person's early life and to highlight ways in which well-being can be supported.

CLINICS CARE POINTS

- Childhood is an important developmental period for TGD children for various reasons, including:
  - The value of enhancing the quality of life for children while they are still children.
  - The value of promoting well-being, positive relationships, and coping skills in order to support children in the transition to adolescence and adulthood with resiliencies in place.
  - Helping children reflect on their gender care needs, prepare for some of the changes that occur with the onset of puberty, and start to reflect on upcoming gender-affirming options (if desired).
- Providers working with TGD children and their families should be well-qualified through general child and family mental health training as well as specific training in the developmental needs of TGD youth.
- Child safety is always a priority and assessment should ensure safety across settings in a child's life. Childhood adversities are common for all children, but even more prevalent for TGD children.
- It is critical for providers to reflect on and address their own biases as well as approach assessment using an intersectionality-informed lens. Further, overt and more subtle interactions can impact children and others during an assessment.
- Providers should be aware that gender needs and gender identity and expression can be fluid for children, and children should be encouraged to appreciate that they will be supported through any gender-related changes they may experience.
- Providers should stay updated on research related to promoting the well-being of TGD youth, which is limited but burgeoning.
- A comprehensive child assessment of gender diverse youth should take into account a child's ecology, and involve important people in a child's life, embrace a holistic approach, and synthesize multiple forms of information. Assessment should focus on promoting well-being as well as decreasing risks and distress.

DISCLOSURE

The authors have no relevant financial disclosures nor conflicts of interest to declare.

REFERENCES

1. Coleman E, Radix AE, Bouman WP, et al. Standards of care for the health of transgender and gender diverse people, version 8. International Journal of Transgender Health 2022;23(S1):S1–260.
2. Bronfenbrenner U. Contexts of child rearing: problems and prospects. Am Psychol 1979;34(10):844–50.
3. Belsky J. Etiology of child maltreatment: a developmental-ecological analysis. Psychol Bull 1993;114(3):413–34.
4. Lynch M, Cicchetti D. An ecological-transactional analysis of children and contexts: the longitudinal interplay among child maltreatment, community violence, and children's symptomatology. Dev Psychopathol 1998;10(2):235–57.
5. Kaufman RT, Tishelman A. In: Keo-Meier C, Ehrensaft D, editors. The gender affirmative model: an interdisciplinary approach to supporting transgender and gender expansive children. American Psychological Association; 2018. p. 173–88, chap Creating a Network of Professionals.
6. Zielinski DS, Bradshaw CP. Ecological influences on the sequelae of child maltreatment: a review of the literature. Child Maltreat 2006;11(1):49–62.
7. Tishelman AC, Haney P, Greenwald O'Brien J, et al. A framework for school-based psychological evaluations: utilizing a 'Trauma lens'. J Child Adolesc Trauma 2010;3(4):279–302.
8. Schnarrs PW, Stone AL, Salcido R Jr, et al. Differences in adverse childhood experiences (ACEs) and quality of physical and mental health between transgender and cisgender sexual minorities. J Psychiatr Res 2019;119:1–6.
9. Thoma BC, Rezeppa TL, Choukas-Bradley S, et al. Disparities in childhood abuse between transgender and cisgender adolescents. Pediatrics 2021;148(2). https://doi.org/10.1542/peds.2020-016907.
10. James SE, Herman JL, Rankin S, et al. The report of the 2015 U.S. Transgender survey. Washington, DC: National Center for Transgender Equality; 2016.
11. Anda RF, Butchart A, Felitti VJ, et al. Building a framework for global surveillance of the public health implications of adverse childhood experiences. Am J Prev Med 2010;39(1):93–8.
12. Masten AS, Cicchetti D. Developmental cascades. Dev Psychopathol 2010;22(3):491–5.
13. Shonkoff JP, Garner AS. Committee on psychosocial aspects of child and family health; Committee on early childhood, Adoption, and dependent care; section on developmental and behavioral pediatrics. The lifelong effects of early childhood adversity and toxic stress. Pediatrics 2012;129(1):e232–46.
14. Hendricks ML, Testa RJ. A conceptual framework for clinical work with transgender and gender nonconforming clients: an adaptation of the Minority Stress Model. Prof Psychol Res Pract 2012;43:460–7.
15. Malpas J, Glaeser E, Giammattei SV. Building resilience in transgender and gender expansive children, families, and communities: A multidimensional family approach. In: Keo C, Ehrensaft MD, editors. The gender affirmative model: An interdisciplinary approach to supporting transgender and gender expansive children. American Psychological Association; 2018. p. 141–56.

16. Olson KR, Durwood L, DeMeules M, et al. Mental health of transgender children who are supported in their identities. Pediatrics 2016;137(3). https://doi.org/10.1542/peds.2015-3223.

17. APA Dictionary of Psychology. American Psychological Association. Available at: https://dictionary.apa.org/psychological-assessment. Accessed June 29, 2023.

18. Ceci SJ, Bruck M. Suggestibility of the child witness: a historical review and synthesis. Psychol Bull 1993;113(3):403–39.

19. Krishnamurthy R, VandeCreek L, Kaslow NJ, et al. Achieving competency in psychological assessment: directions for education and training. J Clin Psychol 2004;60(7):725–39.

20. American Psychological Association. APA task force on psychological assessment and evaluation guidelines. APA Guidelines for Psychological Assessment and Evaluation; 2020.

21. de Vries AL, Cohen-Kettenis PT. Clinical management of gender dysphoria in children and adolescents: the Dutch approach. J Homosex 2012;59(3):301–20.

22. Srinath S, Jacob P, Sharma E, et al. Clinical practice guidelines for assessment of children and adolescents. Indian J Psychiatry 2019;61(Suppl 2):158–75.

23. Pariseau EM, Chevalier L, Long KA, et al. The relationship between family acceptance-rejection and transgender youth psychosocial functioning. Clinical Practice in Pediatric Psychology 2019;7(3):267–77.

24. Parker E, Davis-McCabe C. The sibling experience: growing up with a trans sibling. Aust J Psychol 2021;73(2):188–99.

25. Strang JF, Wallace GL, Michaelson JJ, et al. The Gender Self-Report: a multidimensional gender characterization tool for gender-diverse and cisgender youth and adults. Am Psychol 2023. https://doi.org/10.1037/amp0001117.

26. Rider GN, Berg D, Pardo ST, et al. Using the Child Behavior Checklist (CBCL) with transgender/gender nonconforming children and adolescents. Clin Pract Pediatr Psychol 2019;7:291–301.

27. Brecht A, Bos S, Ries L, et al. Assessment of psychological distress and peer relations among trans adolescents-an examination of the use of gender norms and parent-child Congruence of the YSR-R/CBCL-R among a Treatment-seeking sample. Children (Basel) 2021;8(10):864.

28. Powell MB, Hughes-Scholes CH, Sharman SJ. Skill in interviewing reduces confirmation bias. J Investigative Psychol Offender Profiling 2012;9(2):126–34.

29. Ehrensaft D, Giammattei SV, Storck K, et al. Prepubertal social gender transitions: what we know; what we can learn– a view from a gender affirmative lens. Int J Transgenderism 2018;19(2):251–68.

30. Durwood L, McLaughlin KA, Olson KR. Mental health and self-worth in socially transitioned transgender youth. J Am Acad Child Adolesc Psychiatry 2017;56:116–23.

Complex Psychiatric Histories and Transgender and Gender Diverse Youth

Amy Curtis, MD[a],*, Shanna Swaringen, DO[b], Aron Janssen, MD[c,1]

KEYWORDS

• LGBTQ • Transgender • Youth • Mental health • Minority stress

KEY POINTS

- Gender diverse presentations are normal aspects of development and may not be associated with presence of clinically significant mental health concerns.
- Transgender youth carry unique health risks and needs that are important to consider in the context of the psychiatric assessment.
- Experiences stemming from discrimination and marginalization create unique stressors that may explain higher rates of health-risking behaviors and mental health struggles among transgender youth.
- Complex, co-occurring mental health concerns are important to consider when assessing for gender dysphoria in transgender youth, although they may or may not influence gender goals and/or decisional capacity.
- Assessment and treatment approaches should be adapted based on individual treatment needs while incorporating developmental and communication differences, type and severity of mental illness, pattern of social stressors, and youth and caregiver priorities.

INTRODUCTION

Gender diversity has existed across millennia, cultures, social structures, and human experiences. Exploring gender is a natural part of development, with many children experimenting with gender expression and roles during childhood. Therefore, diverse

---

[a] Department of Psychiatry and Behavioral Sciences, University of Washington School of Medicine. Seattle Children's Hospital, 4800 Sand Point Way NE, Seattle, WA 98105, USA; [b] Division of Psychiatry and Behavioral Health, The Ohio State University College of Medicine. Nationwide Children's Hospital, 700 Children's Drive, Columbus, OH 43205, USA; [c] The Pritzker Department of Psychiatry and Behavioral Health, Associate Professor of Psychiatry and Behavioral Sciences, Northwestern University Feinberg School of Medicine, 446 E Ontario, Chicago, IL 60611, USA
[1] Present address: 746 Michigan Avenue, Evanston, IL 60202, USA
* Corresponding author. 6901 Sand Point Way NE Seattle, WA 98115
E-mail address: amy.curtis@seattlechildrens.org
Twitter: @LGBTDoc (A.J.)

Child Adolesc Psychiatric Clin N Am 32 (2023) 731–745
https://doi.org/10.1016/j.chc.2023.05.011
childpsych.theclinics.com
1056-4993/23/© 2023 Elsevier Inc. All rights reserved.

gendered behaviors and presentations represent normal variations in development and are not inherently reflective of pathologic processes.

Gender diverse identification is also distinct from psychiatric diagnoses. As summarized from the diagnostic criteria in the *Diagnostic and Statistical Manual of Mental Disorders* (Fifth Edition), "gender dysphoria" (GD) refers to the inner sense of distress and related functional impairment stemming from experiencing a gender identity discordant from one's birth-assigned gender.[1] In the absence of impaired functioning or clinically significant distress, one can identify as gender diverse and not meet the clinical threshold for a GD diagnosis. Similarly, one can meet the diagnostic criteria for GD but opt not to pursue social or medical transition. It is important to recognize the harmful impacts of historical care practices and transgender individuals' experiences of bias, discrimination, and barriers to care.

This article focuses on the cause, assessment, and treatment of complex mental health struggles experienced by transgender youth. The first section highlights the importance of considering minority stress in understanding disproportionately high rates of mental illness and health-risking behaviors. Second, the authors review care approaches for transgender youth with complex mental conditions and implications for GD assessment. Finally, tailored treatment approaches and key clinical concepts are reviewed, highlighting the importance of comprehensive approaches in supporting the needs of transgender and gender diverse (TGD) youth.

TRANSGENDER YOUTH AND MINORITY STRESS
Minority Stress Model

Consideration of minority stress is essential when exploring the mental health needs of minoritized populations. Based on work with LGB (lesbian, gay, bisexual) populations, Meyer's Minority Stress Model helps to explain differential health outcomes seen in stigmatized minority groups, with compounding impacts of internal, interpersonal, and structural factors.[2] The model has subsequently been adapted to consider the unique needs of TGD individuals, highlighting elevated rates of adverse experiences and negative health outcomes for TGD populations compared with their cisgender LGB peers.[3] In addition to increased adversities shared with the greater LGBTQ (lesbian, gay, bisexual, transgender, queer/questioning) group, unique stressors for TGD individuals include negative experiences arising from unsupported gender identity and transphobia.

The minority stress model helps to explain higher rates of psychopathology observed in gender and sexual minority populations. External stressors—including overt and covert transphobia and discrimination, social stigma and bias, victimization/bullying, and family rejection—combined with internal stressors—including internalized homophobia and transphobia, GD, difficulty navigating puberty and gender transition, active mental health symptoms, and ongoing effects from past adverse experiences—may collectively contribute to emotional distress and mental health struggles. Discomfort with interpersonal interactions stemming from GD and minority stress can also lead to downstream effects, including social isolation and associated mental health challenges. Concerns related to social acceptance and safety may pressure youth to hide their identity with subsequent, negative psychological impacts.

Discrimination, Rejection, and Victimization

Gender minorities face higher rates of adverse experiences, including family rejection, homelessness, victimization, trauma, academic and employment discrimination, and legal and systems biases.[4] Surveillance studies indicate that TGD youth experience both increased generalized and targeted bullying, with rates of stigma-based bullying and victimization highest for TGD youth of color (YOC).[5] Transgender youth experiencing gender-based victimization are particularly vulnerable to mental health struggles including depression, self-harm, and suicidal ideation.[4]

Although family and peer support are critically important and main predictors of psychosocial outcomes, integral family relationships are also more likely to be disrupted among TGD youth.[6,7] Furthermore, TGD youth are at increased risk of maltreatment, insecure attachment, and increased childhood adverse experiences.[8] Lack of protective social supports can increase susceptibility to stressors, because family disruptions and lack of structured supports are linked with adverse outcomes including mental illness and insecure housing.[6,7]

Discriminatory practices in academic, occupational, and recreational settings are also associated with pervasive negative impacts.[9] Reducing access to safe and affirming spaces, including identity-congruent bathrooms and participation in youth sports, has been associated with harmful health impacts for transgender youth, including increased depression and suicidality.[9,10] Victimization experiences and perceived lack of safety are linked to poorer school performance, chronic absenteeism, and lower graduation and college attendance rates.[5]

Health Care Stigma and Bias

LGBTQ individuals experience multiple health and economic disparities. Historically, diverse sexuality and/or gender identity has been deemed inherently pathologic, subjecting many LGBTQ individuals to invasive and harmful treatment practices. Those with diverse gender identities are at even greater risk of receiving inadequate health care and experiencing bias, discrimination, and humiliation in health care settings. Health care workers are often inadequately trained on LGBTQ-affirming care practices, especially for TGD patients. Invalidating experiences around incorrect name or pronoun use, caregiver confidentiality concerns, and biased care practices can further decrease care engagement. One study on transgender youth revealed concerns that more than one-third of participants had avoided needed medical treatments due to fear of negative interactions surrounding gender identity.[11] Some LGBTQ youth may even avoid disclosing sexuality or gender identity due to safety and confidentiality concerns, despite these being pertinent to the health encounter. Furthermore, navigating burdensome insurance and systemic barriers to medically indicated care can further drive disparities in health outcomes for transgender populations. Ultimately, delays in diagnosis, treatment, and preventive measures are harmful to TGD youth and may result in poorer health outcomes.

Exacerbated by intersecting marginalized identities, gender minority YOC are especially likely to experience health care stigma and its associated impacts. TGD YOC experience greater socioeconomic barriers to accessing health resources, with added limitations on affirming medical care.[9] Additional systemic factors include lack of providers knowledgeable in supporting marginalized populations and rarity of health care staff with shared identity experiences. History of negative health care experiences, in the context of racist and transphobic structural influences, may lead TGD YOC to avoid seeking care for fear of future discrimination. Inadequate preventive care and treatment access contributes to numerous downstream health risks, which are of particular concern in youth with multiple minority identities.[9]

PSYCHOLOGICAL IMPACTS OF MINORITY STRESS

In considering drivers for mental health concerns among TGD youth, influences can be conceptualized as stemming from 3 main categories (**Fig. 1**).

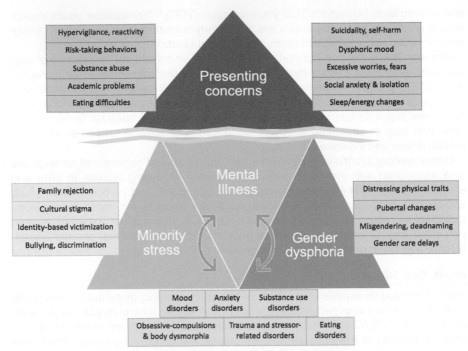

Fig. 1. Three categories of drivers for mental health complaints among transgender youth. Presenting concerns are the "tip of the iceberg" in assessing mental health needs among TGD youth. Any presenting concerns—both internalizing and externalizing—may stem from multiple distinct, yet interrelated, influencing factors. Presenting concerns for TGD youth seeking mental health care can be grouped into 3 main categories: (1) minority stress, (2) mental illness, and (3) gender dysphoria.

1. Mental health concerns secondary to experiences of stigma, marginalization, and gender-based discrimination.
2. Psychopathology related to GD.
3. Psychiatric disorders occurring alongside or integrated with gender concerns, which may or may not be important for understanding gender identity needs.

Given the added risks accompanying minority stress, TGD youth are especially vulnerable to struggles in multiple health and functional domains. It is also important to appreciate that higher rates of mental health concerns among gender minorities tend to normalize in more accepting environments and when receiving appropriate supports.

Stressors unique to gender minority identity can also help to understand disproportionate mental health needs among TGD individuals. Transgender adults suffer from higher rates of mental health disorders than cisgender adults, including depression, suicidality, anxiety, eating disorders, and neurodevelopmental disorders.[12–15] Similar findings are noted in TGD youth, particularly those experiencing numerous adversities, with victimization and rejection increasing risk for multiple mental health sequelae.[9]

Depression and Suicidality

Across literature studies, evidence supports the strong link between adverse experiences, including gender-based victimization/bullying and lack of parent support, and significant mental health struggles, such as depression and suicidal behaviors.[4,16] Numerous studies have demonstrated higher rates of suicidal ideation, suicide attempts, and nonsuicidal self-injury among TGD youth compared with cisgender peers, with literature estimates often ranging from 40% to 60%.[4,16–18] Youth experiencing bullying are more likely to suffer from depression, self-harm, and suicidal ideation, with TGD youth disproportionately impacted.[4,7,19,20]

Anxiety and Posttraumatic Sequelae

Increased rates of anxiety disorders among TGD populations have been conceptualized as an outcome of minority stress.[21] Transgender youth experience higher rates of physical, sexual, and psychological abuse.[22] Earlier trauma combined with later adversities can lead to subsequent trauma-related sequelae including posttraumatic stress, dissociative symptoms, and difficulties regulating emotions.[23] Transgender youth may also experience more social disconnectedness and isolation by way of internalized blame, low self-esteem, and family, peer, and societal rejection.[3,7]

Eating Disorders

Studies demonstrate elevated rates of disordered eating among transgender populations.[24] Many TGD youth experience baseline body dissatisfaction and dysphoria that can be compounded by the onset of puberty.[24–26] TGD youth may engage in restrictive or other compensatory behaviors in efforts to reduce contributors to GD or better align with societal expectations consistent with their identified gender.[26–28] Delays in gender-affirming treatment (GAT) can also lead to the TGD young person's overreliance on maladaptive coping strategies in efforts to optimize gender congruence.[27,29] TGD youth with eating concerns have also been found to be at particularly elevated risk for suicide.[28]

Substance Use and Abuse

LGBTQ youth carry increased risk for substance use and substance use disorders.[20] In addition, transgender teens have higher rates of substance abuse compared with their cisgender peers.[4,18] Adverse experiences, including bullying and violence victimization, have been found to strongly correlate with substance use.[18]

GENDER DYSPHORIA AND COMPLEX PSYCHIATRIC CONDITIONS
Background on Examining Mental Health of Transgender Populations

Gender diverse identities are present across multiple populations, including those with severe and/or persistent mental illness. The authors have reviewed the role of stigma and structural factors in influencing mental health outcomes and experiences of distress secondary to GD. In this section, unique factors in the assessment and management of patients with complex psychiatric conditions presenting with gender-related concerns are reviewed. Specifically, GD is examined in the context of complex psychiatric conditions including bipolar and psychotic disorders. The overlap between gender-related concerns and developmental considerations, such as autism spectrum disorder, is briefly highlighted here but covered in more depth in a separate article in the online version.

Historically, literature on TGD populations have centered on the assumption of gender diversity as illness, including relatively recent classifications schemes within health care and psychiatry. In the mid-twentieth century, it was not uncommon for transgender identity to be seen as an inherent outgrowth of a psychotic disorder.[30,31] By the 1990s, study approaches began to reflect the notion that symptoms of mental illness can coexist with transgender identities and that transgender individuals are not inherently mentally ill.

Practices within gender-affirming care through much of the twentieth century often necessitated a high level of psychological stability in the patient. In a care system requiring mental health conditions be "reasonably well-controlled," TGD individuals with psychiatric disorders, especially those with severe and persistent mental illness (SPMI), have been substantially disadvantaged. Unless individuals successfully concealed their symptoms, there often were insurmountable barriers that prevented access to affirming interventions. As a result, little research has been conducted about the overlap between transgender identity and SPMI, and it was only in the 2010s that larger prospective studies and literature reviews on this overlap emerged.

Overlap of gender dysphoria and chronic mental illness

There are challenges to accurately capturing the data between the overlap of GD and SPMI, which may stem from the small percentage of each population represented by a limited number of studies. As such, there are 3 potential main techniques used to explore the question of diagnostic overlap.

The first approach is to study SPMI rates among those presenting for gender care as part of a scientific study, which represents most of the published literature on this topic to date. The most rigorous efforts collected data longitudinally and systematically using evidence-based and psychometrically validated diagnostic instruments.[32–34] Current literature findings offer limited consensus that SPMI is more likely to occur among those with GD. Although some conditions such as depressive and anxiety disorders are shown to be consistently elevated among studies examining TGD populations, rates of severe and chronic conditions generally reflect those of the greater population. A few studies have found elevated rates of psychosis-related diagnoses in GD study samples.[35,36] No increased rates of bipolar disorder have been demonstrated.[37] Use of this approach has demonstrated increased rates of autism among youth with GD.[38]

The second technique studies rates of GD among individuals with SPMI. Despite several literature reviews noting the potential relevance, there have yet to be published studies using this specific technique with psychotic spectrum or bipolar spectrum disorders.[39,40] For youth with autism, there is evidence of increased rates of gender diversity among the clinically referred population.[40]

The third technique is to use large medical record data to compare expected versus documented rates of the GD and SPMI overlap. Although there are limitations in the interpretation of these data, several studies have used hospital-based claims data to capture large sample sizes.[13,41] Using this methodology, there is some evidence to suggest that TGD patients seeking care are more likely to have a co-occurring psychotic disorder than cisgender peers.

Taken as a whole, apart from the call for further research, the data are mixed. There is no evidence to suggest increased rates of bipolar disorder among individuals with GD, and there is contradictory evidence around rates of psychotic disorders among individuals with GD. In addition, it is hypothesized that higher rates of psychosis-related diagnoses among those with GD could stem from a variety of factors, including misdiagnosis or influence from pathology-driven views of TGD identities, rather than reflective of primary psychotic disorders.[39]

Diagnosing Gender Dysphoria in Complex Conditions

When a patient with SPMI is presenting for assessment, it is important to recognize what is required in an assessment to ensure equitable access to appropriate care.

First, diagnostic clarity around GD may require multiple informants to better understand symptom development over time and across contexts; this is the gold standard in any informed practice, but for individuals with SPMI, whether the individual's GD symptoms persist across illness states and over time must be assessed. That is to say, are symptoms of GD present only when the patient is in an acute psychotic or manic state? Or are the symptoms comparable in more euthymic and/or less psychotic periods? Is the identity stable over time and across states?

Second, after finding diagnostic clarity, one must work collaboratively with the patient and caregivers around a treatment plan. Paramount to treatment planning is a collaborative discussion with the patient and family to elucidate the risks, benefits, and alternatives of any proposed intervention. Although providers should never make assumptions about an individual's capacity to consent, in the population of individuals with SPMI, this missive takes on added importance. Historically, although those with SPMI have been barred access to care, new guidance from World Professional Association of Transgender Health offers a more nuanced approach.[41] There is broad recognition that most individuals with SPMI will retain decision-specific capacity. In addition, it is required that clinicians continue to assess for decisional capacity and to center treatment on ameliorating psychiatric symptoms and restoring capacity if capacity standards are not yet met. Furthermore, clinicians should work collaboratively with their most vulnerable patients to understand and actualize their individual goals. For many individuals with SPMI, there are independent factors that also impair access to care. Unhoused individuals may lack a safe space to transition, store and take medications, or recover from surgery. Those with substance dependency, such as to nicotine, may be able to consent to a procedure but lack access to that procedure due to risks the substance use poses to surgical safety. For individuals with autism, often there are challenges with communication and language that may require more specialized evaluative techniques to best understand that individual's experience.

For these patients, stepped care may not be an option. There will be a cohort of individuals with GD and SPMI who require significant support to achieve or restore decisional capacity. In these cases, there must be collaborative work to incorporate gender-affirming goals into the broader treatment plan and think holistically about how patients may find validation or support. Although not all individuals will be appropriate for medical or surgical interventions, universal efforts should strive for identity validation and affirmation across all contexts.

Outstanding Questions and Research Needs

Although evidence from the longitudinal studies of individuals with GD demonstrate no worsening of SPMI or increased development of SPMI, individuals with GD and SPMI remain a vulnerable population about which little is known.[42–44] With increasing awareness of gender diverse identification among youth, foreseeably a portion of this population will experience SPMI, requiring comprehensive care approaches. As a field, we must work to better understand the unique mental health needs of this important, vulnerable, and resilient population of young individuals. By seeking improved screening and data collection efforts, we can strive to inform more accurately tailored care adaptations, and through the guidance of a trauma-informed approach, create comprehensive care plans to address the unique challenges faced by TGD patients.

Key points: supporting transgender youth with complex mental illness

- Gender diversity is present across all populations and groups, including among those with complex and persistent mental illness.

- Co-occurring mental health needs of TGD youth must not be overlooked.
- Not every psychiatric presentation is related to gender identity.
- Not all gender identity-related concerns persist, and treatment goals may change.
- Psychiatric providers should foster collaborative decision-making efforts with young patients and their caregivers, including use of active listening and perspective-taking strategies while balancing mental health and gender goals.
- Preservation of decision-making capacity for those with complex mental illness is vital, particularly in navigating GAT.

ADAPTIVE ASSESSMENT AND TREATMENT APPROACH
Affirming Psychiatric Assessment of Transgender Youth

It is important to use gender-affirming care principles in approaching psychiatric assessment of TGD youth. The assessment should allow space for the youth to explore their identity, address any relevant co-occurring concerns, and strategize ways to optimize affirming supports and interventions. This evaluation process includes helping the individual and their guardians, if pertinent, fully understand and carefully consider the potential benefits and risks of various gender treatment pathways. On the other hand, narrowing the scope of the psychiatric evaluation to a rigid diagnostic delineation may not offer the most meaningful service to the youth or their family. By using an affirming and patient-centered approach, the evaluation focus can be individualized to the youth's specific circumstances and treatment needs.

Role of the psychiatric provider in supporting transgender youth

- Supporting and affirming the patient's identities, including recognizing and addressing any associated protective and/or risk variables.
- Considering the potential impact of gender concerns, including experiences of GD and unsupported identity, on mental health presentation.
- Helping the patient to identify treatment goals and a care plan that best fits their current needs while balancing youth and caregiver priorities.
- Considering and addressing any co-occurring medical or psychological needs, including those that may influence capacity or gender care decisions.

Youth with complex psychiatric histories in addition to a diagnosis of GD may benefit from a multidisciplinary approach, especially in cases in which safety or medical risks are elevated.[45] Given the heightened risk of mental health challenges, including anxiety, depression, and eating disorders, providers should screen regularly for symptoms that may require additional treatment.

There are few factors that are known to present absolute contraindications or barriers to proceeding with affirming medical interventions, even in the setting of SPMI. Barring acute safety concerns or serious capacity deficits, it is generally recommended to pursue necessary mental health treatment while concurrently supporting gender-affirming care needs.[46] Factors warranting urgent prioritization of crisis stabilization over GAT could include imminent safety risks (significant self-harm, active suicidality, or aggression), acute psychiatric presentations (severe psychosis or mania), concerns for decisional capacity, and/or misaligned gender care goals between patient and caregivers.

It is also important to note that postponing GAT is not necessarily a benign approach, because withholding care may prolong or exacerbate mental health symptoms, including suicidality, driven by GD.[46,47] In this sense, mental health clinicians may unintentionally serve in a "gatekeeper" function. In considering GAT for minors, potential risks and benefits of choosing or not choosing various treatment options should be carefully examined. As the psychiatric provider working with TGD youth and their caregivers, it is important to foster a collaborative conversation in efforts to make a decision that (1) is fully informed, (2) is based on best available evidence, and (3) carries a reasonable expectation of achieving the best overall health outcomes for the individual.

Working to clarify the caregiver's perspective is essential when exploring gender goals, especially given that guardian consent is requisite for any medical or surgical interventions. In addition, understanding family dynamics is a necessary component of case conceptualization. Navigating potential differing treatment priorities between the young person and their caregivers is a component of any psychiatric evaluation but with additional considerations for TGD youth. It is necessary to collaborate with the youth and their support network to create a comprehensive care plan striving for best overall outcomes. Specific patterns of symptoms, while potentially influencing how an individual experiences and/or expresses gender, also factor into the assessment and treatment process. As a whole, any efforts to affirm gender identity, regardless of GAT, can have a profound, positive impact on the well-being and mental health for TGD youth.

Optimizing Resilience and Mitigating Stressors

Treatment approaches in working with TGD youth should prioritize both direct interventions addressing mental and physical health needs and indirect means, including risk mitigation and bolstering resilience. Family acceptance and social connectedness are well-established as important factors influencing health outcomes for TGD youth.[48] Studies have demonstrated that socially transitioned TGD youth with good family support do not seem to have significantly higher inherent rates of psychopathology than cisgender peers.[49]

Because social connectedness is a strong protective factor for TGD youth and predictor of mental health outcomes, it is crucial to consider this when formulating the broader treatment plan.[48,49] Protective factors against negative health outcomes include parent/family engagement, positive parenting practices and affirming approaches, and school connectedness.[50] Increased social support for TGD youth has also been shown to reduce rates of future risk-taking behaviors and victimization.[9] Connecting caregivers to accurate sources of information and linking with parent-focused support systems is associated with improved mental health outcomes in TGD youth.[51]

Practitioners should be mindful that TGD youth may have poor family support or limited access to resources. Several community and national organizations exist for TGD youth, although they may not always be accessible due to geographic or social/family barriers (a resource list can be found in the article "Supporting Transgender Youth Across Psychosocial Systems" in this issue). Strain in the parent-child relationship related to gender may contribute to emotional distancing, which may result in decreased caregiver awareness of a youth's depression or anxiety symptom burden and underreporting of concerns at health care visits.[52] Safe online spaces may also serve as critical means of connection and self-expression for marginalized youth.[53,54]

Ensuring affirming resources in school settings is also a key component of a comprehensive wellness plan for TGD youth. Affirming and inclusive school climates are highly associated with improved experiences and greater sense of safety among LGBTQ students and serve a protective effect against health-risking behaviors including substance use.[5,50] Positive school-based initiatives include access to knowledgeable and trusted adult figures, bully prevention policies, affirming student groups, and LGBTQ-inclusive curriculum.

DISCUSSION AND FUTURE RESEARCH
Improving Health Care Settings and Experiences

Transgender patients frequently report negative and discriminatory experiences in health care settings, which can lead to future care avoidance and health risks.[11] Improving initiatives to educate health care providers and support staff on affirming care, including enhancing trauma-informed approaches, is vital in optimizing health experiences and outcomes for transgender youth and should be prioritized as part of comprehensive efforts to close the health care disparity gap.

Supporting Access to Gender Medical Care

Many studies have linked gender-affirming medical care with positive health and functional outcomes, including decreased suicidality and self-harm, improved psychological and social functioning, and enhanced quality of life among TGD youth.[55–62] Despite these known benefits, TGD youth still face numerous challenges, including lengthy mental health assessments, arbitrary age minimums, caregiver consent consensus, burdensome insurance requirements, and complicated legal restrictions. Furthermore, recent wide sweeping political efforts to restrict medically supported interventions should be critically examined given pervasive literature findings demonstrating mental health benefits of GAT and substantial harms of withholding care.[55–58,60] As these efforts are actively evolving, ongoing surveillance of the potential impact on TGD youth mental health is paramount.[63]

Tailored Assessment and Care Strategies

There is a paucity of research examining the validity of assessment and treatment tools in TGD youth. Robust research efforts examining the mental health needs of TGD youth, such as tracking long-term outcomes or developing best-practice guidelines, remain lacking. TGD populations with SPMI have had even fewer dedicated scientific inquiries. In addition, traditional methods used to treat co-occurring diagnoses (eg, the focus on body positivity and embracing of sex-based body characteristics in the eating disorder population) may be unhelpful and potentially harmful for TGD youth and require reevaluation of benefit and effectiveness.[64]

Some studies do include efforts to improve care in specific TGD populations, including timely interventions to support TGD youth with autism, preventive strategies to mitigate disordered eating risks in GD youth starting GAT, and using a multidisciplinary, team-based care model to support TGD youth with complex needs.[45,63] In addition, it may be helpful to explore tailored GD assessments for TGD populations who may have difficulty with traditional approaches, including those on the autism spectrum or with intellectual disability, and in those experiencing psychosis.

Newer epidemiologic surveys are incorporating screening questions related to gender identity, whereas historical surveys lack the inclusive methods needed to accurately reflect the health needs of TGD communities. Capturing broader population-based data would help to better understand the factors mediating relationships between social stressors and psychiatric symptoms for specialized TGD populations. We recommend continued and expanded surveillance on the experiences of TGD youth to better appreciate and address the unmet social, mental, and physical health needs.

Outstanding research and clinical needs

- Improving health surveillance specific to TGD youth, especially specific subpopulations with added risk factors.

- Studying health outcomes of TGD YOC compared with cisgender and white peers, including better characterizing variables influencing disparities.
- Adapting assessment and treatment approaches to incorporate complex mental health presentations.
- Increasing multidisciplinary provider education efforts on affirming care principles.
- Exploring evidence-based strategies to improve caregiver support of TGD youth, given its known importance for psychological functioning.
- Examining the potential influence of online sources and social media on mental health and well-being, including both protective and risk aspects.
- Monitoring outcomes of sweeping discriminatory legislation and addressing any access barriers to medically supported interventions.

CLINICS CARE POINTS

- Gender diverse presentations are normal aspects of development and may not be associated with the presence of clinically significant mental health concerns.

- Transgender youth carry unique health risks and needs that are important to consider in the context of the psychiatric assessment.

- Experiences stemming from discrimination and marginalization create unique stressors that may explain higher rates of health-risking behaviors and mental health struggles among transgender youth.

- Complex, co-occurring mental health concerns are important to consider when assessing for GD in transgender youth, although they may or may not influence gender goals and/or decisional capacity.

- Assessment and treatment approaches should be adapted based on individual treatment needs while incorporating developmental and communication differences, type and severity of mental illness, pattern of social stressors, and youth and caregiver priorities.

DISCLOSURE

The authors have nothing to disclose.

REFERENCES

1. American Psychiatric Association. Diagnostic and statistical manual of mental disorders: DSM-5. Washington, DC: American Psychiatric Association; 2013.
2. Meyer IH. Prejudice, social stress, and mental health in lesbian, gay, and bisexual populations: conceptual issues and research evidence. Psychol Bull 2003; 129(5):674–97.
3. Hendricks ML, Testa RJ. A conceptual framework for clinical work with transgender and gender nonconforming clients: an adaptation of the minority stress model. Prof Psychol Res Pr 2012;43(5):460–7.
4. Bochicchio L, Reeder K, Aronson L, et al. Understanding factors associated with suicidality among transgender and gender-diverse identified youth. LGBT Health 2021;8(4):245–53.
5. Kosciw JG, Clark CM, Menard L. The 2021 national school climate survey: the experiences of LGBTQ+ youth in our nation's schools. New York: GLSEN; 2022.

6. Morton MH, Dworsky A, Matjasko JL, et al. Prevalence and correlates of youth homelessness in the United States. J Adolesc Health 2018;62(1):14–21.

7. Ybarra ML, Mitchell KJ, Koskiw J. The relation between suicidal ideation and bullying victimization in a national sample of transgender and non-transgender adolescents. In: Goldblum P, Espelage DL, Chu J, et al, editors. Youth suicide bullying: challenges and strategies for prevention and intervention. New York: Oxford University Press; 2014. p. 134–45.

8. Kozlowska K, Chudleigh C, McClure G, et al. Attachment patterns in children and adolescents with gender dysphoria. Front Psychol 2021;11.

9. Call DC, Challa M, Telingator CJ. Providing affirmative care to transgender and gender diverse youth: disparities, interventions, and outcomes. Curr Psychiatry Rep 2021;23(6):33.

10. Price-Feeney M, Green AE, Dorison SH. Impact of bathroom discrimination on mental health among transgender and nonbinary youth. J Adolesc Health 2021;68(6):1142–7.

11. Boyer TL, Sequeira GM, Egan JE, et al. Binary and nonbinary transgender adolescents' healthcare experiences, avoidance, and well visits. J Adolesc Health 2022;71(4):438–45.

12. Connolly MD, Zervos MJ, Barone CJ, et al. The Mental Health of transgender youth: advances in understanding. J Adolesc Health 2016;59(5):489–95.

13. Hanna B, Desai R, Parekh T, et al. Psychiatric disorders in the U.S. transgender population. Ann Epidemiol 2019;39.

14. Nunes-Moreno M, Buchanan C, Cole FS, et al. Behavioral health diagnoses in youth with gender dysphoria compared with controls: a PEDSnet study. J Pediatr 2022;241:147–53.e1.

15. Wanta JW, Niforatos JD, Durbak E, et al. Mental health diagnoses among transgender patients in the clinical setting: an all-payer electronic health record study. Transgend Health 2019;4(1):313–5.

16. Klein A, Golub SA. Family rejection as a predictor of suicide attempts and substance misuse among transgender and gender nonconforming adults. LGBT Health 2016;3(3):193–9.

17. Christensen J, Imhof R, Linder K, et al. Protective factors for transgender and gender non-binary youth experiencing suicidality: a systematic review of the literature. J Adolesc Health 2021;68(2):S35–6.

18. Johns MM, Lowry R, Andrzejewski J, et al. Transgender identity and experiences of violence victimization, substance use, suicide risk, and sexual risk behaviors among high school students — 19 states and large urban school districts, 2017. MMWR Morb Mortal Wkly Rep 2019;68(3):67–71.

19. Gower AL, Rider GN, Coleman E, et al. Perceived gender presentation among transgender and gender diverse youth: approaches to analysis and associations with bullying victimization and emotional distress. LGBT Health 2018;5(5):312–9.

20. Reisner SL, Greytak EA, Parsons JT, et al. Gender minority social stress in adolescence: disparities in adolescent bullying and substance use by gender identity. J Sex Res 2014;52(3):243–56.

21. Busa S, Janssen A, Lakshman M. A review of evidence based treatments for transgender youth diagnosed with social anxiety disorder. Transgend Health 2018;3(1):27–33.

22. Thoma BC, Rezeppa TL, Choukas-Bradley S, et al. Disparities in childhood abuse between transgender and cisgender adolescents. Pediatrics 2021;148(2).

23. Keating L, Muller RT. LGBTQ+ based discrimination is associated with PTSD symptoms, dissociation, emotion dysregulation, and attachment insecurity

among LGBTQ+ adults who have experienced trauma. J Trauma & Dissociation 2019;21(1):124–41.

24. Feder S, Isserlin L, Seale E, et al. Exploring the association between eating disorders and gender dysphoria in Youth. Eat Disord 2017;25(4):310–7.

25. Jones BA, Haycraft E, Murjan S, et al. Body dissatisfaction and disordered eating in trans people: a systematic review of the literature. Int Rev Psychiatry 2015; 28(1):81–94.

26. Nagata JM, Ganson KT, Austin SB. Emerging trends in eating disorders among sexual and gender minorities. Curr Opin Psychiatry 2020;33(6):562–7.

27. Donaldson AA, Hall A, Neukirch J, et al. Multidisciplinary care considerations for gender nonconforming adolescents with eating disorders: a case series. Int J Eat Disord 2018;51(5):475–9.

28. Coelho JS, Suen J, Clark BA, et al. Eating disorder diagnoses and symptom presentation in transgender youth: a scoping review. Curr Psychiatry Rep 2019; 21(11):107–10.

29. Guss CE, Williams DN, Reisner SL, et al. Disordered weight management behaviors, nonprescription steroid use, and weight perception in transgender youth. J Adolesc Health 2017;60(1):17–22.

30. Meerloo JA. Change of sex and collaboration with the psychosis. Am J Psychiatry 1967;124(2):263–4.

31. Siomopoulos V. Transsexualism: disorder of gender identity, thought disorder, or both? J Am Acad Psychoanal 1974;2(3):201–13.

32. Kreukels BPC, Haraldsen IR, De Cuypere G, et al. A European network for the investigation of gender incongruence: the ENIGI initiative. Eur Psychiatry 2012; 27(6):445–50.

33. Wallien MSC, Swaab H, Cohen-Kettenis PT. Psychiatric comorbidity among children with gender identity disorder. J Am Acad Child Adolesc Psychiatry 2007; 46(10):1307–14.

34. de Vries ALC, Doreleijers TAH, Steensma TD, et al. Psychiatric comorbidity in gender dysphoric adolescents. J Child Psychol Psychiatry 2011;52(11): 1195–202.

35. Gómez-Gil E, Trilla A, Salamero M, et al. Sociodemographic, clinical, and psychiatric characteristics of transsexuals from Spain. Arch Sex Behav 2008;38(3): 378–92.

36. Judge C, O'Donovan C, Callaghan G, et al. Gender dysphoria – prevalence and co-morbidities in an Irish adult population. Front Endocrinol 2014;5:87.

37. Dhejne C, Van Vlerken R, Heylens G, et al. Mental health and gender dysphoria: a review of the literature. Int Rev Psychiatry 2016;28(1):44–57.

38. Janssen A, Huang H, Duncan C. Gender variance among youth with autism spectrum disorders: a retrospective chart review. Transgend Health 2016; 1(1):63–8.

39. Barr SM, Roberts D, Thakkar KN. Psychosis in transgender and gender nonconforming individuals: a review of the literature and a call for more research. Psychiatry Res 2021;306:114272.

40. Janssen A, Busa S, Wernick J. The complexities of treatment planning for transgender youth with co-occurring severe mental illness: a literature review and case study. Arch Sex Behav 2019;48(7):2003–9.

41. Dragon CN, Guerino P, Ewald E, et al. Transgender Medicare beneficiaries and chronic conditions: exploring fee-for-service claims data. LGBT Health 2017; 4(6):404–11.

42. de Brouwer IJ, Elaut E, Becker-Hebly I, et al. Aftercare needs following gender-affirming surgeries: findings from the ENIGI Multicenter European Follow-up Study. J Sex Med 2021;18(11):1921–32.
43. Defreyne J, T'Sjoen G, Bouman WP, et al. Prospective evaluation of self-reported aggression in transgender persons. J Sex Med 2018;15(5):768–76.
44. Matthys I, Defreyne J, Elaut E, et al. Positive and negative affect changes during gender-affirming hormonal treatment: results from the European Network for the Investigation of Gender Incongruence (ENIGI). J Clin Med 2021;10(2):296.
45. Coyne CA, Yuodsnukis BT, Chen D. Gender dysphoria: optimizing healthcare for transgender and gender diverse youth with a multidisciplinary approach. Neuropsychiatr Dis Treat 2023;19:479–93.
46. Coleman E, Radix AE, Bouman WP, et al. Standards of care for the health of transgender and gender diverse people, version 8. Int J Transgend Health 2022;23(1):S1–259.
47. Hopkinson RA, Sharon NG. Gender dysphoria and multiple co-occurring psychiatric issues: Compare and contrast. In: Janssen A, Leibowitz S, editors. Affirmative Mental Health Care for Transgender and Gender Diverse Youth. Cham, Switzerland: Springer International Publishing AG; 2018. p. 189–207.
48. Veale JF, Peter T, Travers R, et al. Enacted stigma, mental health, and protective factors among transgender youth in Canada. Transgend Health 2017;2(1):207–16.
49. Olson KR, Durwood L, DeMeules M, et al. Mental health of transgender children who are supported in their identities. Pediatrics 2016;137(3). Published correction appears in Pediatrics 2018 Aug;142(2).
50. Aromin RA. Substance abuse prevention, assessment, and treatment for lesbian, gay, bisexual, and transgender youth. Pediatr Clin North Am 2016;63(6):1057–77.
51. Montano G, Sanders R, Dowshen N, et al. Promoting health equality and nondiscrimination for transgender and gender-diverse youth. J Adolesc Health 2020;66(6):761–5.
52. McGuire FH, Carl A, Woodcock L, et al. Differences in patient and parent informant reports of depression and anxiety symptoms in a clinical sample of transgender and gender diverse youth. LGBT Health 2021;8(6):404–11.
53. Hiebert A, Kortes-Miller K. Finding home in online community: exploring TikTok as a support for gender and sexual minority youth throughout COVID-19. J LGBT Youth 2021;1–18.
54. Selkie E, Adkins V, Masters E, et al. Transgender adolescents' uses of social media for social support. J Adolesc Health 2020;66(3):275–80.
55. Achille C, Taggart T, Eaton NR, et al. Longitudinal impact of gender-affirming endocrine intervention on the mental health and well-being of transgender youths: preliminary results. Int J Pediatr Endocrinol 2020;2020(1).
56. Allen LR, Watson LB, Egan AM, et al. Well-being and suicidality among transgender youth after gender-affirming hormones. Clin Pract Pediatr Psychol 2019;7(3):302–11.
57. Chen D, Berona J, Chan Y-M, et al. Psychosocial functioning in transgender youth after 2 years of hormones. N Engl J Med 2023;388(3):240–50.
58. Colizzi M, Costa R. The effect of cross-sex hormonal treatment on gender dysphoria individuals' mental health: a systematic review. Neuropsychiatr Dis Treat 2016;12:1953–66.
59. Green AE, DeChants JP, Price MN, et al. Association of gender-affirming hormone therapy with depression, thoughts of suicide, and attempted suicide among transgender and nonbinary youth. J Adolesc Health 2022;70(4):643–9.

60. Kuper LE, Mathews S, Lau M. Baseline Mental Health and psychosocial functioning of transgender adolescents seeking gender-affirming hormone therapy. J Dev Behav Pediatr 2019;40(8):589–96.
61. Tordoff DM, Wanta JW, Collin A, et al. Mental health outcomes in transgender and nonbinary youths receiving gender-affirming care. JAMA Netw Open 2022;5(2).
62. Turban JL, King D, Li JJ, et al. Timing of social transition for transgender and gender diverse youth, K-12 harassment, and adult mental health outcomes. J Adolesc Health 2021;69(6):991–8.
63. Pham A, Kasenic A, Hayden L, et al. A case series on disordered eating among transgender youth with autism spectrum disorder. J Adolesc Health 2021;68(6): 1215–9.
64. Hartman-Munick SM, Silverstein S, Guss CE, et al. Eating disorder screening and treatment experiences in transgender and gender diverse young adults. Eat Behav 2021;41:101517.

Common Intersection of Autism and Gender Diversity in Youth: Clinical Perspectives and Practices

John F. Strang, PsyD[a,b,c,d,1],*, Anna I.R. van der Miesen, MD, PhD[e,f,1],
Abigail L. Fischbach, BA[a], Milana Wolff, BS[g], Marvel C. Harris[h],
Sascha E. Klomp, BA[i]

KEYWORDS

- Autism • Autistic • Transgender • Gender diverse • Nonbinary • Gender dysphoria
- Neurodivergence • Gender incongruence

KEY POINTS

- Many youth who identify as gender diverse are autistic; a meta-analysis of available studies on the autism-gender diversity intersection estimated that 11% of gender-diverse individuals are autistic.
- At this point, evidence for how to best provide gender-related care to autistic youth is limited because long-term outcome studies of gender-diverse youth do not disaggregate findings for autistic and nonautistic youth.
- Interdisciplinary care, bridging autism- and gender-related specialties, is needed for youth at the intersection of autism and gender diversity. It is not appropriate for gender care providers, alone, to manage and support the broad care needs of these youth.
- Gender care systems need to be better attuned to autism-related thinking styles and neurodevelopmental neurodiversity by providing appropriate accommodations and supports, which should be codesigned with autistic gender-diverse people.

[a] Gender and Autism Program, Division of Pediatric Neuropsychology, Children's National Hospital, 15245 Shady Grove Suite 350, Rockville, MD 20850, USA; [b] Center for Neuroscience, Children's National Research Institute, Children's National Hospital, Washington, DC, USA; [c] Department of Pediatrics, George Washington University School of Medicine, Washington, DC, USA; [d] Department of Psychiatry and Behavioral Sciences, George Washington University School of Medicine, Washington, DC, USA; [e] Department of Child and Adolescent Psychiatry, Center of Expertise on Gender Dysphoria, Amsterdam University Medical Centers, Location Vrije Universiteit, Amsterdam, the Netherlands; [f] Margaret and Wallace McCain Centre for Child, Youth & Family Mental Health, Campbell Family Mental Health Research Institute, Centre for Addiction and Mental Health, Toronto, Ontario, Canada; [g] College of Engineering and Physical Sciences, University of Wyoming, Laramie, WY, USA; [h] Private Consultant, Hilversum, the Netherlands; [i] Private Consultant, Utrecht, the Netherlands
[1] Co-first authors.
* Corresponding author.
E-mail address: jstrang@childrensnational.org

Child Adolesc Psychiatric Clin N Am 32 (2023) 747–760
https://doi.org/10.1016/j.chc.2023.06.001
1056-4993/23/© 2023 Elsevier Inc. All rights reserved.

childpsych.theclinics.com

THE NATURE OF THE COMMON CO-OCCURRENCE OF AUTISM AND GENDER DIVERSITY

In accordance with international guidance calling for the robust inclusion of autistic gender-diverse experts in research that pertains to the common intersection of autism and gender diversity,[1,2] this article is cocreated and coauthored by an authorship team that equitably balances autistic and nonautistic individuals, as well as gender-diverse and cisgender individuals. Furthermore, the authorship team includes individuals who have experienced a range of gender trajectories and gender-related outcomes.

Prevalence of Autism and Broader Autistic Traits in Gender Diversity

Although this article focuses on the common intersection of autism and gender diversity in youth, many ideas and questions presented here may have some applicability to gender-diverse youth and their care. The field of youth gender care is in its relative infancy, with only 1 longitudinal follow-up study of medical gender care outcomes in adulthood published at the time of writing.[3] Therefore, unanswered questions in the field of intersectional autism and gender diversity are similar to the unanswered questions in the broader fields of youth gender development and gender care.

Many youth who identify as gender-diverse are autistic.[4–7] A meta-analysis of available studies on the autism-gender diversity intersection, which took into consideration the potential for unpublished nonsignificant findings in the field, estimated that 11% of gender-diverse individuals, across the broad age range reflected in the studies, are autistic[8]; this prevalence is much higher than the most inclusive estimates of autism prevalence in the general population (ie, 2.78%).[9] There is also evidence from multiple studies that autistic traits and gender diversity are correlated in the general population.[10–14] Given this linkage, it may not be surprising that autistic traits are proportionally overrepresented in populations of youth who identify as gender diverse, even at subclinical levels.[6,15] For example, an "almost autistic" phenotype of transgender youth has been described clinically, and neuroimaging findings provide initial multimodal behavioral and neural evidence for this subclinical autism grouping.[16]

The autism and gender diversity intersection seems to be common not only among adolescents but also in adulthood,[4,17] suggesting that the intersection is more than an adolescent-period temporary phenomenon, and instead, an intersectional experience that transcends the developmental period of adolescence.

Etiologic Questions and the Influence of an Ableist Context

The intersection of autism and gender diversity is increasingly recognized within clinical and research settings. The intersection has also begun to enter the political fray, with some state-level legislation emerging within the United States that explicitly mentions autism as a reason for restricting gender-related care[18]; furthermore, political and social rhetoric against gender care has begun to reference the common autism intersection.[19,20]

Major advocacy organizations have begun to embrace and discuss the co-occurrence, including the World Professional Association for Transgender Health in its Standards of Care 8, Global Education Institute training offerings, and convention panel sessions.[21–23] Broader LGBTQ+ supportive organizations have been slower to embrace the co-occurrence, with few exceptions.[24]

The current Standards of Care for transgender youth call for broad-based assessment and a clinically supported gender discernment process that unfolds over time for *all* gender-diverse youth.[21] Yet, it has been observed that there is greater clinical scrutinization of gender development in *autistic* gender-diverse youth than nonautistic gender-diverse youth. For example, an etiology or cause of the experience of gender diversity is more often sought among providers working with autistic as compared with nonautistic transgender youth[15,17]; this practice is hinted at in the current Standards of Care for transgender and gender-diverse children and adolescents, which refer to the potential need for "extra support, structure, psychoeducation, and time built into the assessment process" and "a more extended assessment process" for autistic gender-diverse youth.[21] Intensified scrutiny of gender diversity may be more generally accepted in research and clinical work with autistic youth due to societal perspectives and biases regarding autism, such as assumptions that autistic people may have relatively less awareness of their feeling states and are, therefore, at greater risk for errors in decision-making around gender-related care. Some theorists and clinicians have described that common thinking styles in autism (described by these clinicians and researchers as "rigidity" or strong "interests") may predispose autistic youth to decision-making that might not as carefully consider potential future shifts in gender and gender-related needs.[6,25] Yet, for nonautistic transgender youth seeking gender-related care, questions regarding youth developmental processes and the potential for later shifts in gender and gender-related needs are discouraged by some gender care providers and gender diversity advocates, apparently due to interpretations that such questioning denies the authenticity of transgender youth experiences, is transphobic, and/or could lead to inappropriate gatekeeping of gender care.[26]

We, as authors of this article, argue that although the greater "allowances" given to researchers and clinicians to work to understand gender development causes and trajectories in autistic gender-diverse youth may be important for advancing the field, the motivation that permits this scrutiny in autistic youth, but not youth in general, is inherently problematic, as it pathologizes autistic people, viewing them through an ableist lens, and challenges their self-determination and self-efficacy. In a more equitable framework, investigation into gender development, gender trajectories, and the potential that longer-term outcomes for some gender-expansive youth may involve a shift to another gender identity should occur for both autistic *and* nonautistic gender-expansive populations equally. Unfortunately, given the preponderance of one-sided and reactionary viewpoints regarding youth gender care (eg, reactionary stances against careful gender assessment over time), currently, such broader questions (eg, understanding the long-term gender trajectories of transgender youth, generally) are often ignored, or even discouraged.[26]

Overrepresentation of Broader Autistic Traits: Relevance for Clinical Practice

Given that the proportional overoccurrence of autism in gender-diverse youth is present at both the autism diagnostic and autistic trait levels (ie, elevated autistic traits, but falling below diagnostic cutoffs), autism-attuned approaches, accommodations, and supports may be relevant, and even important, for a broad range of gender-diverse youth. In fact, a recent international expert roundtable on the intersection of autism and gender diversity suggested the potential benefit of universal design approaches in gender care, such that autism- and, more broadly, neurodivergence-informed practices are integrated into clinical pathways for all gender-diverse youth.[1]

ETHICAL CONSIDERATIONS IN CARE
Gender Developmental Trajectories in Autistic Youth: Implications for Care

There is intrinsic complexity in youth gender-related decision-making and care. On the one hand, gender and gender diversity can develop and change over time, even in youth with initial surety regarding gender and gender-related medical decisions.[27,28] On the other hand, delays in care decisions may equate to less optimal physical outcomes (and potentially poorer mental health) for individuals who will continue to experience gender diversity long-term. There is not much information on the gender developmental trajectories of youth experiencing gender diversity, and developmental trajectories of gender for *autistic* gender-diverse youth are unstudied. What is known is that the proportional overoccurrence of intersecting autism and gender diversity exists in multiple nations and societies and across a broad age range (including in adulthood).[8]

Findings from the 2 existing clinical and linked research programs specializing in intersecting autism and gender diversity (co-first author J.F.S., Director of the Gender and Autism Program in Washington, DC, USA, and co-first author A.I.R.v.d.M., Clinician Researcher with the Center of Expertise on Gender Dysphoria in Amsterdam, the Netherlands) suggest that time can help young people in general to best discern their needs regarding gender, whether they be social, medical, and/or legal,[27,29] and this is true also for autistic youth, specifically.[27,30] One of these studies identified that a substantial proportion of youth ($\sim$30%), autistic and nonautistic, showed shifts in their gender-related medical requests over time; this study was conducted in the US clinic, which followed the Dutch care model of more extended evaluation spread out over time to determine needs.[27] Interestingly, there were no differences in the likelihood of autistic versus nonautistic youth experiencing shifts in requests. Providing autistic young people time to consider options and to mature appropriately is included as a recommendation in an international Delphi consensus study of experts on the autism gender diversity co-occurrence,[31] as well as in the current Standards of Care for gender-diverse and transgender individuals.[21] Yet, there are critics who express concerns that slower access to gender-related medical care for autistic youth might be unethical. For example, for autistic transgender youth who show a consistency of gender diversity and broad gender-related needs over time, extra delays (ie, beyond those experienced by nonautistic transgender youth) in medical decision making might be driven by ableist assumptions by parents and providers regarding autistic self-awareness and integrity of decision making. Unfortunately, at the time of writing this article, the evidence base for medical decision making for gender-diverse youth, generally, is limited, with only 1 longitudinal adult outcome study that statistically tested differences over time in a group of youth who made gender-related medical decisions in early adolescence.[3] This study had restrictive inclusion criteria at baseline, included only 55 individuals at long-term follow-up, and included only one adult-period follow-up/outcome assessment (ie, in young adulthood). Importantly, it is unclear how well the findings of this study extrapolate to autistic youth.

To the best of the first authors' knowledge, our gender programs (J.F.S. in the United States and A.I.R.v.d.M. in the Netherlands) are the only programs internationally that possess databases of autistic gender-diverse patients, diagnosed autistic with gold-standard procedures, who are followed into adulthood. The Dutch clinic used gold-standard autism measures in a cohort of gender referrals from the early 2000s and has followed up with more than half of them in adulthood.[32] In addition, the Washington, DC, clinic has a cohort of autistic gender-diverse youth, diagnosed and well-characterized through gold-standard autism measures from assessments in the mid to late 2010s, who are now adults. Nearly all (more than 92%) of the DC cohort have follow-ups in adulthood.[33] Pooling across these 2 databases, which together include more than 40 autistic individuals with follow-up gender-related data, a large majority of the autistic transgender individuals at follow-up continued to be gender diverse.[32,33] Even if all of the individuals who were not available for follow-up hypothetically shifted to a cisgender identity later on (which we do not know), more than half of the combined cohort would show ongoing gender diversity in adulthood.[32,33] Importantly, the Dutch portion of the cohort received gender care as minors during the early 2000s, a time when referral patterns to gender clinics were in some ways different[34]; therefore, it is not clear that the outcomes within the Dutch sample would generalize to the autistic gender-diverse youth seen in clinics currently.

Of the available studies on detransition, we are aware of 2 that specifically report rates of autism diagnosis among the detransitioners recruited.[28,35] In these studies, the definition of "detransition" is somewhat inconsistent but broadly refers to the stopping or reversing of a social or medical gender transition. Unfortunately, these 2 studies do not present whether the rates of regret versus nonregret among the detransitioners were similar or different among the autistic participants. This may be an especially important consideration among autistic adults, because health care access and usage is often reduced,[36,37] likely due to executive function and independence skill challenges; we have certainly experienced clinical cases in which an autistic person stops their medical transition due to reasons other than a shift in gender identity or the onset of regret. We still present, as follows, the rates of diagnosed autism as reported in these studies of detransition, but further work is required to understand whether autism is under-represented among detransitioners with regret; equivalent to the base rates of autism in gender-diverse populations, generally; or overrepresented among detransitioners with regret. In the 2 studies reporting autism diagnoses rates in detransitioners, 20% of 237 detransitioners identified from an international social media recruitment (representing a mix of US, European, and other respondents[28]) had an autism diagnosis and 10% of 100 detransitioners identified from primarily US-focused social media (representing primarily US respondents[35]) had an autism diagnosis. It must be noted that informal descriptions from representatives of detransitioner groups reporting an overrepresentation of autism within the detransitioner groups might simply reflect the underlying base rates of autism among gender-diverse people.[38] There are also narrative descriptions from within social media communities indicating that some autistic detransitioners feel that their autism contributed to their initial decisions to medically transition.[39] However, there is no information on how common this experience is, or whether those reporting it were clinically versus self-diagnosed autistic.

Underpinnings of Gender Diversity in Autism: Does It Matter?

Some autistic people have described an essential link between the autistic experience and the autistic person's experience of gender; 2 identity terms have emerged to explain this link: autigender and gendervague.[40,41] The description that autism itself might influence the gender experience is important to consider for clinical practice. Previously, clinical guidance has suggested that if the gender experience emerges related to a young person's neurodivergence, the gender identity is, therefore, suspect in terms of authenticity.[6,25] Yet, an understanding that the autistic experience itself might color the experience and interpretation of gender suggests that this might be a specific pathway to gender diversity, not autistic "confusion." Adding complexity, we do not have any information on whether autism-related gender experiences are any more or less likely to be stable versus fluid over time.

Neurodivergence-Related Considerations for Gender Care Decisions

When there is uncertainty in decision making regarding youth gender care, care decisions may be driven by conscious—or unconscious—feelings or interpretations, which may vary by individuals, providers, health care systems, communities, cultures, and nations. Neurodivergence, and autism specifically, may elicit a range of feelings and perspectives in people, from neurodiversity affirming to assumptions about self-awareness or decision-making capacities. These perspectives can be varied and complex. It may be helpful for clinicians and parents to explore the feelings, perspectives, and assumptions they have regarding autism and neurodivergence.

It is also essential to consider the heterogeneity of neurodivergence and the heterogeneity within autism itself. Not all autistic people have a similar profile of thinking styles, just as not all nonautistic people have the same strengths or challenges. Therefore, a person-specific approach, which seeks to understand a young person's neuropsychological profile, including strengths, challenges, risks, and resilience factors, should inform how autism—or, more broadly, neurodivergence—may be supported and accommodated in care decisions for gender-diverse youth. To obtain truly informed consent and assent with gender-diverse youth contemplating medical intervention, we recommend a clinical process that helps the young person and their family (1) understand the various potential short- and long-term outcomes (eg, general satisfaction, regret, a mix of the 2)—outcomes that cannot be predicted—and (2) consider and weigh the implications of the unknowns. The therapeutic processes and supports needed to facilitate the young person's understanding and weighing of risks versus benefits should be informed by careful knowledge of the young person's neuropsychological profile of strengths, challenges, and learning and thinking styles. For example, if a young person struggles with big-picture thinking and future thinking, those skills should be supported and developed to the best extent possible to allow for a truly informed consent/assent regarding medical treatments. Equally, however, we are often confronted by the dilemma in which a gender-diverse autistic young person may always struggle with future thinking skills—even with intervention and accommodations—and yet their presenting and voiced needs regarding gender are intense and urgent. In supporting these complex decisions, a more formal ethical decision-making process, shared with the young person, their family, and the care team, may be helpful. We are aware of one such decision-making tool designed for use with gender-diverse youth, specifically.[42]

CLINICAL PRACTICES: PRIORITIES AND UNKNOWNS
The Need for Interdisciplinary Care

The systems in which youth receive health care often segregate care provision among providers and specialties. The Standards of Care for transgender and gender-diverse youth call for *interdisciplinary* care that involves coordination and collaboration between mental health and medical care providers.[21] We would argue that, for autistic youth, the integration of care across gender providers, autism-informed mental health providers, and professionals supporting the education, transition to adulthood, independence, and social needs of the young person is, in most cases, essential. Importantly, gender care providers and programs often do not have specialization in these broader care needs of autistic gender-diverse youth. Furthermore, other care providers (eg, autism specialists and mental health providers) may be reluctant to provide psychosocial, developmental, and/or psychiatric care and supports to autistic youth who are *also* gender diverse; we have heard explanations from such providers that they do not feel sufficiently specialized in the care of gender-diverse youth and that they feel *out of their depth* in supporting these young people; this can result in autistic gender-diverse youth "falling through the cracks" in terms of their broader care needs.

We have observed that many of these young people are served primarily—or sometimes exclusively—by gender-specialized providers, who may struggle to understand and appropriately prioritize the autistic transgender person's broader care needs. And, even when gender care providers recognize and advocate for the broader care needs of their autistic—and more broadly, neurodivergent—patients, providers are often not available or have multiyear waitlists due to the dearth of autism-specialized providers. Or, as described earlier, broader care providers may be reluctant to work with these young people due to a lack of specialization in gender development. This striking care gap for gender-expansive youth with broad developmental and/or mental health needs has been highlighted in a commentary on one of the largest gender care programs internationally.[26] We would argue that given the broad care and support needs that autistic gender-diverse youth typically require, even a gender care provider well-trained in autism-related care is insufficient to support a young person alone. This insufficiency is because the types of supports and interventions needed by these youth are diverse and a single provider wearing multiple clinical hats simultaneously with a client is inappropriate (eg, providing directive social skill and/or cognitive behavioral interventions *while at the same time* supporting the more open-ended gender evaluation and discernment process).[43] Solutions would require new models of care that expand access to the broad spectrum of needed resources through interdisciplinary collaborations that bridge multiple care practices (eg, autism, neuropsychology, psychiatry, gender care, educational specialties). We are aware of one program, internationally, that has worked to develop such an interdisciplinary approach.[43]

Autism Diagnosis and Supports

Unfortunately, the autistic identities and autism-related needs of young people at the intersection of autism and gender diversity are often missed or ignored; this may relate to the complexity of diagnosing autism in gender-diverse youth. Our preliminary work has identified that autism is often diagnosed later in gender-diverse youth compared with cisgender youth.[44] Although the factors driving later autism diagnosis in gender-diverse youth have not been studied, we surmise that they may include (1) provider training in diagnosing the cisgender male version of autism (which may lead to late or missed diagnoses in cisgender girls,[45] as well as in gender-diverse youth[44]); (2) the apparent common intersection of higher intelligence quotient (IQ), autism, and gender diversity,[46] and findings that youth with higher verbal IQs may be diagnosed autistic later[47]; (3) youth gender-related experiences and needs obfuscating underlying autism (eg, social differences attributed to gender minority stressors instead of neurodevelopmental differences); and (4) a subset of gender-diverse youth who are at the cusp of the autism diagnosis.[16,48]

We have also observed that for some providers, some youth, and some parents, there is a primary focus on the gender diversity of the young person over autism; this may be related to perceptions or assumptions by families and individuals that autism supports will be more burdensome, challenging, and abstract. Such perceptions and assumptions may derive from how LGBTQ+ identities versus autistic identities are viewed in society. Regarding youth gender care, some providers, youth, and families view the supports as rather concrete, such as through more-or-less straightforward medical pathways; in contrast, there is no specific medical approach for supporting autism. Finally, considering the developing body during the youth and teen years, gender diversity-related needs may also have more concrete *timelines* and feel more urgent to youth, families, and providers. We caution in these situations that autism-related diagnostics and supports not be forgotten or de-emphasized, even in the midst of time-urgent gender-related decision-making. In fact, the 2 (ie, gender-related discernment and autism-related characterization and supports) are often interlinked, given the need to assess the young person's broad skills for future thinking, codified in the current Standards of Care for gender-diverse youth.[21]

A late autism diagnosis may increase risks, potentially due to the missed opportunities for earlier supports and interventions as well as earlier autistic identity formation and self-understanding.[49,50] Because many gender-diverse youth are diagnosed autistic later than their cisgender peers,[44] it may be important for providers working with autistic gender-diverse youth to develop enriched care pathways for late-diagnosed youth and their families, which can intensify supports for autism and help families get connected with late diagnosis-related resources.

Executive Function and Autistic Gender-Diverse Youth

Autistic youth often experience challenges with executive function, including in the areas of flexibility, working memory, initiation, task completion, organization, and planning.[51] Executive function challenges in autism predict later adult adaptive outcomes.[52,53] Among transgender youth, even when controlling for autism symptoms, executive function differences in big-picture (ie, gestalt) thinking are significantly related to suicidality.[48] Qualitative research with autistic transgender youth identifies the extra burden executive function challenges create for the youth, especially as related to gender discernment and gender affirmation/transition processes.[54] Executive function-related barriers (and broader neurodivergence-related barriers) to moving forward with gender-related discernment and transition, as described by autistic transgender youth and young adults, include challenges in the following areas[54,55]:

1. Figuring out the steps for moving forward with gender-related needs.
2. Navigating gender-related care systems due to difficulties with organization and planning skills.
3. Communicating about and advocating for gender-related needs.
4. Managing sensory and/or social aspects of health care settings that may be overwhelming/overloading.
5. Keeping track of and remembering gender-related goals and health care appointments.

Mental Health

The intersection of autism and gender diversity is associated with a greater risk for clinical anxiety, depression, and suicidality among transgender and autistic youth, independently.[48] Little is known about the nature of mental health challenges in autistic gender-diverse youth. Initial research suggests that some types of executive function challenges may be associated with worse mental health.[48] Specifically, challenges with big-picture/gestalt thinking and executive function gender barriers were associated with poorer mental health among autistic and nonautistic youth.[48]

Gender Discernment in Autistic Gender-Diverse Youth

As described previously, little is known about gender developmental trajectories in gender-diverse youth, generally, or in autistic gender-diverse youth, specifically. What we have learned from the available clinical studies is that autistic gender-diverse youth may benefit from exposure to real-world exemplars as part of their gender discernment.[56] Contemplating gender diversity over time (eg, future thinking regarding gender) can be extremely challenging for autistic youth. Providing opportunities to meet and interact with various and diverse role models of individuals with many different types of gender journeys and outcomes may help to make decision making more concrete.[56]

Importantly, some autistic people may be less influenced by social conventions. Conventions regarding gender may also be of less concern for some.[54] Unconventional gender expressions in autistic gender-diverse young people (eg, a full beard worn by an autistic transgender woman) may be interpreted by others (eg, family, providers) as evidence against an authentic gender-diverse identity. Yet, autistic people may be less concerned with such social gender expressions in general, so assumptions regarding the authenticity of the inner gender experience based on external expressions of gender may be inappropriate. It must also be noted that based on our clinical observation, there are some autistic gender-exploring youth who, after exploring gender-diverse expressions (or meeting other transgender people), determine that a gender-diverse/transgender identity does not fit them.

Medical Decision Making

There is currently no autism-specific evidence regarding gender-related medical care decisions in youth. Unfortunately, none of the longitudinal studies of gender-affirming care included information as to whether autistic youth were part of the cohorts, and if so, whether autistic youth showed similar trajectories and outcomes to nonautistic youth.[3,57-60] The current Standards of Care include guidance on medical care decisions in youth, laying out a set of assessment targets for young people considering gender-affirming treatments.[21] It will be critical to test how the Standards of Care work for autistic gender-diverse youth.

Clinicians and families may feel uncomfortable moving forward with medical interventions in youth who struggle with future thinking and planning. However, there may be considerable enthusiasm from the young person to start treatments. These can be challenging situations, clinically, balancing the perspectives of the team and parents as well as the urgent feelings of the young person. Accommodations and supports for future thinking (eg, visual timelines), opportunities for the young person to meet individuals across the spectrum of gender outcomes (eg, consistent gender diversity over time, attenuating gender diversity over time, fluid gender diversity), and autism-informed psychoeducation regarding what is known and unknown in gender care and outcomes may be appropriate.

CLINICS CARE POINTS: THE EVIDENCE BASE

The following list includes 9 care points for youth at the intersection of autism and gender diversity that have some degree of evidence based on the results from *more than one* study. There is a great deal more evidence for diagnostics and supports for autistic youth, specifically, and this broader empirical literature is relevant to autistic gender-diverse youth, as well. Here, only those care points that are specifically related to the intersection of autism and gender diversity are listed.

1. There is a proportional overoccurrence of autism and, separately, elevated autistic traits among gender-diverse people.[4,8,15]
2. This proportional overoccurrence of intersecting autism and gender diversity appears in youth and adults.[4,8]
3. Autistic gender-diverse youth often face greater mental health challenges than autistic youth or gender-diverse youth independently.[7,48,61]
4. Autistic gender-diverse youth (in qualitative research) have often reported that autism-related challenges can impact their ability to navigate their gender-related needs (eg, executive function challenges making it harder to navigate care

systems).[54,56,62] Gender care systems need to be better attuned to autism-related thinking styles by providing appropriate accommodations and supports.[54,56,62]

5. Necessary training for providers working with youth at the intersection of autism and gender diversity and recommendations for gender-related evaluations with these youth appear in 2 expert consensus clinical guidelines.[21,31] Conclusions across these 2 clinical guidelines include:

  a. Training and expertise in autism and other neurodevelopmental presentations, or direct collaboration with an autism/developmental disability expert, is recommended when gender providers work with autistic gender-diverse youth.

  b. A more extended gender-related assessment process may be necessary for some autistic gender-diverse youth.

  c. Gender-related assessments should be tailored to the autistic young person's neurodevelopmental profile (eg, these "youth may require extra support, structure, psychoeducation, and time built into the assessment process").

  d. Consideration is recommended for the potential impact of communication differences, concrete or less flexible thinking, self-awareness differences, and challenges with future thinking and planning skills on (1) gender evaluations as well as (2) the ability of the young person to deeply consider the long-term implications and potential outcomes related to gender care decisions.

  e. As part of gender-related assessments required for gender-related medical care decisions, it is recommended to work to understand whether apparent gender diversity and gender diversity-related needs arise from common autism-related features and are transient.

FUTURE DIRECTIONS

Researchers and research funders must attend to the proportional overrepresentation of autism among gender-diverse populations. At present, clinical research in this field is extremely limited, yet many autistic youth are urgently requesting gender-related supports, including gender-related medical care. There is a dearth of information as to whether these treatments function similarly or differently in autistic youth, and whether autistic youth show similar or different gender trajectories over time when compared with nonautistic youth. One problem that must be overcome is the stigmatization of autism that remains in some gender-related research and advocacy circles. The fact that at the time of this publication none of the major longitudinal studies of gender-diverse youth development or gender care have characterized and reported the presence of autism—and more broadly, autistic traits—in the youth cohorts[3,57–60] is a lost opportunity that must be corrected moving forward. In fact, future gender-diverse youth research may need to intentionally oversample autistic youth within study designs to allow for equitable statistical modeling of this relatively large and at-risk subset of youth. Such oversampling approaches have been proposed and accomplished by members of this author team.[16,27,48,63] Furthermore, to be ethical, research in this field must be centered on the perspectives and priorities of autistic individuals across the gender spectrum, including those who have experienced consistent gender diversity over time, as well as those who have experienced shifts in their gender and gender-related needs.[2]

DISCLOSURE

J.F. Strang was a coauthor of the Child and Adolescent chapters of the Standards of Care 8 revision through the World Professional Association for Transgender Health (WPATH). J.F. Strang and A.I.R. van der Miesen are both faculty members with the WPATH Global Education Institute and coleads of the specialized WPATH training program for care for individuals at the intersection of autism, broader neurodivergence, and gender diversity. This research was supported by the National Institutes of Health Clinical and Translational Science Award (KL2TR001877, J.F. Strang).

REFERENCES

1. Gratton FV, Strang JF, Song M, et al. The intersection of autism and transgender and nonbinary identities: community and academic dialogue on research and advocacy. Autism Adulthood 2023. https://doi.org/10.1089/aut.2023.0042.
2. Strang JF, Klomp SE, Caplan R, et al. Community-based participatory design for research that impacts the lives of transgender and/or gender-diverse autistic and/or neurodiverse people. Clin Pract Pediatr Psychol 2019;7(4):396.
3. de Vries ALC, McGuire JK, Steensma TD, et al. Young adult psychological outcome after puberty suppression and gender reassignment. Pediatrics 2014; 134(4):696–704.
4. Warrier V, Greenberg DM, Weir E, et al. Elevated rates of autism, other neurodevelopmental and psychiatric diagnoses, and autistic traits in transgender and gender-diverse individuals. Nat Commun 2020;11(1):1–12.
5. Hisle-Gorman E, Landis CA, Susi A, et al. Gender dysphoria in children with autism spectrum disorder. LGBT Health 2019;6(3):95–100.
6. de Vries ALC, Noens ILJ, Cohen-Kettenis PT, et al. Autism spectrum disorders in gender dysphoric children and adolescents. J Autism Dev Disord 2010;40(8): 930–6.
7. Strauss P, Cook A, Watson V, et al. Mental health difficulties among trans and gender diverse young people with an autism spectrum disorder (ASD): findings from Trans Pathways. J Psychiatr Res 2021;137:360–7.
8. Kallitsounaki A, Williams DM. Autism spectrum disorder and gender dysphoria/ incongruence. a systematic literature review and meta-analysis. J Autism Dev Disord 2022. https://doi.org/10.1007/s10803-022-05517-y.
9. Maenner MJ, Shaw KA, Bakian AV, et al. Prevalence and characteristics of autism spectrum disorder among children aged 8 years - autism and developmental disabilities monitoring network, 11 Sites, United States, 2018. MMWR Surveill Summ 2021;70(11):1–16.
10. George R, Stokes MA. Gender identity and sexual orientation in autism spectrum disorder. Autism 2018;22(8):970–82.
11. Kallitsounaki A, Williams D. Mentalising moderates the link between autism traits and current gender dysphoric features in primarily non-autistic, cisgender individuals. J Autism Dev Disord 2020;50(11):4148–57.
12. Kallitsounaki A, Williams DM, Lind SE. Links between autistic traits, feelings of gender dysphoria, and mentalising ability: replication and extension of previous findings from the general population. J Autism Dev Disord 2021;51(5): 1458–65.
13. Munoz Murakami LY, van der Miesen AIR, Nabbijohn AN, et al. Childhood gender variance and the autism spectrum: evidence of an association using a child behavior checklist 10-item autism screener. J Sex Marital Ther 2022;48(7): 645–51.
14. Nabbijohn AN, van der Miesen AIR, Santarossa A, et al. Gender variance and the autism spectrum: an examination of children ages 6–12 years. J Autism Dev Disord 2019;49(4):1570–85.

15. van der Miesen AIR, de Vries ALC, Steensma TD, et al. Autistic symptoms in children and adolescents with gender dysphoria. J Autism Dev Disord 2018;48(5): 1537–48.

16. Strang JF, McClellan LS, Li S, et al. The autism spectrum among transgender youth: default mode functional connectivity. Cereb Cortex 2023. https://doi.org/10.1093/cercor/bhac530.

17. Walsh RJ, Krabbendam L, Dewinter J, et al. Brief report: gender identity differences in autistic adults: associations with perceptual and socio-cognitive profiles. J Autism Dev Disord 2018;48(12):4070–8.

18. Autistic Self Advocacy Network. Statement: ASAN Condemns Restrictions on Gender-Affirming Care. March 22 2023. Available at: https://autisticadvocacy.org/2023/03/asan-condemns-restrictions-on-gender-affirming-care/.   Accessed June 3, 2023.

19. Rowling J.K. J.K. Rowling Writes about Her Reasons for Speaking out on Sex and Gender Issues. JK Rowling blog. 2020. Available at: https://www.jkrowling.com/opinions/j-k-rowling-writes-about-her-reasons-for-speaking-out-on-sex-and-gender-issues/. Accessed June 3, 2023.

20. Devega C. There is no secret plan: First they came for trans people. Salon. March 13 2023. Available at: https://www.salon.com/2023/03/13/there-is-no-secret-plan-first-they-came-for-trans-people/. Accessed June 3, 2023.

21. Coleman E, Radix AE, Bouman WP, et al. Standards of care for the health of transgender and gender diverse people, version 8. Int J Transgend Health 2022; 23(sup1):S1–259.

22. Strang JF, van der Miesen AIR, Lawson W, et al. Neurodiversity Workshop. World Professional Association for Transgender Health Global Education Initiative; 2022. Available at: https://www.wpath.org/gei. Accessed June 3, 2023.

23. Strang JF, van der Miesen AIR, Janssen A, et al. The Intersection of Autism and Gender Diversity: The Lives of Transgender/Gender Diverse Neurodiverse Individuals. Conference Proceedings of the World Professional Association for Transgender Health Symposium. November 3–6, 2018. Buenos Aires, Argentina.

24. The Trevor Project. Research Brief: Mental Health Among Autistic LGBTQ Youth. April 29, 2022. Available at: https://www.thetrevorproject.org/research-briefs/mental-health-among-autistic-lgbtq-youth-apr-2022/. Accessed June 3, 2023.

25. Parkinson J. Gender dysphoria in Asperger's syndrome: a caution. Australas Psychiatry 2014;22(1):84–5.

26. Barnes H. Time to think: the inside story of the collapse of the Tavistock's gender service for children. London: Swift Press; 2023.

27. Cohen A, Gomez-Lobo V, Willing L, et al. Shifts in gender-related medical requests by transgender and gender-diverse adolescents. J Adolesc Health 2023;72(3):428–36.

28. Vandenbussche E. Detransition-related needs and support: a cross-sectional online survey. J Homosex 2021;1–19. https://doi.org/10.1080/00918369.2021.1919479.

29. de Vries ALC, Cohen-Kettenis PT. Clinical management of gender dysphoria in children and adolescents: the Dutch approach. J Homosex 2012;59(3):301–20.

30. van der Miesen AIR. Contemporary Complexities in Transgender Care: Disentangling the Intersections Among Gender Diversity, Autism, and Mental Health. [PhD thesis]. Vrije Universiteit Amsterdam; 2021.

31. Strang JF, Meagher H, Kenworthy L, et al. Initial clinical guidelines for co-occurring autism spectrum disorder and gender dysphoria or incongruence in adolescents. J Clin Child Adolesc Psychol 2016;47(1):1–11.

32. van der miesen AIR., van Wieringen IM, Strang JF, et al. A Long-Term Follow-up of Autistic Transgender Children and Adolescents into Young Adulthood. Conference Proceedings of the European Professional Association for Transgender Health Symposium. April 26–28, 2023; Killarney, Ireland.

33. Clawson A, Strang JF. The gender and autism program: a new neuropsychology service for gender-expansive youth. Rockville (MD): Children's National Hospital Center for Autism Spectrum Disorders Didactic Series; 2023.

34. Arnoldussen M, Steensma TD, Popma A, et al. Re-evaluation of the Dutch approach: are recently referred transgender youth different compared to earlier referrals? Eur Child Adolesc Psychiatry 2019. https://doi.org/10.1007/s00787-019-01394-6.

35. Littman L. Individuals treated for gender dysphoria with medical and/or surgical transition who subsequently detransitioned: a survey of 100 detransitioners. Arch Sex Behav 2021;50(8):3353–69.

36. Mason D, Ingham B, Urbanowicz A, et al. A systematic review of what barriers and facilitators prevent and enable physical healthcare services access for autistic adults. J Autism Dev Disord 2019;49(8):3387–400.

37. Weir E, Allison C, Baron-Cohen S. Autistic adults have poorer quality healthcare and worse health based on self-report data. Mol Autism 2022;13(1):23.

38. Barnes H, Cohen D. 'How do I go back to the Debbie I was?'. British Broadcasting Corporation. November 26, 2019. Available at: https://www.bbc.com/news/health-50548473. Accessed June 2, 2023.

39. Detransition Subreddit - r/detrans. Reddit. Available at: https://www.reddit.com/r/detrans/. Accessed June 2, 2023.

40. Brown LXZ. Gendervague: At the Intersection of Autistic and Trans Experiences. The National LGBTQ Task Force Blog. Available at: https://www.autistichoya.com/2020/05/gendervague-at-intersection-of-autistic.html. Accessed June, 2023.

41. Rivera L. What is AutiGender? The Relationship Between Autism & Gender: An Autistic Perspective. Neurodivergent Rebel. Available at: https://neurodivergentrebel.com/2021/01/06/what-is-autigender-the-relationship-between-autism-gender-an-autistic-perspective/. Accessed June 2, 2023.

42. de Snoo-Trimp J, de Vries A, Molewijk B, et al. How to deal with moral challenges around the decision-making competence in transgender adolescent care? Development of an ethics support tool. BMC Med Ethics 2022;23(1):96.

43. Strang JF, Fischbach AL, Rao S, et al. Gender and Autism Program: A Novel Clinical Service Model for Gender-Diverse/Transgender Autistic Youth and Young Adults. [Manuscript submitted for publication]. 2023.

44. McQuaid GA, Ratto AB, Jack A, et al. Gender, assigned sex at birth, and gender diversity: Windows into diagnostic timing disparities in autism. [Manuscript preprint] 2023;doi:10.31234/osf.io/kc6ax.

45. McDonnell CG, DeLucia EA, Hayden EP, et al. Sex differences in age of diagnosis and first concern among children with autism spectrum disorder. J Clin Child Adolesc Psychol 2020;1–11. https://doi.org/10.1080/15374416.2020.1823850.

46. Thomas TR, Tener AJ, Pearlman AM, et al. Dimensional gender diversity is associated with greater polygenic propensity for cognitive performance and interacts with other genetic factors in predicting health outcomes. medRxiv 2022;2021. https://doi.org/10.1101/2021.11.22.21266696, 11.22.21266696.

47. Harrop C, Libsack E, Bernier R, et al. Do biological sex and early developmental milestones predict the age of first concerns and eventual diagnosis in autism spectrum disorder? Autism Res 2021;14(1):156–68.

48. Strang JF, Anthony LG, Song A, et al. In addition to stigma: cognitive and autism-related predictors of mental health in transgender adolescents. J Clin Child Adolesc Psychol 2021;1–18. https://doi.org/10.1080/15374416.2021.1916940.
49. Oredipe T, Kofner B, Riccio A, et al. Does learning you are autistic at a younger age lead to better adult outcomes? A participatory exploration of the perspectives of autistic university students. Autism 2023;27(1):200–12.
50. Estes A, Munson J, Rogers SJ, et al. Long-term outcomes of early intervention in 6-year-old children with autism spectrum disorder. J Am Acad Child Adolesc Psychiatry 2015;54(7):580–7.
51. Demetriou E, Lampit A, Quintana D, et al. Autism spectrum disorders: a meta-analysis of executive function. Mol Psychiatry 2018;23(5):1198–204.
52. Pugliese CE, Anthony LG, Strang JF, et al. Longitudinal examination of adaptive behavior in autism spectrum disorders: influence of executive function. J Autism Dev Disord 2016;46(2):467–77.
53. Wallace GL, Kenworthy L, Pugliese CE, et al. Real-world executive functions in adults with autism spectrum disorder: profiles of impairment and associations with adaptive functioning and co-morbid anxiety and depression. J Autism Dev Disord 2016;46(3):1071–83.
54. Strang JF, Powers MD, Knauss M, et al. "They thought it was an obsession": trajectories and perspectives of autistic transgender and gender-diverse adolescents. J Autism Dev Disord 2018;48(12):4039–55.
55. Strang JF, McClellan LS, Raaijmakers D, et al. The gender-diversity and autism questionnaire: a community-developed clinical, research, and self-advocacy tool for autistic transgender and gender-diverse young adults. Autism Adulthood 2023;5(2):175–90.
56. Strang JF, Knauss M, van der Miesen AIR, et al. A clinical program for transgender and gender-diverse neurodiverse/autistic adolescents developed through community-based participatory design. J Clin Child Adolesc Psychol 2020;1–16. https://doi.org/10.1080/15374416.2020.1731817.
57. Olson KR, Durwood L, Horton R, et al. Gender identity 5 years after social transition. Pediatrics 2022;150(2). https://doi.org/10.1542/peds.2021-056082.
58. de Vries ALC, Steensma TD, Doreleijers TAH, et al. Puberty suppression in adolescents with gender identity disorder: a prospective follow-up study. J Sex Med 2011;8(8):2276–83.
59. Chen D, Berona J, Chan Y-M, et al. Psychosocial functioning in transgender youth after 2 years of hormones. N Engl J Med 2023;388(3):240–50.
60. Kuper LE, Stewart S, Preston S, et al. Body dissatisfaction and mental health outcomes of youth on gender-affirming hormone therapy. Pediatrics 2020;145(4). https://doi.org/10.1542/peds.2019-3006.
61. Mahfouda S, Panos C, Whitehouse A, et al. Mental health correlates of autism spectrum disorder in gender diverse young people: evidence from a specialised child and adolescent gender clinic in Australia. J Clin Med 2019;8. https://doi.org/10.3390/jcm8101503.
62. Cooper K, Butler C, Russell A, et al. The lived experience of gender dysphoria in autistic young people: a phenomenological study with young people and their parents. Eur Child Adolesc Psychiatry 2022. https://doi.org/10.1007/s00787-022-01979-8.
63. Strang JF, Wallace GL, Michaelson JJ, et al. The gender self-report: a multidimensional gender characterization tool for gender-diverse and cisgender youth and adults. Am Psychol 2023. https://doi.org/10.1037/amp0001117.

Individual Affirming Care
Psychological and Social Approaches to Trans and Gender-Diverse Youth

Erin L. Belfort, MD, DFAACAP[a],*, Brandy Brown, DSW, LCSW[b]

KEYWORDS

- Transgender and gender-diverse (TGD) adolescents • Gender-affirming care
- Individual therapy

KEY POINTS

- Clinicians are likely to see transgender and gender-diverse (TGD) youth in their clinical practices and must be familiar with terminology and gender-affirming treatment models, which are described in this article.
- Psychological and social supports are important for the well-being of the youth, regardless of a young person's desire for medical and/or surgical treatments.
- Multidisciplinary care models provide effective supports for TGD youth and their families to make collaborative and fully informed treatment decisions over time.
- Self-examination and reflection of one's own biases as a clinician are important to working effectively with TGD youth and their families.

INTRODUCTION
History

Medical treatment for Transgender and Gender-Diverse (TGD) youth began in the early 2000s, after a clinic in Amsterdam introduced the initial protocol, often referred to as The Dutch Protocol.[1]

This is a treatment pathway that includes a period of suppressing puberty, initiation of gender-affirming hormone treatment, and gender-affirming surgeries. This treatment was brought to the United States in 2007 when Boston Children's Hospital opened the first pediatric gender program in the United States.[2] At this time, most major children's hospitals have a dedicated pediatric gender program. These programs follow the same guidelines; however, there is a lack of consensus in treatment approaches, including diagnosis and treatment recommendations.[3]

[a] Maine Medical Center, Tufts University School of Medicine, 66 Bramhall Street, Portland, ME 04102, USA; [b] Maine Medical Center, Tufts University School of Medicine, The Gender Clinic, 1577 Congress Street, 2nd Floor, Portland, ME 04102, USA
* Corresponding author.
E-mail address: erin.belfort@mainehealth.org

Child Adolesc Psychiatric Clin N Am 32 (2023) 761–773
https://doi.org/10.1016/j.chc.2023.05.006
1056-4993/23/© 2023 Elsevier Inc. All rights reserved.

Over the past decade, research and best practices for the care of TGD youth have increased. The World Professional Association for Transgender Health published the most recent Standard of Care (SOC8), in 2022.[4] In the SOC8, providers qualified to conduct a comprehensive biopsychosocial assessment have training in adolescent identity development and family dynamics when determining appropriateness for gender-affirming medical interventions. Additional information regarding the recommendations in SOC8 are listed elsewhere in this issue; however, in addition to medical treatments, both psychological and social supports are important for long-term well-being of TGD youth, which is the focus of this article.

The American Psychological Association published an ethically based guideline for practice with TGD people in 2015. This guideline covers basic principles related to (a) foundational knowledge and awareness; (b) stigma, discrimination, and barriers to care; (c) life span development; and (d) research, education, and training.[5] With regard to youth, clinicians are reminded that work with gender-questioning (GQ) youth (those youth who have not developed a TGD identity) should allow for exploration of identity and an understanding that not all GQ youth will affirm a TGD identity.

For those working with prepubertal children, there have historically been 3 major mental health treatment models: (a) the "live in your own skin" model, (b) the watchful waiting model, and (c) the gender-affirmative model.[6] The first approach assumes that a child is unlikely to have a solid gender identity and has a treatment goal of preventing them from asserting a transgender identity in the future, thus reducing future experiences with stigma, and therefore, mental health comorbidities.[7] This treatment model has been scrutinized and likened to conversion therapy, which aims to change an individual's sexual orientation or gender identity to conform to the social majority. Conversion therapy, practiced by mental health professionals, members of the clergy or faith traditions, or laypeople, has been deemed unethical by all major medical and psychological professional organizations, including American Psychological Association, American Psychiatric Association, American Academy of Child & Adolescent Psychiatry, the American Academy of Pediatrics, and the National Association of Social Workers.[8-12] These practices have clear evidence of harm and no research evidence to support their utility. The consensus of these professional organizations and others emphasizes the normal and expected variation of sexual orientation and gender identities, which exist across cultures and time.[13] The watchful waiting model was used in developing "The Dutch Protocol" for medical treatment; the goal is to provide time to explore and develop gender identity before permanent changes occur. Within this model, it is recommended that a child be allowed to explore their identity but to wait for any transition steps until adolescence. The gender-affirmative model takes the prior approach a step further and encourages children to assert their gender, with adults providing support, which may include social transition in childhood as well as medical transition in adolescence.

The gender-affirmative model is the only model that embraces social transition in childhood. Social transition is the process whereby an individual presents and is respected as their affirmed gender. This may include changes in dress, name, and pronoun and "coming out" or sharing this information with friends and family. A social transition can occur at any developmental stage; however, children often transition with thoughtful consideration from their parents. Adolescents may socially transition with their parents or may choose to explore transition with their peers initially, involving parents later in the process. In either case, mental health providers should be ready to support young people and their families through the process of affirmative gender exploration and/or social transition. Historically, the main concern that is often presented against embarking on a social gender transition is whether a child will persist in their identity over time. A recent study of 317 children who went through a prepubertal binary social transition noted that although 7.3% of these youth had at least one retransition during the 5-year period, only 2.5% ultimately identified as cisgender.[14] These data suggest that clinicians should be aware of and prepared to support all authentic outcomes (including retransition), whereby an individual may shift their understanding of identity and socially transition to a different gender identity after they have already completed a social transition. This may be to their previous identity/sex assigned at birth or to a nonbinary identity.

BACKGROUND

Research has consistently identified high rates of health and mental health disparities among TGD people of all ages, including higher rates of both internalizing and externalizing disorders.[15] In one large sample study comparing treatment-seeking TGD youth with cisgender male and female youth, TGD youth demonstrated higher levels of anxiety, depression, risk of suicide, and self-harm. They also were more likely to have experienced emotional abuse and prior suicide attempts and to report a less supportive family than their cisgender counterparts.[16] One potential limitation of the existing published data is that various gender identities are often studied as a cohort when there may exist differences within and between subgroups of the population. For example, some studies have suggested lower levels of mental health comorbidities among gender nonbinary persons compared with binary transgender persons.[17]

These disparities are multifactorial in origin, likely related to a combination of external structural factors, environmental social stressors, and internal stressors related to one's gender minority status. One model for understanding these disparities is the minority stress theory, which suggests that individuals within stigmatized or marginalized groups experience unique stressors owing to their minority status and their experience with prejudice, stigma, and discrimination.[18] Initially proposed as a way to conceptualize the disparities experienced by sexual minorities, the theory was further adapted to include gender minorities.[19,20] Several studies have linked the higher rates of mental health conditions that TGD youth experience to minority stress.[21,22]

Structural factors, including discrimination and biases within health care systems and within individual providers, contribute to TGD experiencing challenges receiving necessary health care services or having poor experiences, which may lead to avoidance of future.[23] As providers, it is imperative to understand historical and structural factors leading to poor access to care. For example, homosexuality was not removed from the Diagnostic and Statistical Manual of Mental Disorders (DSM) as a clinical psychiatric diagnosis until 1974, and mental health providers have long served a "gatekeeping" role for medical treatments accompanied by the perception of additional barriers for TGD persons receiving necessary care. As other studies have highlighted, the avoidance of seeking health care and feeling treated poorly in health care facilities are commonly reported experiences among TGD people.[24]

Considerations of context are important in our clinical work, and the COVID-19 pandemic has increased disparities for TGD people.[25] Access to culturally sensitive and informed mental health care was problematic before 2019 and has worsened in recent years. In the current sociopolitical climate where many states are pursuing legislative efforts to prohibit gender-affirming treatment for TGD youth, access is an important consideration.[26] Barriers to care are particularly many for youth with multiply stigmatized intersectional identities (ie, transgender youth of color). A large 2020 to 2021 survey study, The Trevor Project, reported that more than half (54%) of LGBTQ youth who reported wanting mental health care in the past year did not receive it. Cost of services, necessity of parental permission, concerns about provider bias, and cultural factors were highlighted as obstacles to care.[27]

As important as knowing our historic context as providers within a system is our own self-reflection and examination practice of our internalized biases, beliefs, and language practices. We would argue that our own inward self-examination work as individual providers is necessary in working with a marginalized patient population. Furthermore, it is our responsibility to advocate within our systems for structural changes and improvements to ameliorate some of these historic and ongoing barriers to care for TGD persons.

Other external stressors, such as experiencing discrimination, bullying, harassment, and interpersonal violence, are also more prevalent among TGD people. Lack of social supports and acceptance of one's identity within family, school, or larger community contexts can contribute to poorer outcomes. Internalized stigma, such as internalized homophobia or transphobia, can greatly impact one's sense of value, capacity, and well-being.

One survey-based study of individuals 15 years and older who identified as transgender or transfeminine examined perceived, anticipated, and enacted stigmas as a result of gender identity and sexual behavior and its relationship with psychological distress. Severe psychological distress, past year suicidal ideation, and suicide attempt were associated with higher levels of perceived stigma related to both gender identity and sexual behavior.[24] An adapted Testa and colleagues model of gender minority stress includes the addition of more proximal risk factors, such as internalized transphobia, negative expectations, body dysphoria, and identity confusion, which help us conceptualize mental health disparities among TGD people.[28]

Gender-Affirming Care Model of Care for Transgender and Gender-Diverse Youth

There is a large and increasing body of literature supporting the gender-affirming care model of treatment. Affirming care models, which may include the provision of puberty-blocking medications and/or gender-affirming hormones, are associated with improved mental health outcomes. One study of 104 youths found the gender-affirming medical treatments were associated with an improvement in symptoms of depression and suicidality over 12 months.[29] A survey study of more than 27,000 transgender adults found those who had undergone a gender-affirming surgical procedure in the 2 years before the survey reported lower levels of psychological distress, past-year smoking, and past-year suicidal ideation.[30] More recently, in 2023, Olsavsky and colleagues[31] demonstrated the importance of *both* psychological/social supports in addition to biomedical gender-affirming treatments.

DISCUSSION

Our introduction and background sections offer some context to the mental health disparities and needs for TGD youth. We have suggested that it is imperative for providers to understand the history of structural contributors to disparities as well as to understand our own biases and gaps in knowledge in order to understand the individual needs of the child/adolescent and what psychological and/or social interventions may be necessary. Whether a specialized clinician in a gender clinic setting or a generalist in an outpatient or inpatient setting, the clinical work and language are rapidly evolving over time, which is a humbling and sometimes overwhelming experience. Embracing this change as life-long learners striving for cultural humility is an important aspect of the work.

In our discussion, we hope to focus on the why, where, how, and what of individualized treatment with TGD youth and to offer themes worth exploring with youth in our clinical work.

The Why

Adolescence in particular is a complex time in child development with rapid brain growth (frontal lobe myelination) and the accompanying social, emotional, and cognitive changes. Paired with hormonal changes of puberty and the emergence of mental health disorders during these years, adolescence can be a tumultuous time, particularly for those questioning sexuality and/or gender identity. Individual therapy can be a safe place to explore these complexities and the emerging sense of self, competence, and purpose.

Helping the youth create a coherent sense of *self* and an understanding of the relationship of *self to other* are common themes of individual sessions. Ultimately, much of our individual therapeutic work with youth is helping them define for themselves and create a life worth living, with joy, purpose, and meaningful and healthy relationships with others.

As with any clinical concern, we recommend starting with a thorough psychiatric/psychological assessment of the youth as the starting place for an informed biopsychosocial formulation of the young person. In addition to the usual psychiatric review of systems, which informs mental health diagnoses, the initial assessment process also explores the youth's sexual development, gender and sexual identity journeys and future treatment goals, family/peer/school/work interpersonal functioning and dynamics, and discovery of strengths and areas of resilience. Notably, not all TGD youth meet criteria for Gender Dysphoria, which is a clinical diagnosis necessitating impairment in functioning and distress as well as the time criterion of at least 6 months. Often families and clinicians alike conflate the concepts of gender identity (ie, transgender identity) with Gender Dysphoria, and it is helpful to distinguish the two and quantify the level of functional impairment and distress in those meeting criteria for Gender Dysphoria. In order to meet criteria for Gender Dysphoria in Adolescents or Adults (F64.0), an individual will have a prolonged (minimum of 6 months) duration of incongruence between experienced and assigned gender, along with clinically significant distress or impairment in function (*DSM-5*). Gender Dysphoria in Childhood (F64.2) has a different set of criteria, based primarily on the observational information obtained from caregivers. Gender Dysphoria may present in childhood and persist in adolescence through adulthood, or it may present in adolescence or later, with few signs in early childhood, often occurring after secondary sex characteristics have developed in the context of puberty. Understanding the factors associated with the timing of a young person's gender-diverse expression and/or declaration of another identity is important when working with the patient and their family members.

Given common cooccurring psychiatric and psychological vulnerabilities that often accompany gender dysphoria, it is worth paying particular attention to history of trauma (including harassment, bullying, victimization, and similar events), evaluation of suicide risk, evaluation for eating-disordered behavior, and assessment for autism spectrum disorder. The overall biopsychosocial formulation of the youth informs our treatment recommendations, which may include various modalities of psychotherapy as well as psychopharmacologic interventions for such mental health comorbidities, such as depression or anxiety, when they need to be prioritized.[32]

Individual therapy modalities are often a crucial part of supporting TGD youth and are the focus of this article. Although other modalities of treatment are outside the scope of this article (refer to the separate article dedicated to family system interventions), we would argue that family systems interventions are important and complementary services in addition to (or in place of) individual therapy modalities. Younger children, for example, may benefit more from family systems interventions whereby the source of conflict or confusion is generated within the family system and not necessarily within the child. In these cases, supporting families through decisions around prepubertal social transition and considerations of puberty-blocking medications, as the child enters puberty, if/when appropriate, are helpful.

Family interventions are sometimes avoided owing to lack of clinician training in systemic treatment models and resultant discomfort working with family systems, which present us with multiple agendas and perspectives. In addition, clinicians may incorrectly assume a family is unwilling to change or to work toward family acceptance. Sometimes well-intentioned providers fall prey to the narrative that the child is a victim and parents/guardians are villains, leading to the exclusion of the family from the work, which can be misguided and potentially harmful. Having a clear understanding among all involved clinicians (if there are multiple) supporting a youth about the roles and goals as well as ongoing good communication is crucial in best supporting TGD youth. There is an inherent need to balance emerging adolescent autonomy with the need for parental consent for medical treatment of minors, which necessitates family involvement in the care.

The Where

Whether providing outpatient, inpatient, or residential treatment services, it is the responsibility of both the organization and the clinician to create a safe, welcoming, and nonjudgmental space for the therapeutic work to occur. At the systems level, attention to signage (ie, bathroom signs), posters, or artwork in public spaces (ie, pride flags), provider name tag badges that include pronouns, and ensuring that forms and paperwork have inclusive language are important considerations. Training of all staff members around providing sensitive care for all patients is crucial. Many electronic medical records now include areas for affirmed name and pronouns, gender identity, and sexual orientation labels, which make it less likely for TGD patients to get misgendered in clinical settings. For clinicians, e-mail signatures and customizable name tags in telehealth visits allow the easy editing of one's name, credentials, and pronouns.

Many TGD youth who are referred for psychotherapy do not require professional support. It is important to determine the purpose of the referral and establish collaborative goals at the onset of treatment. We have seen an increase in referrals for specialized gender evaluation and treatment that may best be understood as a byproduct of family and/or provider discomfort, rather than patient need. Young people are exploring gender identity options at earlier ages and may assert several different identities as they come to better understand themselves. These youth may struggle with their identity formation and require exploratory psychotherapy, and others may seek out these services; however, the fact that they are exploring their identity should be seen as a normal part of adolescence, rather than a psychological problem requiring intervention. An ongoing consultative model through a connection with a gender-affirming mental health provider may be all that is necessary to support these youth with appointments approximately 2 to 3 times per year. At these appointments, therapeutic options are explored and recommended as needed. Parents and outpatient providers often report that having an option to connect and collaborate at regular intervals allows them to feel comfortable supporting their TGD youth as they continue to explore their identities; this gives the clinician the opportunity to provide supportive family psychotherapy, provide psychoeducation, and share resources. We recommend that psychotherapy providers assess whether their TGD client requires a treatment plan with psychotherapy at the time of referral and, if not, to consider ways to increase access/reduce barriers to therapeutic services if they are needed in the future.

Outside of the realm of psychotherapy, there are many interventions that can increase support and improve resilience of TGD youth. Encouraging connection with other TGD people and/or the LGBTQ+ community can help cultivate a sense of belonging for youth, create safe spaces to explore gender identity without further marginalization, and provide opportunities for youth to connect with adult role models. Youth may also find themselves as role models or mentors for others. This may be through formal support groups, social gatherings, and/or community activism. These social connections may be found in person as well as online. In addition to community supports, there are many self-help resources that TGD youth can use as they explore their gender identity and goals. These resources include a range of Web sites, phone applications, social media channels, and self-help workbooks. The role of the clinician may be to familiarize themselves with these resources and help TGD youth navigate these spaces safely.

The How

The stance of the clinician, the "how" we are with our patients, is particularly important in working with TGD or other marginalized youth. We have discussed the importance of self-reflection and examination of one's own biases and beliefs as well as awareness of one's own areas of privilege and marginalization as foundational work. There may be times in working with an individual youth when it is appropriate and therapeutic to offer a considered aspect of self-disclosure. This is done in the service of better joining and creating a safe space for a youth and makes power differentials and historical structural biases more explicit. An acknowledgment that our society in general remains a binary place regarding gender and that there remain heteronormative and cisgender norms in our culture can be important discussion points. A self-disclosure if one is part of majority groups (ie, white, cisgender, heterosexual) to acknowledge that there are areas where the therapist does not have shared lived experience can help a youth feel more comfortable in discussing topics that may be rooted in shame. Ultimately, whether a youth's therapist is alike or dissimilar is often based on assumptions (sometimes incorrect ones), and exploration of transference and countertransference together can facilitate the creation of a therapeutic space.

It is important that a clinician not use self-disclosure as a way to excuse a lack of competency. Youth are often told by their providers that they do not "specialize in gender" as a way to limit the expectations they can have from their provider. This is particularly damaging in rural communities, where mental health resources are already limited. We argue that any therapist working with adolescents should have an understanding of identity formation and development to leverage as they increase their competency related to the unique needs of TGD youth. Young people should not be led to believe that a therapeutic space cannot be held for them unless they seek subspecialty services.

Although the evidence base is steadily increasing, there are many unknowns and areas of controversy in the field of gender medicine, particularly in the treatment of minors. We find we must balance the existing knowledge and expertise from the literature and our own clinical experience over time with the unknowns. Much of working with adolescents is neither black nor white but rather gray, and a nuanced exploration often necessitates humility on the part of the clinician. We lean on the work of Harlene Anderson, LCSW, who writes about the importance of the stance of "not knowing."[33] In working with TGD youth, this involves deferring expertise about one's identity back to the patient. The explicit message is "you are the expert in you, in your identity and your lived experience." The clinician can use curiosity and not-knowing to better understand the youth's identity and to help cocreate an integrated narrative about past, present, and future. Drs Aron Janssen and Scott Leibowitz[34] offer a conceptualization of our role as mental health providers working with TGD youth as "collaborative path pavers."

The What

Exploration of comorbidities

Suicidal ideation and self-harm are areas that clinicians should routinely screen for as they work with TGD youth. In a study comparing youth referred for gender and those who were not, children with gender dysphoria were 5 times more likely to endorse self-harm and suicidality, and the rate of this endorsement increased as they got older.[35] Although an initial screening during the biopsychosocial evaluation is important, clinicians should continue to reevaluate and be prepared for crisis intervention and ongoing safety planning. Referral to local crisis assessment teams and emergency rooms may be important as well as education around LGBTQ+-specific resources, such as the Trevor Project, a not-for-profit, crisis-counseling resource (thetrevorproject.org).

Mental health stabilization and World Professional Association for Transgender Health criteria

Youth may seek gender-affirming medical and surgical intervention and will therefore require assessment and subsequent referral (sometimes referred to as a letter of referral) to appropriate medical providers.[4] This includes diagnosing gender dysphoria and addressing any coexisting mental health concerns that may have interfered with the clarity of the young person's identity. In addition, a course of psychotherapy, or psychotropic medications, may be recommended before the referral for medical treatment in order to treat coexisting concerns to alleviate symptoms that may interfere with the patient's ability to understand treatment options and reasonable expectations, and then provide educated and informed consent. In some cases, coexisting concerns should be managed before a referral for medical treatment. At other times, these concerns may be concurrently treated. For TGD youth, the process of assessment often involves family therapy and collaboration with other medical and mental health providers. Other medical treatments that do not lead to irreversible consequences, such as menstrual suppression for appropriate youth, may be used in conjunction with therapy, as noted in SOC8.

Self-diagnoses trends (autism spectrum disorder, dissociative identity disorder, bipolar disorder, and so forth)

A newer challenge to assessment and individual treatment has been the increase in self-diagnosis of severe mental health conditions and personality disorders. Although there is limited research on these self-diagnosis trends, we, along with our colleagues in the field, have noticed an increase in young people seeking confirmation of diagnoses that they have learned about from peers and on social media. Patients are frequently seeking confirmation of their self-determined diagnoses of ADHD, Tourette, Borderline Personality Disorder, Dissociative Identity Disorder, and Autism Spectrum Disorder. On the positive side, these disorders are being destigmatized as people learn more about them and symptoms are normalized. There is likely a percentage of people who are undiagnosed who will benefit from bringing up their symptoms to discuss with their providers. However, prolonged and repetitive exposure via social media (ie, TikTok) to severe symptomology and conditions increased during the COVID-19 pandemic, raises the question of mass sociogenic illness for some conditions.[36] Careful assessment is warranted, and individualized therapeutic treatment plans, which identify and validate a young person's understanding of their unique symptoms rather than focusing on diagnostic clarification, may be useful in partnering with youth to address and/or resolve the symptoms that they bring forward.

Psychological themes that may emerge in individual therapy

Adolescence is a period of identity consolidation. Developmentally, adolescents work to consolidate a healthy and coherent sense of self and sense of self in relationship to others. Individual therapy supports can be an important part of helping TGD youth develop a narrative that is integrated, that generates pride and self-esteem, and that supports healthy attachments with others.

In individual therapy work with TGD youth, many themes arise that are worth exploring. Helping youth understand their experiences of discrimination and stigma within their families and within the larger cultural and societal context is important. This may involve exploration of internalized biases, such as internalized homophobia or internalized transphobia as well. TGD youth often need to process current sociopolitical events and discourse as it relates to their emerging identities and sense of autonomy. Dialectics (borrowed from Dialectical Behavioral Therapy, in this case) can be helpful for youth to understand longer-term social justice trajectories and trends with the recent distress, which many are experiencing in very personal and profound ways. For some, mobilization into action in the form of social media social justice movements or joining a supportive group, such as a Gay Straight Alliance, at their school, can feel empowering and help identify community. For others, the focus necessitates more self-care and minimization of news and social media consumption. Helping youth identify and mobilize family, school, and social supports is an important part of overall wellness.

Starting from a stance of nonjudgment and curiosity helps the clinician support the youth's exploration of their identity over time. Discussion of their hopes and goals regarding social, medical, and/or surgical transitions helps identify realistic expectations and offers education and support if there are unrealistic expectations or aspects yet unconsidered. Appreciating the young person's understanding and awareness of societal stereotypes on gender roles is also helpful as they navigate their own decisions to express themselves. Challenging rigid ideas around these gender roles may be important as they think through the medical treatments that may lead others in society to perceive and treat them differently over time. Clinicians can help youth troubleshoot and navigate safety concerns and interpersonal conflicts that may arise over time.

Treatment models

Clinicians may use traditional psychotherapy techniques as they support TGD youth through the process of gender exploration, identity integration, management of comorbidities, and overall stabilization. Depending on the individual youth's presentation, multiple modalities may be appropriate and helpful, including family therapy interventions, psychodynamic therapy, behavioral therapy models, such as Cognitive Behavioral Therapy (CBT) and Dialectical Behavioral Therapy. As has been well borne out in psychotherapy research, likely the most important factor is the quality of the therapist-patient relationship.

A framework that has been developed is the Transgender Resilience Intervention Model (TRIM), which is an expansion from the minority stress model.[37] Although TRIM can be used to develop future interventions for transgender people, this model provides a way for clinicians to adapt individual interventions they are already familiar with, that are known to target resilience, including those from positive psychology and those targeting self-compassion, self-worth, and self-acceptance.

Although the data are limited, there are several adaptations that have been made to center techniques on the specific needs of sexual and gender minorities. One such treatment option is the AFFIRM model, using CBT content grounded in an affirming, youth-centric orientation.[38] This treatment modality has shown promising efficacy to reducing depression in transgender youth.

Other treatment options may be for the clinician to adopt a different framework of practice, such as can be seen with the gender-affirming life span approach. This framework provides the clinician with 5 key areas to incorporate in psychotherapy: "(a) developing gender literacy, (b) building resiliency, (c) moving beyond the binary, (d) exploring pleasure-oriented sexuality, and (e) making connections to medical providers."[39] This framework combines psychoeducation, advocacy, and individual treatment in an affirming approach grounded in interdisciplinary practice that can be used throughout the different stages of an individual's life.

Future directions

Digital mental health interventions may be one potential future direction. LGBTQ youth in particular may prefer to seek mental health supports in online (compared with offline) spaces. A small study of the AFFIRM Online model, using 8 sessions of asynchronous online CBT modules, was shown to improve depressive symptoms and have high acceptability among participants.[40]

SUMMARY

Whether a clinician works at a specialized gender clinic or as a generalist in outpatient or inpatient settings, one is likely to encounter TGD youth in their clinical work. Having foundational knowledge and training about language/terminology and awareness of the unique challenges faced by TGD youth and their families is important. This involves understanding the structural and societal stigma and biases faced by TGD folks, historical and current obstacles to medical and mental health care and understanding of the significant mental health disparities in the LGTBQ community, including elevated rates of suicidality and suicide. To work effectively with TGD youth (or any marginalized group), clinicians must additionally engage in ongoing inward self-reflective practices to understand our own internalized biases and beliefs. As lifelong learners who embrace cultural humility, we must remain vigilant to changing clinical challenges over time.

TGD youth are often best served in the context of a multidisciplinary team providing gender-affirming care. We recommend starting with a thorough biopsychosocial formulation of the youth in the context of their family/school/community, which informs the development of a collaborative treatment plan. The treatment plan may involve psychiatric care to support mental health comorbidities as well as individual and/or family therapy interventions. The treatment plan may also involve referral to medical or surgical colleagues for gender-affirming care interventions. For mental health providers, discussion about roles and modalities of care are important such that if there are multiple providers involved (ie, Psychiatrist, Social Worker, Psychologist) all understand the roles and are communicating effectively.

CLINICS CARE POINTS

- There are significant mental health disparities for transgender and gender-diverse youth, who have higher rates of mental health disorders, including suicidality compared with their cisgender and/or heterosexual peers.

- Clinicians must understand the societal and structural contributors to these mental health disparities and self-reflect on one's own biases and beliefs to most effectively support transgender and gender-diverse youth.

- Psychological and social interventions are important components of the overall treatment plan for transgender and gender-diverse youth.

- Clinicians should consider their own clinical stance and treatment model in working with transgender and gender-diverse youth. Multidisciplinary teams are often most effective in supporting transgender and gender-diverse youth and their families navigating treatment decisions.

- The evidence base supports the crucial importance of family acceptance for transgender and gender-diverse youth, and clinicians can support youth through family therapy and individual therapeutic treatment modalities.

DISCLOSURE

The authors have no relevant financial disclosures nor conflicts of interest to declare.

REFERENCES

1. de Vries ALC, McGuire JK, Steensma TD, et al. Young adult psychological outcome after puberty suppression and gender reassignment. Pediatrics 2014; 134(4).
2. Spack NP, Edwards-Leeper L, Feldman HA, et al. Children and adolescents with gender identity disorder referred to a pediatric medical center. Pediatrics (Evanston) 2012;129(3):418–25.
3. Vrouenraets LJ, Fredriks AM, Hannema SE, et al. Early medical treatment of children and adolescents with gender dysphoria: an empirical ethical study. J Adolesc Health 2015;57(4):367–73.
4. Coleman E, Radix AE, Bouman WP, et al. Standards of care for the health of transgender and gender diverse people, Version 8. Int J Trans Health 2022;23(S1): S1–260.
5. American Psychological Association. Guidelines for psychological practice with transgender and gender nonconforming people. Am Psychol 2015;70(9):832–64.
6. Ehrensaft D. Gender nonconforming youth: current perspectives. Adolesc Health Med Ther 2017;8:57–67.
7. Zucker KJ, Wood H, Singh D, et al. A developmental, biopsychosocial model for the treatment of children with gender identity disorder. J Homosex 2012;59(3): 369–97.
8. American Psychological Association. APA Resolution on Gender Identity Change Efforts. https://www.apa.org/about/policy/resolution-gender-identity-change-efforts.pdf. Accessed May 3, 2023.
9. Psychiatry.org. Policy Statement on Conversion Therapy and LGBTQ Patients. https://www.psychiatry.org/getattachment/3d23f2f4-1497-4537-b4de-fe32fe8761bf/Position-Conversion-Therapy.pdf. Accessed May 3, 2023.
10. AACAP.org. American Academy of Child & Adolescent Psychiatry Conversion Therapy Policy Statement. https://www.aacap.org/aacap/Policy_Statements/2018/Conversion_Therapy.aspx. Accessed May 3, 2023.
11. Rafferty J, AAP Committee on psychosocial aspects of child and family health, AAP committee on adolescence, AAP section on lesbian, gay, bisexual, and

transgender health and wellness. Ensuring comprehensive care and support for transgender and gender-diverse children and adolescents. Pediatrics 2018; 142(4). e20182162.

12. Socialworkers.org. National Association of Social Workers, National Committee on LBGT Issues Position Statement. Available at: https://www.socialworkers.org/LinkClick.aspx?fileticket=yH3UsGQQmYI%3D&portalid=0. Accessed May 3, 2023.

13. Anton BS. Proceedings of the American psychological association for the legislative year 2009: minutes of the annual meeting of the council of representatives and minutes of the meetings of the board of directors. Am Psychol 2010;65: 385–475.

14. Olson K, Durwood L, Horton R, et al. Gender identity 5 years after social transition. Pediatrics 2022. https://doi.org/10.1542/peds.2021-056082.

15. van der Miesen Anna IR, Steensma TD, de Vries ALC, et al. Psychological functioning in transgender adolescents before and after gender-affirmative care compared with cisgender general population peers. J Adolesc Health 2020; 66(6):699–704.

16. Stewart SL, Van Dyke JN, Poss JW. Examining the mental health presentations of treatment-seeking transgender and gender nonconforming (TGNC) youth. Child Psychiatry Hum Dev 2021. https://doi.org/10.1007/s10578-021-01289-1.

17. Jones BA, Bouman WP, Haycraft E, et al. Mental health and quality of life in nonbinary transgender adults: a case control study. International J Transgenderism 2019;20(2–3):251–62.

18. White Hughto JM, Reisner SL, Pachankis JE. Transgender stigma and health: a critical review of stigma determinants, mechanisms, and interventions. Soc Sci Med 2015;147:222–31.

19. Hendricks ML, Testa RJ. A conceptual framework for clinical work with transgender and gender nonconforming clients: an adaptation of the minority stress model. Prof Psychol Res Pract 2012;43(5):460–7.

20. Meyer IH. Prejudice, social stress, and mental health in lesbian, gay, and bisexual populations: conceptual issues and research evidence. Psychol Bull 2003; 129(5):674–97.

21. Chavanduka TMD, Gamarel KE, Todd KP, et al. Responses to the gender minority stress and resilience scales among transgender and nonbinary youth. J LGBT Youth 2021;18(2):135–54.

22. Chodzen G, Hidalgo MA, Chen D, et al. Minority stress factors associated with depression and anxiety among transgender and gender-nonconforming youth. J Adolesc Health 2019;64(4):467–71.

23. Kcomt L, Gorey KM, Barrett BJ, et al. Healthcare avoidance due to anticipated discrimination among transgender people: a call to create trans-affirmative environments. SSM - Population Health 2020;11:100608.

24. Maksut JL, Sanchez TH, Wiginton JM, et al. Gender identity and sexual behavior stigmas, severe psychological distress, and suicidality in an online sample of transgender women in the United States. Ann Epidemiol 2020;52:15–22.

25. Akré E, Anderson A, Stojanovski K, et al. Depression, anxiety, and alcohol use among LGBTQ people during the COVID-19 pandemic. Am J Public Health 2021;111(9):1610–9.

26. Hughes LD, Kidd KM, Gamarel KE, et al. These laws will be devastating": provider perspectives on legislation banning gender-affirming care for transgender adolescents. J Adolesc Health 2021;69(6):976–82.

27. Green AE, Price-Feeney M, Dorison S. Breaking barriers to quality mental health care for LGBTQ youth. New York, New York: The Trevor Project; 2020.
28. Coyne CA, Poquiz JL, Janssen Aron, et al. Evidence-based psychological practice for transgender and non-binary youth: defining the need, framework for treatment adaptation, and future directions. Evidence-Based Practice in Child and Adolescent Mental Health 2020;5(3):340–53.
29. Tordoff DM, Wanta JW, Collin A, et al. Mental health outcomes in transgender and nonbinary youths receiving gender-affirming care. JAMA Netw Open 2022;5(2): e220978.
30. Almazan AN, Keuroghlian AS. Association between gender-affirming Surgeries and mental health outcomes. JAMA Surg 2021;156(7):611–8.
31. Olsavsky A, Grannis C, Bricker J, et al. Associations among gender affirming hormonal interventions, social support, and transgender adolescents' mental health. J Adolesc Health 2023. https://doi.org/10.1016/j.jadohealth.2023.01.031.
32. Ryan C. & Futterman D., Lesbian & Gay Youth: Care & Counseling. New York: Columbia University Press, 1998. Available at: https://familyproject.sfsu.edu/sites/default/files/Mental_Health_Assessment%20Protocol.pdf. Accessed May 15, 2023.
33. Anderson H. Then and now: a journey from "knowing" to "not knowing". Contemp Fam Ther 1990;12:193–7.
34. Janssen A, Leibowitz S, et al. Affirmative mental health care for transgender and gender diverse youth. A clinical Guide. 1st edition. Springer International Publishing : Imprint: Springer; 2018. https://doi.org/10.1007/978-3-319-78307-9.
35. Aitken M, VanderLaan DP, Wasserman L, et al. Self-harm and suicidality in children referred for gender dysphoria. J Am Acad Child Adol Psychiat 2016;55: 513–20.
36. Olivera C, Stebbins GT, Goetz CG, et al. TikTok tics: a pandemic within a pandemic. Movement Disorders 2021;8(8):1200–5.
37. Matsuno E, Israel T. Psychological interventions promoting resilience among transgender individuals: transgender resilience intervention model (TRIM). Counsel Psychol 2018;46(5):632–55.
38. Austin A, Craig S, D'Souza S. An AFFFIRMative cognitive behavioral intervention for transgender youth: Preliminary effectiveness. Prof Psychol Res Pract 2017; 49(1):1–8.
39. Spencer KG, Berg DR, Bradford NJ, et al. The gender-affirmative life span approach: a developmental model for clinical work with transgender and gender-diverse children, adolescents, and adults. Psychotherapy 2021;58(1): 37–49.
40. Craig SL, Leung VWY, Pascoe R, et al. AFFIRM online: utilising an affirmative cognitive-behavioural digital intervention to improve mental health, access, and engagement among LGBTQA+ youth and young adults. Int J Environ Res Public Health 2021;18(4):1541.

Family-Based Psychosocial Care for Transgender and Gender-Diverse Children and Youth

Caitlin Ryan, PhD, ACSW[a], Antonia Barba, LCSW[b],*,
Judith A. Cohen, MD[c]

KEYWORDS

- Transgender/gender diverse youth • Family focused treatment
- Psychosocial intervention • Psychological maltreatment • Trauma-informed care
- Family Acceptance Project • Trauma-focused CBT

KEY POINTS

- Family support plays a critical role in a child's treatment and recovery from trauma, thus, clinicians should make every effort to engage and include parents in the care of traumatized transgender and gender-diverse (TGD) youth.
- All TGD youth and their families should learn about family rejecting and affirming behaviors and their impact on a child's risk and well-being.
- Parents who are rejecting and ambivalent can change their behavior to become more supportive and affirming of their TGD child.
- Providers can engage parents in treatment by aligning with their cultural values and desire for their child to be healthy and safe.
- Existing integrated evidence-based treatment of TGD children and youth, such as the Family Acceptance Project-Trauma-Focused Cognitive Behavioral Therapy integrated treatment model is recommended for the care of TGD children and youth who have experienced trauma.

INTRODUCTION

Family focused psychosocial treatment is critical for transgender and gender-diverse (TGD) children and adolescents given the early ages of identifying and the increasingly

[a] Family Acceptance Project, San Francisco State University, 423 Capp Street, San Francisco, CA 94110, USA; [b] Inform Transform, 250 Bronxville Road, Bronxville, NY 10708, USA; [c] Allegheny Health Network, Drexel University College of Medicine, 4 Allegheny Center, 8th Floor, Pittsburgh, PA 15212, USA
* Corresponding author.
E-mail address: antonia.barba@gmail.com

Child Adolesc Psychiatric Clin N Am 32 (2023) 775–788
https://doi.org/10.1016/j.chc.2023.03.002
1056-4993/23/© 2023 Elsevier Inc. All rights reserved.

childpsych.theclinics.com

hostile social environment for TGD youth,[a] and their families. Moreover, parental and caregiver inclusion is a core component of most evidence-based trauma treatments of children and adolescents for many reasons, including that (1) youth typically live with and depend on parents and caregivers and thus clinicians need to understand their culture, perception of their needs and problems, and current parenting practices; (2) parents and caregivers are in a key position to affect the emotional and behavioral changes, so clinicians need to engage them in using positive parenting strategies and minimize negative ones; (3) after trauma, youth benefit when parents and caregivers understand their trauma experiences and become more supportive about them. Parental inclusion in treatment is even more critical for TGD youth, who experience high rates of chronic identity-related family rejection (psychological maltreatment), often accompanied by other forms of maltreatment or other traumas.

Evidence-based interventions provide therapeutic guidance for parents and youth to gain new skills, acknowledge and process what has occurred, and develop more supportive relationships. When including parents in trauma-focused interventions, it is important to consider where the parents and youth are with regard to their attitudes and beliefs about their gender identity, and trauma experiences. Families can learn to support their TGD youth and enhance their safety when culturally relevant guidance is provided, when care is inclusive and respectful of the child's diverse identities, and when trauma-focused intervention is implemented collaboratively between the clinician, parent, and child, honoring the respective expertise of each. Of note, because many TGD youth are in out-of-home settings, different adults may provide parental roles for youth.

TRAUMA AND TRANSGENDER AND GENDER-DIVERSE YOUTH

Trauma exposure is all too common, with more than 65% of US youth experiencing at least one trauma before adulthood, and a third experiencing multiple traumas.[1] TGD youth additionally experience bullying and family rejection related to their gender identity, gender expression, and/or sexual orientation. As youth are increasingly sharing their diverse gender identities earlier in development, family rejection related to these identities also may begin early in the child's development. Family rejection often consists of a chronic pattern of overt and/or covert messages of being "not good enough" or "less than" other family members, as well as behaviors such as being left out of family gatherings, being made to attend religious services or pray to change their gender identity, not being able to attend support groups for TGD youth, and receiving constant pressure to dress, act, groom, and/or be different.[2] All of these experiences can have a traumatic impact similar to or worse than other traumatic experiences.

The American Professional Society on Abuse of Children defines "psychological maltreatment" as "a repeated pattern or extreme incident(s) of caregiver behavior that thwart the child's basic psychological needs...and convey a child is worthless, defective, damaged goods, unloved, unwanted, endangered, primarily useful in meeting another's needs, and/or expendable".[3] The Family Acceptance Project (FAP) has identified and measured over 50 family rejecting behaviors in response to a youth's Lesbian, Gay, Bisexual, Transgender, Queer or Questioning (LGBTQ) identity and gender expression.[4,5] These rejecting behaviors attempt to change, prevent, deny, or minimize the child's LGBTQ identity and gender expression and communicate the parent's disapproval, anger, disgust, and disappointment with the youth's identity and

---

[a] The term "youth" refers to children and adolescents.

gender expression. They are experienced as rejection by the youth and contribute to suicidal behavior, depression, illegal drug use, and sexual health risks. A common characteristic of psychological maltreatment is that these behaviors are so common that they are hidden in plain sight. Family rejecting behaviors are learned, transmitted intergenerationally, and enforced by cultural and religious beliefs. TGD youth may perceive rejecting experiences as the cost of staying connected to their family and/or their cultural world.[6] Although ongoing efforts to change and prevent a child's gender identity are typically viewed by parents as efforts to help their child fit in and be accepted by others, they are harmful to the youth and represent a form of psychological maltreatment.[6] It is important to recognize that TGD youth who experience family rejection may also experience parental physical or sexual abuse and/or neglect, and these are associated with elevated risk for cumulative negative impact on health and mental health over the course of the youth's lifetime (**Fig. 1**).

The adverse impacts of trauma compound with increased duration and intensity of the traumatic exposure.[7] TGD youth exposed to acute and chronic traumas have an increased risk of posttraumatic stress disorder, depression, suicidality, substance abuse, anxiety, and a variety of medical disorders. Furthermore, the chronic and pervasive nature of identity-related trauma experienced by TGD youth leads to complex trauma presentations, which—in addition to typical post-traumatic stress disorder (PTSD) symptoms—may include significant affective dysregulation, difficulty with interpersonal relationships, and negative self-image.[8] Assessment is critical to recognize trauma exposure and impact among TGD youth.

ASSESSMENT

Given the high prevalence of childhood trauma, all TGD youth should be screened to identify exposure to potentially traumatic events and the presence of trauma symptoms. If endorsed by a youth or parent, the clinician should follow with a more comprehensive trauma assessment, including the use of standardized assessment tools for youth and parents and clinical interviews to develop a deeper understanding of the youth's trauma history. Assessment should include the following: the frequency and severity of trauma symptoms; impacts on social, emotional, and cognitive functioning; and the presence of strength and protective factors that may promote resiliency. Clinicians may also find it helpful to engage and gather information from other adults involved in the youth's care, including extended family, teachers, and therapists.

It is important to screen for all forms of trauma, particularly those prevalent among youth and families in the clinician's community and TGD youth. Clinicians should conduct assessments separately with the youth and parent to promote safety and honesty and to protect the youth from potential exposure to rejection and harm during the assessment.[8] Youth who are open about their TGD identity and/or sexual orientation may readily identify traumas related to their gender identity and expression, including bullying and harassment at school and in the community. When a youth has disclosed their TGD identity, the clinician can use open-ended questions to explore any perceived or experienced connection between their identity and their trauma experience. Clinicians may also wish to use a screener with developmentally-appropriate questions to explore the connection between trauma and gender identity.[b]

---

[b] The authors specifically recommend the use of the screener "Identifying the Intersection of Trauma and Sexual Orientation and Gender Identity: Part II: The Screener" from The National Child Traumatic Stress Network. This document is available at https://www.nctsn.org/resources/identifying-the-intersection-of-trauma-and-sexual-orientation-and-gender-identity-the-screener.

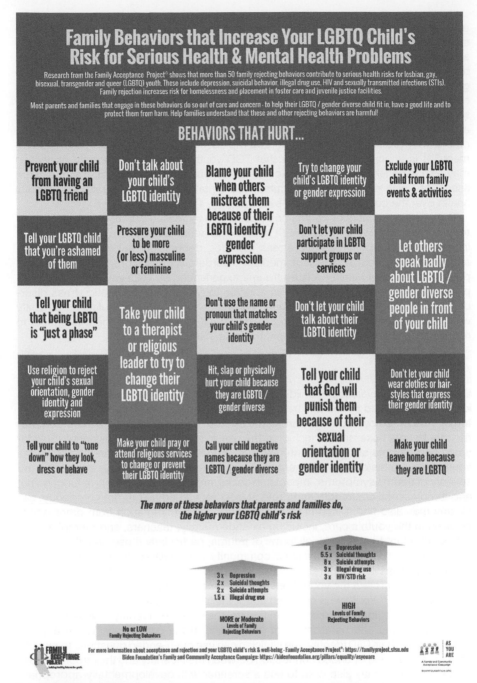

Fig. 1. Family rejection poster from FAP's multilingual four-poster series.

Effectively engaging and assessing TGD youth and their families requires meeting them where they are and learning about cultural context. Clinicians should consider exploring the family's cultural, racial, ethnic, and religious backgrounds, including their beliefs and perceptions about LGBTQ and gender-diverse identities and the caregiver's reactions to their TGD children. The FAP family support model offers several assessment tools that can be used to augment the trauma assessment process. These tools employ an open-ended, culturally grounded approach to learning about the youth and parents' knowledge, attitudes, and behaviors related to LGBTQ identity and gender expression, the youth's level of openness about their identity, and the youth's experience with family rejecting and affirming behaviors. The following FAP assessment tools are available in the appendix of the TF-CBT LGBTQ Implementation Manual:[c]

- Youth and Family Questionnaires: FAP's questionnaires are used separately with youth and parents to ask about cultural backgrounds, to elicit knowledge, attitudes, beliefs, and perceptions related to sexual orientation, gender identity, and gender expression, and to assess family reactions to TGD youth in the context of culture, religion, and community.
- Youth and Parent Social Support Maps: FAP's support maps help to identify family members, peers, and additional individuals in the child's and parent's social worlds, including those who know of the youth's TGD identity and provide sources of support for the youth and caregivers. Youth and parents can use the social support maps to identify and expand their support network and to support confidentiality.
- Gender Scales: FAP's gender scales provides a simple resource to help youth and caregivers initiate conversation about the youth's gender expression using a non-judgmental framework that is especially helpful for caregivers with lower literacy skills and cognitive abilities.

Clinicians can also explore family behaviors using FAP's multilingual *Healthy Futures* posters[4][d] as visual aids to create a behavior index with youth. Youth may be asked to rate their parent's level of acceptance and describe their response to their identity, then asked to identify specific rejecting behaviors they experience, along with the frequency and duration of these rejecting behaviors. Youth are then asked if their parent has expressed support or acceptance and to identify specific supportive behaviors, again noting duration and frequency. The youth is also asked about other family reactions to their TGD identity and how those behaviors have impacted them. This approach creates an inventory of family reactions that can be used to inform the approach to treatment and processed individually with youth and parent, as well as conjointly, later in treatment.

When initially engaging parents and caregivers through assessment, clinicians should prioritize rapport building through a culturally attuned approach and recognize that parents of TGD youth may not have anyone with whom they can safely speak about their child's trauma or gender diversity. Clinicians should strive to create a validating and non-judgmental space using the following strategies: observation and alignment with parents' language; avoiding the use of offensive or inappropriate terms; asking parents to share their hopes and dreams for their child; and inquiring about parents' understanding of their child's identity and any associated fears or worries, particularly as they relate to cultural and religious values and beliefs. At this point, it is recommended that clinicians engage parents in creating an inventory of family

---

[c] The manual Implementing TF-CBT for LGBTQ Youth and their Caregivers is available at https://tfcbt. org/tf-cbt-lgbtq-implementation-manual. Updated versions can be obtained directly from the Family Acceptance Project via email at fap@sfsu.edu.

[d] The Family Acceptance Project Healthy Futures posters are available online in 11 languages and cultural versions in four sizes at https://familyproject.sfsu.edu/posters.

behaviors using the process described above. This procedure helps parents and caregivers begin to understand the importance of family support and the fact that despite being motivated by caring for their child and wanting their health and happiness, the way they may respond to their child (eg, isolating them from TGD friends, not allowing participation in support groups for TGD youth, or pressuring them to change their gender expression) is experienced as rejection and contributes to mental health risks. FAP's youth and parent/caregiver questionnaires[9] provide language and guidance for this assessment.

CONSIDERATIONS

Providers and organizations treating traumatized children and families must provide safe and affirming environments to facilitate their trauma recovery. For TGD youth, that means cultivating environments and therapeutic relationships in which youths are seen and validated as the gender they know themselves to be.[10] Gender-affirming spaces employ gender-inclusive language when engaging youth and families, avoid assumptions about gender identity based on external appearance, provide gender-inclusive or all-gender bathrooms, display diverse and representational media and resources, and inform staff and clients about non-discrimination policies and practices.

Organizations should ensure a safe and confidential process for asking all youth and families about sexual orientation and gender identity and expression, including pronouns and name used, during the initial engagement. This process should take into account legal or ethical issues relevant to evaluating and treating TGD youth, including confidentiality rights, policies for documenting and sharing sensitive information across treatment teams, and access to the youth's medical records. All personnel should take active steps to prevent the involuntary disclosure of the youth's identity, as such disclosure could result in maltreatment, abuse, rejection, and further traumatization.[11] Youth and families should be made aware of confidentiality protocols and limitations, including how the disclosure of sensitive identity-related information is managed, as part of an informed consent process. It is recommended that information related to the youth's sexual orientation and gender identity *not* be documented in their medical record unless it is known by anyone who may access the record without the youth's expressed consent.

When engaging youth and families, consider ways to ensure that youth feel respected and safe to disclose their identity. Follow disclosure with validation and assessment of the degree to which youth are open to sharing their identity with others involved in their care. Clinicians should respect and support a youth's decision and right to come out when and to whom they choose, and can assist them either by creating plans to share this information with relevant treatment team members (ie, composing an email communicating preferred name and pronouns) or assuring them of steps being taken to maintain confidentiality.

If a youth is not open about or does not wish to disclose their identity with their family, explore their rationale, including their perceived risk of maltreatment or rejection if their family were to learn of their identity. Validate their concerns and explore to what extent peer or social perceptions grounded in cultural biases or stereotypes may be influencing beliefs about their family's reaction. It can be helpful to explore the potential benefits of disclosure, such as letting go of their worries about discovery and having a more trusting relationship with their parent or caregiver, particularly when the clinician suspects the parent may know or be accepting of their child's identity. If the youth is firmly opposed to sharing their identity, or the clinician suspects disclosure could result in maltreatment, rejection, or further traumatization, it is recommended that they support the youth's autonomy and right to confidentiality and develop a plan to limit sharing aspects of the youth's traumatic experience that may disclose their identity when working with their parent.[8]

Because family support is a critical aspect of trauma treatment and plays such a significant role in reducing risk factors and promoting future well-being for TGD youth, including helping parents understand the components of gender-affirming care, it is imperative that clinicians not exclude or give up on rejecting or ambivalent parents. All parents and caregivers can benefit from a culturally attuned, non-judgmental space where they can have concerns validated and receive guidance on how to support their traumatized TGD child and continue working with parents struggling with their child's identity to foster connection and increase their ability to advocate for their child's safety and wellness. Given the often complex nature of a youth and family's trauma history and experience, be flexible and allow additional time to address confidentiality and ongoing safety concerns related to the youth's identity. Family treatment can proceed, even in the case of youth who are not open about their identity, and with parents who are rejecting, provided it is grounded in the child and family's cultural world.

EVIDENCE-BASED INTERVENTIONS AND INTEGRATED FAMILY ACCEPTANCE PROJECT-TRAUMA-FOCUSED COGNITIVE BEHAVIORAL THERAPY MODEL

The FAP is a research, education, intervention, and policy initiative that helps diverse families learn to support their LGBTQ children to reduce health risks and promote well-being in the context of their families, cultures, and faith communities. FAP's work includes the first comprehensive research on LGBTQ youth and families and the first evidence-informed family support model for use in educational and treatment approaches for prevention, wellness, and care for LGBTQ children and adolescents.[12–14] In participatory mixed methods research, FAP researchers identified more than 100 specific behaviors that parents and caregivers use to express rejection and acceptance of their LGBTQ children and measured how these behaviors contribute to health risks and well-being.[5] FAP worked with diverse families and LGBTQ youth to develop intervention strategies and research-based resources to help families to decrease rejection and increase support and acceptance for their LGBTQ children. FAP's family support model [e] includes comprehensive family assessment, psychoeducation, parenting skills, and culturally grounded peer support **(Fig. 2)**.[15]

Trauma-Focused Cognitive Behavioral Therapy (TF-CBT),[7] is an evidence-based treatment of youth aged 3 to 18 who have significant symptoms related to any trauma and their parent/caregiver. TF-CBT consists of nine components provided in parallel individual sessions to the youth and their parent, with several planned conjoint sessions. The components are summarized by the acronym PRACTICE (Psychoeducation; Parenting Skills; Relaxation Skills; Affective Modulation; Cognitive Processing; Trauma Narration and Processing; In vivo Mastery; Conjoint Sessions; and Enhancing Safety). The content is available for traumatic grief and can be applied to complex trauma and specific patient populations. TF-CBT has strong evidence of efficacy from 24 randomized controlled trials and several effectiveness trials,[f] including for LGBTQ youth,[16] for improving PTSD as well as other trauma-related outcomes that often arise from experiencing ongoing, chronic, or complex trauma.

An integrated FAP-TF-CBT approach was created through a recent SAMHSA-funded National Child Traumatic Stress Network Learning Community targeting TF-

---

[e] More information about the FAP model is available at https://familyproject.sfsu.edu.

[f] More TF-CBT information is available at https://tfcbt.org and https://tfcbt2.musc.edu.

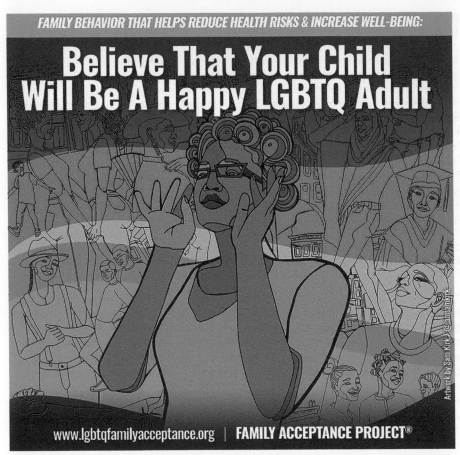

Fig. 2. Family Acceptance Project meme— Believe—about here. Artwork by © 2020 Sam Kirk.

CBT applications for trauma-impacted LGBTQ youth.[8,15] As TF-CBT typically does not include the perpetrators of the trauma, one of the most significant modifications to the approach was to include rejecting parents and caregivers of LGBTQ youth in this application. In addition to applications developed during the learning community to tailor TF-CBT strategies to the needs of LGBTQ youth, the integrated model provides the following: additional focus on family assessment; psychoeducation about the impact of family rejection, rejecting behaviors, and supportive and affirming behaviors; preparing parents to serve as strong advocates for their TGD youth; and the optional exercise of parents preparing an apology letter to share during the conjoint sessions after trauma narration and processing. Through these integrated components, TGD youth who experience family rejection and/or other traumas and their parents and caregivers learn about the impact of these respective traumas, gain skills for coping with trauma reminders and memories, acknowledge and process the impact of these experiences, and move forward together in more supportive and safer family relationships. Details about the integrated model are available in the TF-CBT for LGBTQ Youth and Families Implementation Manual (https://tfcbt.org/tf-cbt-lgbtq-implementation-manual/). The following section describes the core components of the integrated model that clinicians can use in any setting, that is, safety, psychoeducation, and parenting skills, regardless of whether they implement the full TF-CBT model in trauma-focused therapy.

APPROACH

The approach to family treatment with traumatized TGD is intended to be a flexible, non-prescriptive series of potential treatment options designed to be utilized as part of a collaborative and culturally attuned therapeutic process. It is recommended that support be offered to youth and parents separately and concurrently to promote safety and allow each family member a confidential space to explore without risk of harm or re-traumatization. Practitioners should employ clinical judgment when selecting interventions and prioritize those that (1) most align with the youth and family's experience and needs; (2) promote the youth's safety and well-being; and (3) strengthen the parent–child relationship. Psychosocial care for TGD youth helps parents and caregivers learn to support and advocate for their children. This treatment has become especially important in light of widespread politicized efforts to block access to care, which have deepened anxiety and distress for TGD youth and their families.

ENHANCING SAFETY

Creating safety for TGD youth is an active and ongoing process involving the youth, their family, and the treatment team. Clinicians should utilize information gathered during the assessment to identify recurring traumas, trauma reminders, and ongoing threats to the youth's safety, including those connected to their sexual orientation and/or gender identity and expression. Clinicians work with youth to develop a safety plan comprised of safety and coping strategies that correspond to specific risks and trauma reminders, identifying areas where they may require additional support and advocacy from family and other supportive adults. Clinicians may find it useful to review the FAP Social Support Maps with youth and parents to identify members of their support network who are aware and affirming of the youth's gender identity and consider ways to enlist their involvement. It is important to examine past and current unsafe responses to dangerous or triggering situations and work with the youth to identify safer and healthier alternatives, particularly if these behaviors put them at risk and create stress within the family. Unsafe coping strategies can be reframed as the youth's best efforts to survive prior traumatic circumstances. Though protective in the past, they may no longer be useful or necessary. Clinicians may facilitate the youth's exploration of new coping skills and safety strategies through practice and role-playing while providing concurrent space for parents to express concerns and identify ways they can aid and reinforce their child's developing safety plan. Model patience with youth and parents, and continue to revisit and adjust the plan over time as treatment continues. If feelings of frustration arise, provide reassurance that behavior change takes time, particularly when patterns of behavior have been in place for some time, and explore barriers that may be impacting the youth's ability to effectively utilize their plan.

PSYCHOEDUCATION AND PARENTING SKILLS

Traumatized youth and their parents benefit from receiving targeted information about the impact of trauma on their functioning, as it may normalize troubling reactions and ongoing struggles as an expected response to dangerous and overwhelming circumstances. When offering psychoeducation about the specific traumas the youth has experienced, clinicians should explore any potential connection to the youth's gender identity, sexual orientation, and gender expression and how those experiences have impacted the youth's feelings, behaviors, cognitions, and self-image. The intent is not to assume that all trauma experienced by TGD youth is connected to their identity, but rather to facilitate the youth's safe exploration of the meaning of their trauma experiences. For example, in some cases, youth may have avoided reporting abuse or harassment due to a fear of having their identity outed, blamed themselves and their gender expression for their experienced abuse, or normalized rejecting family behaviors and attempts to change their identity as "just the way things are." Clinicians should listen carefully for identity-related misinformation, confusion, and gaps in knowledge and respond with individualized culturally grounded information about sexual orientation and gender identity development and expression, sexual health, and healthy relationships (**Fig. 3**).

Similarly, when engaging parents of TGD youth, the clinician will explore their understanding of gender identity development and how it may be related to their child's trauma experience. Be mindful that while visibility and representation of TGD people have increased, parents may feel confused about how gender identity is expressed in childhood. Clinicians may find it helpful to further explore information shared during

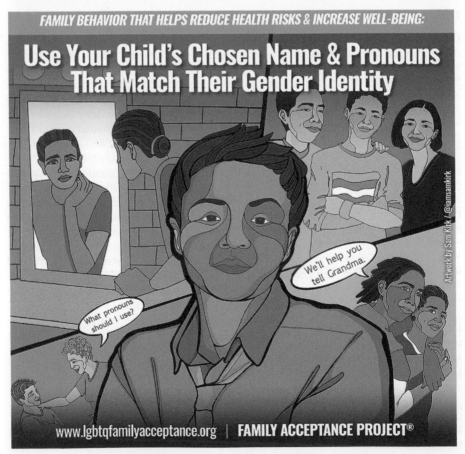

Fig. 3. Family Acceptance Project meme—Using Names and Pronouns—about here. Artwork by © 2020 Sam Kirk.

the assessment, such as parents' beliefs about TGD people and how they are viewed within their culture or faith community. Provide validation and space to ask questions, followed by information about gender and sexual orientation as it relates to their child's identity.

It is recommended that clinicians share information about rejecting and affirming family behaviors with both youth and parents. Even parents who perceive themselves as accepting or are experienced as such by their children can benefit from building awareness of the importance of family behaviors and their connection to youth's safety and risk factors. Begin by teaching youth and parents about how accepting and rejecting behaviors are connected to the youth's well-being. FAP provides an array of tools, including multicultural family education booklets, written visual aids (such as their multilingual *Healthy Futures* posters), and graphics, that can be used to help families learn about the range of rejecting and accepting behaviors. These tools highlight how the amount and frequency of each behavior may contribute to serious health risks or protect against harm and promote wellness.[5] Clinicians may use the inventory of rejecting and affirming behaviors gathered during the assessment to introduce specific behaviors present in the family, explore how these behaviors have been experienced by the youth, and discuss how they may contribute to or exacerbate the youth's trauma response. Youth and parents alike may be surprised to learn that particular family behaviors perceived to be innocuous and normalized within the family culture, are, in fact, harmful and have been linked to an increased risk of negative health outcomes.[5] Support parents through this process by exploring and affirming the intentions behind these behaviors and validating expressed fears, worries, and concerns for their child. Parents' behaviors are often motivated by caring and a desire for their children to be safe and fit in. It is important to communicate to parents that (1) small changes in the ways they respond to their TGD children can make an important difference in that child's health and well-being, and (2) their words, actions, and behaviors can have a profound impact on their child's physical and emotional functioning.[14]

Parents and caregivers of TGD youth can greatly benefit from support aimed at building their capacity to recognize and respond to their child's safety concerns and trauma-related challenges. Upon learning about the negative impact of rejecting and accepting behaviors, some parents may quickly make changes to increase support for their TGD children, while others may struggle and require more time to make changes. It is imperative for clinicians working with ambivalent and struggling parents to actively create a space where they feel supported and validated and their cultural and religious values are respected. Allowing the parents to express worries and concerns without fear of judgment provides a foundation to begin teaching parenting skills that support and affirm their TGD child.

FAP's approach to parent engagement, psychoeducation, and skills building shifts the focus from morality to the health and well-being of their child and targets parents' underlying values, rather than their beliefs.[2] All offered interventions should be aligned with the family's core cultural values and desire for their child to be healthy and safe. Clinicians are encouraged to view parents and families as potential allies who have the capacity to support their TGD children and wish the best for their children.

It can be challenging to address active parental rejection related to a youth's gender identity and expression, such as name-calling, demeaning comments about the youth's identity, exclusion from family events, or allowing a child to be ridiculed or belittled by extended family. Clinicians will have gathered an inventory of these behaviors, including those having the most significant impact on the youth, during the assessment phase. It is critical to address these behaviors directly with parents, demonstrate how these behaviors contribute to suicidality, depression, and other health risks, and work with them to make changes in the way they relate to their children. Begin by providing a rationale for making small changes to behaviors that are aligned with the family's cultural and religious values and/or their hopes and dreams for their child. Address immediate concerns such as reducing the risk of suicide or drug and alcohol abuse. Explore the parents' beliefs and concerns about their child's gender identity, for example, believing that their identity is a choice rather than an inherent trait. Validate the parents' feelings and intentions, then reinforce the connection between parental behaviors and their child's well-being. Consider any experienced improvements in the strength of the parent–child relationship as well.

Parents and caregivers struggling with having a TGD child can benefit from building skills in key areas, including basic communication skills for talking with their child and specific communication skills like neutral, respectful, and non-harmful language for discussing their child's gender identity and expression. Advocacy skills are a key family accepting behavior and parental advocacy can strengthen the parent–child bond and help protect against health risks[13] as parents become more involved in their child's social world. Parents need to know how to stand up for their TGD child, even if they disagree about their identity. This can pose challenges as not all parents are natural advocates; they may not know how to effectively advocate for their child or be aware of their child's rights, or they may have fears or cultural proscriptions against challenging authority figures. Explore and identify advocacy behaviors that could positively impact the child's sense of safety and reduce the likelihood of triggering traumatic responses, for example, standing up for their TGD child within their family, religious congregation, school, or community. Help-seeking skills are also important for the families of TGD youth, as parents may be unsure about how and where to find support and assistance for themselves and their child.

In addition to the support provided in treatment, parents can benefit significantly from connecting to culturally grounded peer support, a component of FAP's family support model. Parents of TGD children often experience their own "coming out" process with regard to sharing their child's identity with extended family members, religious congregations, and community at large. These experiences can subject parents to stigma, judgment, and blame. Connecting with other families, parents, and caregivers who share their cultural identities can reduce parents' isolation and provide the opportunities for learning from other parents who have been there. Clinicians can present family/parent support spaces as an opportunity to expand their social support network with peers who share their cultural and religious beliefs and may have experienced similar worries, concerns, and challenges in learning to support and affirm their TGD children. Families can utilize FAP's online resource center (https://lgbtqfamilyacceptance.org) to find support services for culturally diverse TGD youth and families that are available virtually and in their local community.

Throughout your work, remember that parents who are ambivalent or rejecting of their child's TGD identity can learn to change how they respond to their TGD child to help reduce their child's health risks and increase connectedness. FAP uses a harm reduction framework that uncouples acceptance from support. This approach helps parents who are struggling with their child's identity to change family rejecting behaviors and engage in supportive behaviors that help protect against risk and increase their TGD child's well-being, even when they believe that being transgender and/or gender diverse is wrong.[14]

Parents and caregivers who do not accept their child's TGD identity can still listen to their child and learn about their needs, require other family members to treat their child with respect, and stand up for their child when they are mistreated due to their gender identity and expression. Clinicians can support parents and caregivers in moving away from an all-or-nothing view of having to choose between their child and their culture and faith by staying focused on parents' underlying values, their love for their child, and their desire for their child to live a safe and healthy life.

CLINICS CARE POINTS

- Understand that family support is a crucial aspect of trauma treatment and make every effort to engage parents in treatment, including those who are ambivalent about or rejecting of their child's gender identity and expression.
- Screen TGD youth for all forms of trauma including those prevalent among TGD youth using developmentally appropriate questions and tools.
- Connect TGD youth and families with culturally-grounded peer support to reduce isolation and expand their social network.
- For TGD youth with significant trauma symptoms, clinicians should be familiar with and provide evidence-based trauma-focused treatments such as integrated FAP-TF-CBT.

DISCLOSURE

Dr J.A. Cohen receives grant funding from NIMH, United States, SAMHSA, United States and NICHD, and TF-CBT royalties from Guilford Press, Up To Date, and the Medical University of South Carolina. Dr C. Ryan and Ms A. Barba have nothing to disclose.

REFERENCES

1. Copeland WE, Keeler G, Angold A, et al. Traumatic events and posttraumatic stress in childhood. Arch Gen Psychiatry 2007;64(5):577–84.
2. Glassgold J. and Ryan C., The role of families in efforts to change, support, and affirm sexual orientation, gender identity and expression in children and youth, In: Haldeman D.C., *The case against conversion "therapy": evidence, ethics and alternatives*, (pp. 89-107). 2022, APA Books; Washington, DC.
3. Brassard M.R., Hart S.N., Baker A.L., et al., American professional Society on the abuse of children Monogram on psychological maltreatment, 2019, American Professional Society on the Abuse of Children, New York, NY. Available at: https://www.apsac.org.
4. Ryan C. Poster guidance and Healthy Futures poster series. Marian Wright Edelman Institute, San Francisco State University, 2019a. Available at: https://familyproject.sfsu.edu/poster. Accessed April 29, 2022.
5. Glassgold J. and Ryan C., The role of families in efforts to change, support, and affirm sexual orientation, gender identity and expression in children and youth, In: Haldeman D.C., *The case against conversion "therapy": evidence, ethics and alternatives*, (pp. 89-107). 2022, APA Books; Washington, DC.
6. Ryan C. Family rejection is a health hazard for LGBTQ children and youth. J Am Acad Child Adolesc Psychiatr 2020;59(10):S336.
7. Cohen JA, Mannarino AP, Deblinger E. Treating trauma and traumatic grief in children and adolescents. 2nd edition. New York: Guilford Press; 2017.

8. Cohen JA, Mannarino AP, Wilson K, et al. Trauma-focused cognitive behavioral therapy LGBTQ Implementation Manual. Pittsburgh (PA): Allegheny Health Network; 2018. Available at: https://tfcbt.org/tf-cbt-lgbtq-implementation-manual/.

9. Ryan C. Parent/caregiver and youth questionnaires. Family Acceptance Project. Marian Wright Edelman Institute, San Francisco State University; 2022. fap@sfsu.edu.

10. Clarke M, Farnan A, Barba A, et al. Gender-affirming care is trauma-informed care. Los Angeles (CA): National Center for Child Traumatic Stress; 2022.

11. Barba A, Mooney M, Giovanni K, et al. Identifying the Intersection of trauma and sexual orientation and gender identity Part I: key considerations. Los Angeles (CA): National Center for Child Traumatic Stress; 2021.

12. Ryan C. Generating a revolution in prevention, wellness and care for LGBT children and youth. Temple Political Civ Rights Law Rev 2014;232:331–44.

13. Ryan C, Russell ST, Huebner DM, et al. Family acceptance in adolescence and the health of LGBT young adults. J Child Adolesc Psychiatr Nurs 2010;23(4): 205–13.

14. Ryan C. The Family Acceptance Project's model for LGBTQ youth. J Am Acad Child Adolesc Psychiatr 2019;58(10):S28–9.

15. Cohen JA, Ryan C. The trauma-focused CBT and family acceptance Project: an integrated framework for children and youth. Psychiatr Times 2021;38(6):15–7.

16. Cohen JA. (2020). Trauma-Focused Cognitive Behavioral Therapy for LGBTQ youth across systems of care. Presented at the AACAP Virtual Conference, Washington, DC, Systems of Care Special Programs Institute, Fortuna L, Larson J & Bellonci C, Chairs, October 19, 2020.

Gender-Affirming Medical Treatments

Puja Singh, MD*, Ximena Lopez, MD

KEYWORDS

- Transgender • Gender diverse • Gender dysphoria • Gender incongruence
- Hormone therapy • Gender-affirming care • Puberty suppression
- Gender-affirming surgery

KEY POINTS

- Gender-affirming hormone therapy such as estrogen and testosterone is associated with improved mental health outcomes in transgender youth.
- Child and adolescent psychiatrists, and other mental health professionals, should be up to date on the effects of sought gender-affirming medical and surgical treatments when assessing for decision-making capacity.
- It is recommended that for transgender minors, a multidisciplinary approach that involves mental health providers supports the assessment of the readiness to start puberty suppression or hormone therapy.
- Overall puberty suppression and hormone therapy are generally safe and well tolerated in transgender and gender diverse youth; however, there are important factors that require additional investigation.

INTRODUCTION

Evaluation for gender-affirming treatment in youth is a multidisciplinary effort.[1] Such treatment includes mental health care, social support, hormone therapy, and/or surgical treatment (for adolescents, chest surgery exclusively). Collaboration with the appropriate professionals responsible for each specific aspect of care will help maximize a successful outcome. The goal of this article is to provide an overview of the gender-affirming hormone therapy aspect to this multidisciplinary care. See Belfort and Brown's article's, "Individual Affirming Care: Psychological and Social Approaches to Trans and Gender Diverse (TGD) Youth," in this issue for additional information on those interventions.

Historically, medical interventions for individuals with gender dysphoria or incongruence such as hormone therapy were typically reserved for adults, even though many

Pediatric Endocrinology Division, UT Southwestern Medical Center, 5323 Harry Hines Boulevard, Dallas, TX 75390, USA
* Corresponding author.
E-mail address: Puja.singh@utsouthwestern.edu

Child Adolesc Psychiatric Clin N Am 32 (2023) 789–802
https://doi.org/10.1016/j.chc.2023.05.007
1056-4993/23/© 2023 Elsevier Inc. All rights reserved.

adults remember their adolescence as a difficult time.[2] The analysis of the 2015 US Transgender Health Survey supports offering gender-affirming hormones to transgender and gender diverse (TGD) adolescents rather than waiting until adulthood.[3] Survey analysis showed that those who had received gender-affirming hormone therapy during adolescence (age 14–17 years) had better mental health outcomes such as lower odds of psychological distress, binge drinking, illicit drug use, and suicidal ideation compared to those who had received gender-affirming hormones in adulthood (age ≥ 18 years).[3] A case report published in 1998 from the Netherlands introduced the concept of use of puberty suppression to allow for gender exploration.[4] The case highlighted an individual assigned female at birth with a male gender identity, who was treated with puberty suppression followed by hormone therapy.[4] This case showed that puberty suppression can be an additional tool for aiding in diagnosis and treatment of young adolescents with gender incongruence or dysphoria by "buying time" with a reversible treatment before any hormone therapy or surgery, which have irreversible effects, is started. This led to the development of a protocol, referred to as "the Dutch protocol," which after a comprehensive psychological evaluation, considered treatment of adolescents with puberty suppression after the onset of puberty, followed by sex hormone therapy (around age 16 years), and gender-affirming surgery as adults (at or after age 18 years).[5,6]

Because of the high prevalence of psychological vulnerability of many individuals with gender incongruence/gender dysphoria, these individuals should have access to mental health care before, during, and after transitioning. Protocols have been developed to help provide gender-affirming medical interventions to transgender adolescents to align their bodies with their gender identities. The Endocrine Society Guidelines and World Professional Association for Transgender Health (WPATH) Standards of Care (SOC8) recommend appropriately assessed transgender adolescents be offered gonadotropin-releasing hormone analogs (GnRHas) for puberty suppression, often referred to as "puberty blockers" after the onset of puberty.[7,8] By delaying pubertal development, youth can explore gender identities without the pressure of dysphoria that can result from gender-incongruent physical development. In adolescents who request sex hormone treatment, this is initiated with a gradually increasing dose schedule after a multidisciplinary team confirms persistence of gender dysphoria or gender incongruence, and sufficient mental capacity to provide informed consent, as this is a partly irreversible treatment.[7]

BENEFITS OF GENDER-AFFIRMING MEDICAL TREATMENTS IN TRANSGENDER AND GENDER DIVERSE YOUTH

Studies done in the adult transgender population show improvement in psychological function from endocrine and surgical interventions.[9] There has been increasing research and studies showing the mental health benefits of medical intervention in transgender youth. The outcomes demonstrate an association between medical intervention and decreased rates of depression, anxiety, body dysphoria, and suicidal risk in individuals receiving gender-affirming care including puberty suppression and gender-affirming hormones.[10–14] When interpreting the studies, it is important to note that the evidence is evolving, and that the evidence cannot come from double-blind randomized control trials (as this would be unethical). Regardless of the level of evidence, what is clear is that the growing literature on the subject points to the importance of treating appropriately assessed young people.

In one study, those receiving gender-affirming interventions (puberty suppression or gender-affirming hormones) were associated with 60% lower odds of moderate to severe depressive symptoms and 73% lower odds of self-harm or suicidal thoughts after 1 year of treatment compared to youth who did not receive interventions.[10] Depressive symptoms and suicidality were 2-fold to 3-fold times higher in youth who did not receive puberty suppression or gender-affirming hormones.[10] Risks of depression and suicidality are decreased with gender-affirming medications and multidisciplinary care, even in as short of a time frame as 1 year.[11] One study reported large improvements in body dissatisfaction, improvement in anxiety symptoms, and improvement in self-reported depressive symptoms in transgender youth receiving gender-affirming care at a multidisciplinary clinic at 1 year follow-up.[11] When compared to individuals who wanted puberty suppression but did not receive it, a study using retrospective survey data showed treatment with pubertal suppression was associated with lower odds of suicidal ideation, decreased lifetime suicidal ideation, and severe psychological distress.[12] Another study in TGD adolescents showed that puberty suppression and psychological support led to further improvements in global functioning when compared to psychological support alone.[15] One study assessed adolescents before and after starting gender-affirming hormone treatment.[13] Before starting gender-affirming hormone treatments, TGD youth endorsed at least one item on suicidality on a screening instrument. However, with initiation of gender-affirming hormone therapy, there was a significant decrease in suicidal ideation and significant increase in well-being scores.[13] For better outcomes, it is important to optimize both medical and social factors. One study showed that both social support from family members and friends and gender-affirming hormonal interventions (ie, puberty blockers, testosterone, estradiol) can have improvement in mental health outcomes in TGD adolescents.[16] Family support was associated with fewer depressive symptoms and less nonsuicidal self-injury, and support from friends was associated with less suicidality and fewer anxiety symptoms.[16]

Longitudinal studies in transgender youth support similar findings.[11,14] One study followed transgender youth at a site in New York over 5 year period, and suicidal ideation decreased over time as well as improvement in quality of life.[14] This was observed in both transfeminine and transmasculine identified participants, though with stronger effect size in transfeminine participants.[14] The largest longitudinal prospective cohort study to date with 315 participants assessed psychosocial functioning after starting gender-affirming hormones over a 2 year period in TGD youth.[17] Findings show that gender-affirming hormone therapy was associated with an increase in appearance congruence, improvement in life satisfaction, as well as a decrease in depression and anxiety scores.[17] The improvement in appearance congruence (assessed using the Transgender Congruence Scale in this study) supports the general concept that by inducing physical changes that are gender specific, gender-affirming hormones (GAH) helps a transgender person feel that their body is congruent. This study was also the first to directly link improvements in appearance congruence with mental health improvements. Additionally, those started on gender-affirming hormones in early puberty compared to later puberty had improved outcomes.[17]

For youth who receive gender-affirming care, there are associations with long-lasting benefits into late adolescence and early adulthood. A recent long-term follow-up study over 6 years in the Netherlands showed that gender-affirming medical therapy in adolescents led to improvements in self-perceived physical appearance and global self-worth as young adults.[18] In another longitudinal study of individuals who received puberty suppression and sex hormone therapy as adolescents followed by gender-affirming surgery as adults, results showed that gender dysphoria had resolved, and improvement of well-being was comparable to peers.[5] None of the individuals in the study regretted the decision to begin puberty suppression, sex hormone therapy, or receive gender-affirming surgery. Psychological functioning improved over time, and quality of life, satisfaction with life, and subjective happiness were comparable to same age peers in the general population.[5] Regardless, discussion of regret and the multitude of identity experiences or mental health outcomes that any given individual may have in the future is important at the time of consent.

The use of puberty suppression leads to a decrease of endogenous secondary sexual characteristics, and this can have implications on future gender-affirming surgeries. When compared to controls who did not receive puberty suppression, transmasculine individuals had less breast development and therefore a lower rate of mastectomies were performed.[19] For transfeminine individuals, puberty suppression leads to less penile development and length. As such, penoscrotal skin may not be sufficient to construct a neovagina, and an alternative technique such as the use of intestinal tissue might be needed.[19] All of this should be kept in mind when counseling patients before and during treatment.

PUBERTY SUPPRESSION

For many adolescents with gender dysphoria/gender incongruence, physical changes from puberty can be distressing and unbearable. Initiation of pubertal suppression at the start of early puberty may lead to improved psychological outcomes as described above. By suppressing puberty, this allows the adolescent to explore options and live in one's experienced gender prior to deciding on gender-affirming sex hormone therapy and/or surgery.[7] Use of puberty suppression in pubertal TGD youth is recommended to improve symptoms of dysphoria.[7,8]

Pubertal physiology includes 2 main events: gonadarche and adrenarche. Gonadarche begins with pulsatile secretion of gonadotropin releasing hormone (GnRH) from the hypothalamus leading to activation and secretion of follicle-stimulating hormone (FSH) and luteinizing hormone (LH) from the pituitary gland. These hormones, also referred to as gonadotropins, then act on endogenous gonads (ovaries or testis) leading to production of estrogen or testosterone, respectively. Tanner staging is used to note progression of puberty clinically, with Tanner II denoting the onset of puberty (**Boxes 1** and **2**). In female puberty, breast budding followed by an increase in breast and fat tissue is the first sign of puberty. This is followed by pubertal growth spurt and menarche (onset of menstrual periods) 2 to 3 years later. Height growth ends around 2 years after menarche.[20,21] For male puberty, testicular growth to a volume of 4 mL is first sign of puberty (stage Tanner II).[20,21] It is important to note that pubic hair, axillary odor, or axillary hair is controlled by the adrenal glands in a process called adrenarche. This can occur before, at the same time, or after gonadarche and it is not different in

---

Box 1
Tanner or Pubertal Stages Breast Development

1. Prepubertal

2. Breast bud stage. Elevation of breast and papilla as small mound, enlargement of areola diameter

3. Enlargement of breast and areola, no separation of contours

4. Areola and papilla projection to form secondary mound above level of breast

5. Mature breast contour

Adapted from[20,21]

> **Box 2**
> **Tanner or Pubertal Stages Male External Genitalia**
>
> 1. Prepubertal. Testes volume less than 4 mL
>
> 2. Scrotum and testes enlargement. Testes volume 4 to 6 mL, testicular length greater than 2.5 cm
>
> 3. Penile growth first in length and some increase in breadth, testes volume 8 to 12 mL
>
> 4. Further penile growth in length and breadth, glans development, and darkening of scrotal skin. Testes volume increases 12 to 15 mL
>
> 5. Genitalia adult in size and shape. Testicular volume increases 15 to 25 mL
>
> *Adapted from*[20,21]

assigned males versus assigned females at birth. Therefore, adrenarche is not used to signal "true puberty" (male or female gonadarche).

Puberty suppression treatment can be started once the individual is at least stage Tanner 2 on pubertal examination. Puberty suppression would not provide any benefit, and it is not recommended before puberty starts. Timing of onset endogenous male or female puberty is highly variable, and it is influenced mostly by genetic factors.[20,21] Normal onset ranges typically between ages 8 to 13 years in female puberty and 9 to 14 years in male puberty.[20] Therefore, it is impossible to predict exactly when puberty will start, and the onset will be determined by a physical examination by an experienced health provider. Blood levels of sex hormones increase from a "prepubertal" to a "pubertal" range gradually with puberty: LH, FSH, as well as testosterone for male puberty and estrogen for female puberty. Nevertheless, these can remain in the prepubertal range in early stages of puberty (Tanner II–III) and therefore, the physical examination is more reliable than a blood test to detect the onset of puberty.[20,21] It is important to note that estrogen is also produced in male puberty by the testis, and testosterone in female puberty by the ovaries, but in smaller amounts versus the other sex assigned at birth.[20]

The first-line treatment for pubertal suppression is GnRH analogs or agonists (GnRHa). In puberty, pulsatile GnRH secretion from the hypothalamus signals the pituitary to make LH and FSH. Although GnRH has a short half-life, GnRHas are less susceptible to degradation by enzymes.[21] When first started on GnRHa treatment, there is an initial increase of gonadotropins (LH, FSH), but as treatment is continued it leads to downregulation of the gonadotropin–gonadal axis.[21] This is initially because desensitization of GnRH receptors in the pituitary gland, followed by a decrease in the number of GnRH receptors.[21]

Long-acting GnRHa and depot formulations are the preferred treatment options.[20] These are also the medications approved by the FDA for pediatric patients for central precocious puberty for over 40 years.[22] Depot medication comes in 1, 3, and 6 months injections. There is also the option of 1 year implant (histrelin-acetate), and some reports show that the implant can suppress puberty axis for 2 years or more.[23] Monitoring of transgender youth on GnRHa therapy includes assessment of Tanner stage and growth velocity every 6 months, monitoring for evidence of pubertal progression, and evaluation of FSH and LH levels, as well as levels of endogenous sex steroids.[20] The overall effect of GnRHas is a decrease in pituitary stimulation of the ovaries or testis with a reduction of endogenous sex steroids (estrogen or testosterone), which is reversible after discontinuation of treatment.[24,25] If the individual no longer wishes to continue with transition, GnRHa treatment can be discontinued, leading to resumption of spontaneous pubertal development at a normal rate.[26]

There are also a few studies about the use of progestins (progesterone-based hormones) for blocking endogenous puberty in late pubertal youth. This is an option when GnRHas are not covered by insurance or are too expensive. However, efficacy was not as good when compared to GnRHa.[25]

Adverse Effects of Pubertal Suppression

GnRHas are relatively safe with rare severe acute or chronic adverse effects. One commonly reported adverse effect is injection site reactions such as redness and swelling in up to 9% of patients. Local pain is reported by 10% to 20% of patients.[27] Transiently, GnRHas will promote pubertal changes for 1 month, as initially the first dose stimulates pituitary LH and FSH secretion. As a result, initiation of treatment may lead to mood changes, emotional lability, vaginal bleeding (particularly in those with advanced puberty), acne, testicular pain.[25] Long-term treatment might lead to relative changes in body composition, such as decrease in lean body mass and increase in body fat percentage.[23] In terms of fertility outcomes, those treated with GnRHa have intact gonadal function if treatment is discontinued, but fertility will likely be compromised if endogenous puberty is halted in early stages of puberty and not allowed to complete.[23] One hypothetical concern regarding puberty suppression is that it may limit individuals' sexual exploration, but there is no research in this field. In individuals assigned male at birth, early GnRHa use will limit secondary sexual characteristics including phallus growth, and potentially limit future outcomes of gender-affirming surgery such as vaginoplasty.[19]

Many studies are investigating adverse effects on bone health. Because of lack of sex steroids once started on GnRH agonists, there can be effects in bone mineral accruement which normally occurs during puberty. However, exposure to exogenous sex steroids with gender-affirming hormone treatment or onset of endogenous puberty should lead to at least partial recovery of such skeletal effects.[25] A recent study demonstrated that use of GnRH agonists decreased markers of bone turnover in TGD youth and decreased measures of bone mineral density.[28] Although bone mineral density improves with sex hormone therapy, in this study TGD youth did not reach pretreatment Z-scores for bone mineral density after 24 months of treatment.[28] One study showed that in those assigned male at birth, estrogen treatment did not lead to a significant improvement of bone mineral density, perhaps due to a relative initial low dose of estrogens.[29] In comparison, individuals assigned female at birth, there was greater improvement in bone mineral density with testosterone.[29] In summary, these data suggest that the negative effect of GnRHa on bone density will largely depend on how long this treatment is prolonged into late adolescence without sex hormones (testosterone or estrogen). In other words, the risk will be lower the sooner testosterone or estrogen treatment is initiated and there is more concern on transfeminine patients on estrogen (vs transmasculine patients on testosterone). Furthermore, overall the effects are modest (few patients develop osteoporosis), and the long-term clinical consequences such as risk for fractures are unknown.

The effects of prolonged GnRH agonist therapy on brain development such as brain maturation, cognition, and psychological performance are unknown though there is ongoing research in the field. The brain undergoes many changes during puberty, and sex steroids play an important role in this development and maturation.[30] One case study found lack of significant variation in brain white matter for transgender female receiving GnRH analog treatment.[30] Another study from Amsterdam compared executive functioning in adolescents receiving GnRHa versus adolescents not receiving GnRHa to age-matched controls.[31] In this study, there was no significant effect of GnRHas on executive functioning of TGD youth receiving GnRHas compared to untreated TGD adolescents.[31] There is a need for more longitudinal studies to determine the effect of GnRH analog therapy in these developmental stages.

HORMONE THERAPY

As many of the changes from starting hormone therapy are irreversible, it is important that adolescents reach a reasonable level of competence regarding medical decision making. The most recent WPATH Standard of Care guidelines recommend starting hormone therapy in the adolescent who has expressed marked and sustained gender diversity/incongruence over time, is able to provide informed consent/assent, has emotional and cognitive maturity, does not have mental health concerns interfering with diagnostic clarity, is informed of reproductive effects and has reached Tanner stage 2.[8] Both the medical health provider and mental health provider play an important role in assessing readiness of the adolescent to start sex hormone therapy and assessing ability to consent.[7] Family support is crucial. A regimen of "pubertal induction" is typically used, similar to what is used in (cisgender) adolescents unable to undergo puberty for other medical reasons. During pubertal induction, testosterone or estradiol is given in gradual increasing doses mimicking normal (male or female) puberty.[7] As pubertal induction begins, the medical health provider and mental health provider should monitor the adolescent's psychological response. When starting puberty induction, there is careful monitoring for both desired and undesired effects.[7] The goal of hormone therapy is to replace endogenous sex hormone levels that are consistent with the individual's gender identity with the induction of desired secondary sex characteristics.[7] Most of the physical changes occur gradually over 2 years, but the timeline can vary.

Feminizing Hormone Therapy

Estrogen formulations include oral, transdermal, or intramuscular 17β-estradiol.[7] Measurement of serum estradiol levels is used to monitor dose of oral, transdermal, and intramuscular estradiol, where the goal is maintaining estradiol levels within the normal female range after a regimen of gradual increasing doses over 6 months to 2 years. The Endocrine Society provides recommendations for a faster puberty induction regimen for those patients who present late in puberty (Tanner stage IV–IV) and who are typically older, and a slower regimen for those who present in early puberty (Tanner II–III) and typically received puberty suppression before hormone therapy.[7]

Endogenous testosterone needs to be suppressed to allow for estrogen to induce the desired secondary sex characteristics. Physiologic doses of estrogen alone are not enough to suppress testosterone levels into the normal "female" range and adjunctive therapy is required.[7] Options include GnRHa or "antiandrogens" that block the effect of testosterone. Common anti-androgen agents include spironolactone, which is a diuretic and directly inhibits testosterone action.

Effects

Physical changes are seen in the first 3 to 12 months of estrogen and anti-androgen therapy. These changes include decreased spontaneous erections, decreased oiliness of skin, decreased body hair and facial hair, increased breast tissue growth (maximal breast development is usually 2 years after initiation of hormones), and redistribution of fat mass.[7] On long-term treatment, individuals will have atrophy of prostate gland and testicles. One area of major concern for transgender females is breast development. There is a great range of variability. Anecdotally, some transgender females report improvements in mood, sexual desire, and breast development with use of progesterone. However, there are not enough studies regarding its use in hormone regimens for transgender females, and current evidence does not indicate that they enhance breast development.[7,8]

Adverse effects

It is important to obtain thorough medical history to determine if there are any risk factors to starting estrogen therapy, although these are extremely rare in youth, and includes history of thrombotic events (such as deep vein thrombosis or pulmonary embolism).[8] Tobacco use is associated with increased risk of venous thrombosis, and patients should be counseled regarding this risk prior to starting estrogen as it can further increase risk.[8] There is a particularly increased risk of thromboembolic events specifically with ethinyl estradiol (vs 17β-estradiol), so it is not recommended in any transgender treatment regimen.[7] Oral routes of administration are thought to be more thrombogenic due to its "first pass effect" in the liver, verses transdermal or injected routes.[7] Therefore, for those with nonmodifiable risk factors (history of thrombophilia, history of thrombosis, family history of thromboembolism), transdermal estrogen in combination with anticoagulants may decrease risk of thromboembolism.[8] Estrogen also decreases testicular volume and sperm production.[7] Prolonged treatment can lead to infertility.[32]

If on spironolactone, an anti-androgen agent, serum electrolytes with special attention to potassium are monitored. If there is an elevation in potassium, electrolytes may normalize with cessation of medication and with resumption at a lower dose.[33] Individuals should also have bone mineral density assessment, particularly in those not compliant with hormone therapy. Estrogen can cause elevation of prolactin levels or enlargement of the pituitary gland.[7] Often, prolactin level returns to normal range with reduction or discontinuation of estrogen. Some studies showed that transgender females on estrogen had favorable lipid changes, such as increased high-density lipoprotein and decreased low-density lipoprotein concentrations.[7] Another study found that individuals on estrogen therapy had no significant changes in body mass index (BMI) or blood pressure[33] (**Table 1**).

Table 1
Feminizing effects in transgender females

Effect	Onset	Maximum
Redistribution of body fat	3–6 mo	2–3 y
Decrease in muscle mass and strength	3–6 mo	1–2 y
Softening of skin/decreased oiliness	3–6 mo	Unknown
Decreased sexual desire	1–3 mo	3–6 mo
Decreased spontaneous erections	1–3 mo	3–6 mo
Male sexual dysfunction	Variable	Variable
Breast growth	3–6 mo	2–3 y
Decreased testicular volume	3–6 mo	2–3 y
Decreased sperm production	Unknown	> 3 y
Decreased terminal hair growth	6–12 mo	> 3 y
Scalp hair	Variable	-
Voice changes	None	-

From Hembree, W.C., et al., Endocrine Treatment of Gender-Dysphoric/Gender-Incongruent Persons: An Endocrine Society* Clinical Practice Guideline. The Journal of Clinical Endocrinology & Metabolism, 2017. 102(11): p. 3869-3903, by permission of Oxford University Press[7]

Masculinizing Hormone Therapy

There are various androgen preparations to induce masculinization in transgender males including intramuscular (IM) or subcutaneous (SC), subcutaneous pellets, and transdermal routes of administration (gel or patches). A new oral formulation has been recently approved for adults in the United States but there is no experience in its use for transgender care.[34] IM and SC testosterone is usually dosed every 1 to 2 weeks, and some patients note cyclic variation in effects. Pubertal induction in transgender youth is typically done with IM or SC formulations because it allows for smaller initial doses and accurate gradual increase in doses versus transdermal testosterone, which provides a maintenance adult dose.[7] Transdermal testosterone is more expensive and often not covered by insurance in the United States.

Effects

Treatment with testosterone leads to clitoromegaly, voice deepening, amenorrhea (which can occur within few months of testosterone treatment but can take up to a year), increase in body hair on face and body, decrease in fat mass, increased muscle mass, increased acne, increased libido, and male pattern baldness (if genetically predisposed).[7] Once on therapy, there is close monitoring to make sure the individual is in goal range, as supraphysiologic levels increase the risk for adverse events. Initially, additional agents can be used to achieve menstrual cessation. One option is the use of GnRHa in combination with testosterone in early hormone therapy. Progestins and oral contraceptives can also be used to achieve menstrual cessation.[8]

Adverse effects

In TGD youth, pregnancy and attempting to become pregnant are the only absolute contraindications to testosterone therapy, and relative contraindications include severe hypertension, polycythemia (elevated hemoglobin and hematocrit), and sleep apnea.[8] Individuals on testosterone therapy often have an increase in hemoglobin and hematocrit levels to the male normal range.[33] Follow-up visits for patients on testosterone therapy includes laboratory and clinical evaluation, such as weight gain, signs of uterine breakthrough bleeding, and acne.[8] Testosterone will decrease fertility, but does not cause infertility.[35] There are multiple reports of pregnancy occurring in transmasculine patients after as well as during testosterone treatment.[36] Therefore, education about pregnancy prevention while receiving testosterone should be provided, even in the absence of menses.

In terms of body habitus, one study reported a significant increase in BMI percentiles and z-scores in individuals on testosterone when compared to BMI-matched cisgender females at both short- and long-term follow-up.[37] Clinicians also should evaluate cardiovascular risk factors such as lipid profiles. Studies show that testosterone therapy in transgender males leads to a more atherogenic lipid profile, such as higher triglycerides, higher total cholesterol, higher low-density lipoprotein cholesterol, and lower high-density lipoprotein cholesterol.[7,33] Thus far, long-term studies have not shown an increased risk for cardiovascular mortality[7] (**Table 2**).

MENSTRUAL SUPPRESSION

Menstrual vaginal bleeding can cause dysphoria in transmasculine or nonbinary individuals.[38] Puberty suppression and testosterone will induce desired menstrual suppression. Occasionally, patients who are not ready for puberty suppression or testosterone might benefit from a treatment to suppress menstrual bleeding. This can be achieved with daily oral contraceptives taken continuously (skipping the placebo week), daily oral progesterone or progestins (ie, Aygestin), intramuscular injections of

Table 2
Masculinizing effects in transgender males

Effect	Onset	Maximum
Skin oiliness/acne	1–6 mo	1–2 y
Facial/body hair growth	6–12 mo	4–5 y
Scalp hair loss	6–12 mo	-
Increased muscle mass/strength	6–12 mo	2–5 y
Fat redistribution	1–6 mo	2–5 y
Cessation of menses	1–6 mo	-
Clitoral enlargement	1–6 mo	1–2 y
Vaginal atrophy	1–6 mo	1–2 y
Deepening of voice	6–12 mo	1–2 y

From Hembree, W.C., et al., Endocrine Treatment of Gender-Dysphoric/Gender-Incongruent Persons: An Endocrine Society* Clinical Practice Guideline. The Journal of Clinical Endocrinology & Metabolism, 2017. 102(11): p. 3869 to -3903, by permission of Oxford University Press [7]

depo-progesterone every 3 months, or an intrauterine device. These are typically well tolerated with no irreversible effects, although mood worsening has been reported particularly with oral progestin-based treatments.[38] Patients on testosterone can take 6 to 12 months to achieve menstrual suppression and can also benefit from these treatments during this time, or occasionally during "breakthrough' bleeding that can occur while on testosterone treatment.[38]

FERTILITY PRESERVATION

Discussions regarding fertility are strongly recommended. These discussions should be started during counseling for initiation of GnRHa, and prior to initiation of sex hormones.[8] In early pubertal youth, treatment with GnRHa will impair spermatogenesis and oocyte maturation. This is reversible if GnRHas are stopped before starting hormone therapy. Therefore, for those who wish to preserve fertility potential, one option is delay or discontinue GnRHa therapy to advance gamete maturation. However, this may not be the preferred option as mature sperm production is seen in later stages of puberty and this would imply the development of significant secondary sex characteristics which would cause dysphoria.[7] Prior to starting sex hormone therapy, fertility options should be reviewed, even if the individual is not particularly interested in the issue at time of treatment.

Options for individuals assigned male at birth who have undergone enough endogenous puberty include sperm preservation and can consider sperm banking prior to gender-affirming hormone therapy.[8,32] The timing of such interventions should be prior to hormone therapy ideally, or after stopping hormone therapy to allow for rise of sperm counts.[8] For those who received GnRHa in early pubertal stages and puberty was not resumed, testicular biopsy followed by cryopreservation is an option as an experimental procedure under a research study, with the hope that maturation of premature testicular tissue will be achieved in vitro in the future.

For individuals assigned female at birth, reproduction options include oocyte (egg) or embryo freezing. In the future, a surrogate woman or themselves could carry frozen gametes and embryo to pregnancy.[8] Again, the timing of such reproductive options should be prior to hormone therapy. However, stopping testosterone may lead to adequate recovery of ovaries to release eggs, but this depends on patient's age and duration of testosterone therapy.[8] Data from adults show that pregnancy can occur after long-term testosterone therapy and even while on testosterone.[36] Therefore, youth who are started on testosterone after undergoing a complete endogenous (female) puberty seem to be at lower risk for fertility implications. For individuals assigned female at birth who received pubertal suppression in an early stage of puberty, there is not enough data to know if fertility preservation can be done after being on GnRHa and testosterone for a prolonged period of time.

CHEST DYSPHORIA AND MASTECTOMIES

Breast development can cause significant chest dysphoria in transgender males. Many transgender males bind their chest to appear more masculine and to have a flat chest. However, this has negative health outcomes such as pain, weakness, skin infection, rib fractures, and light headedness.[39] Not all transgender individuals pursue surgical procedures, but often procedures are desired to better align the individual's physical body with their experienced gender and there are high satisfaction rates for those undergoing mastectomies (breast removal).[39] Of note, some transgender male individuals experience worsening chest dysphoria after treatment starts, perhaps due to a wider disparity between masculine appearance and female chest appearance.[39] In one cohort study, comparison of postsurgical and nonsurgical youth suggested that chest reconstruction had a positive impact.[39] Per WPATH SOC 8, chest masculinization surgery can be considered in a select group of mature minors when clinically and developmentally appropriate as determined by a multidisciplinary team experienced in adolescent and gender development, and the duration or current use of testosterone therapy should not preclude surgery if otherwise indicated.[8]

GENDER-AFFIRMING MEDICAL TREATMENTS FOR NONBINARY YOUTH

Most of the studies evaluating gender-affirming medical treatments in adolescents do not include a significant number of nonbinary identified patients. Furthermore, nonbinary patients might desire embodiment treatments that are not completely male or female while endocrine treatments are "binary." Nevertheless, nonbinary youth also experience dysphoria and might benefit from puberty suppression, hormone therapy, or chest surgery.[40] Adherence to standards of care practice with mental health involvement to assess readiness to initiate any of these treatments is particularly relevant for nonbinary adolescents as the lack of research cautions a careful approach and follow-up.[40]

SUMMARY

The care for TGD youth has advanced significantly with the use of puberty suppression and hormone therapy with an improvement in psychosocial outcomes. Standards of care per Endocrine Society and WPATH encourage the use of a multidisciplinary team for best practice. Medical affirming therapies in combination with mental health care improve outcomes such as decreased rates of depression, anxiety, body dysphoria, and suicidal risk. There is still ongoing research on the long-term follow-up of TGD youth, but studies thus far have shown the benefits extend into adulthood.

CLINICS CARE POINTS

- It is recommended that TGD youth receiving gender-affirming medical treatments undergo a multidisciplinary approach involving care from mental health providers.

- Child and adolescent psychiatrists providing care to these youth should ideally know more about the medical and surgical treatments when assessing for decision-making capacity.
- Puberty suppression can be useful to suppress endogenous sex hormones temporarily until decision-making capacity for more irreversible treatments is achieved, and it is associated with decreased negative mental health outcomes.
- Gender-affirming hormones (estrogen or testosterone) are associated with improved mental health outcomes in youth in several types of studies, both cross-sectional and longitudinal.
- Overall puberty suppression and hormone therapy are safe and well tolerated with low risk of adverse effects in TGD youth.
- Gender-affirming medical treatments can have fertility implications and options for preservation should be offered when available.
- Nonbinary youth also might benefit from gender-affirming medical treatments but the lack of research cautions for a careful approach.

DISCLOSURE

The authors have nothing to disclose.

REFERENCES

1. American Psychiatric Association. *Diagnostic and statistical manual of mental disorders: DSM-5™*. 5th edition. Arlington (VA): American Psychiatric Publishing, Inc; 2013. xliv, 947-xliv, 947.
2. Gooren L, Delemarre-Van de Waal H. The feasibility of endocrine interventions in juvenile transsexuals. J Psychol Hum Sex 1996;8(4):69–74.
3. Turban JL, King D, Kobe J, et al. Access to gender-affirming hormones during adolescence and mental health outcomes among transgender adults. PLoS One 2022;17(1):1–15.
4. Cohen-Kettenis PT, Van Goozen SHM. Pubertal delay as an aid in diagnosis and treatment of a transsexual adolescent. Eur Child Adolesc Psychiatr 1998;7(4): 246–8.
5. De Vries ALC, Mcguire JK, Steensma TD, et al. Young adult psychological outcome after puberty suppression and gender reassignment. Pediatrics 2014; 134(4):696–704.
6. de Vries ALC, Cohen-Kettenis PT. Clinical management of gender dysphoria in children and adolescents: the Dutch approach. J Homosex 2012;59(3):301–20.
7. Hembree WC, Cohen-Kettenis PT. Gooren L.,et al., Endocrine treatment of gender-dysphoric/gender-incongruent persons: an endocrine Society* clinical practice guideline. J Clin Endocrinol Metab 2017;102(11):3869–903.
8. Coleman E, Radix AE, Bouman WP, et al. Standards of care for the health of transgender and gender diverse people, version 8. Int J Transgend Health 2022; 23(sup1):S1–259.
9. White Hughto JM, Reisner SL. A Systematic review of the effects of hormone therapy on psychological functioning and quality of life in transgender individuals. Transgender Health 2016;1(1):21–31.
10. Tordoff DM, Wanta JW, Collin A, et al. Mental health outcomes in transgender and nonbinary youths receiving gender-affirming care. JAMA Netw Open 2022;5(2): e220978.

11. Kuper LE, Stewart S, Preston S, et al. Body dissatisfaction and mental health outcomes of youth on gender-affirming hormone therapy. Pediatrics 2020;145(4): e20193006.
12. Turban JL, King D, Carswell JM, et al. Pubertal suppression for transgender youth and risk of suicidal ideation. Pediatrics 2020;145(2):e20191725.
13. Allen LR, Watson LB, Egan AM, et al. Well-being and suicidality among transgender youth after gender-affirming hormones. Clin Pract Pediatr Psychol 2019;7(3):302–11.
14. Achille C, Taggart T, Eaton NR, et al. Longitudinal impact of gender-affirming endocrine intervention on the mental health and well-being of transgender youths: preliminary results. Int J Pediatr Endocrinol 2020;2020(1):8.
15. Costa R, Dunsford M, Skagerberg E, et al. Psychological support, puberty suppression, and psychosocial functioning in adolescents with gender dysphoria. J Sex Med 2015;12(11):2206–14.
16. Olsavsky AL, Grannis C, Bricker J, et al. Associations among gender-affirming hormonal interventions, social support, and transgender adolescents' mental health. J Adolesc Health 2023;72(6):860–8.
17. Chen D, Berona J, Chan Y-M, et al. Psychosocial functioning in transgender youth after 2 Years of hormones. N Engl J Med 2023;388(3):240–50.
18. Arnoldussen M, Van Der Miesen AIR, Alberse AME, et al. Self-perception of transgender adolescents after gender-affirming treatment: a follow-up study into young adulthood. LGBT Health 2022;9(4):238–46.
19. Van De Grift TC, Van Gelder ZJ, Mullender MG, et al. Timing of puberty suppression and surgical options for transgender youth. Pediatrics 2020;146(5): e20193653.
20. Sperling MA. In: Sperling MA, editor. Sperling pediatric Endocrinology. Fifth Edition. Philadelphia, PA: Elsevier; 2021.
21. Koenig R, Rosen CJ, Williams RH, et al. Williams Textbook of Endocrinology. 14th edition. Philadelphia: Elsevier; 2020.
22. Leuprolide Acetate Depot-PED, Injection. Vol 2010. McKesson Health Solutions LLC; 2010
23. Schagen SEE, Delemarre-van de Waal HA, Hannema SE, et al. Efficacy and safety of gonadotropin-releasing hormone agonist treatment to suppress puberty in gender dysphoric adolescents. J Sex Med 2016;13(7):1125–32.
24. Mejia-Otero JD, White P, Lopez X. Effectiveness of puberty suppression with gonadotropin-releasing hormone agonists in transgender youth. Transgender Health 2021;6(1):31–5.
25. Panagiotakopoulos L. Transgender medicine - puberty suppression. Rev Endocr Metab Disord 2018;19(3):221–5.
26. Clemons RD, Kappy MS, Stuart TE, et al. Long-term effectiveness of depot gonadotropin-releasing hormone analogue in the treatment of children with central precocious puberty. Am J Dis Child 1993;147(6):653.
27. Sun Pharmaceutical Industries, Inc. Leuprolide acetate injection [prescribing information]. Cranbury; 2014.
28. Vlot MC, Blankenstein MA, Heijboer AC, et al. Effect of pubertal suppression and cross-sex hormone therapy on bone turnover markers and bone mineral apparent density (BMAD) in transgender adolescents. Bone 2017;95:11–9.
29. Klink D, Caris M, Heijboer A, et al. Bone mass in young adulthood following gonadotropin-releasing hormone analog treatment and cross-sex hormone treatment in adolescents with gender dysphoria. J Clin Endocrinol Metab 2015;100(2): E270–5.

802   Singh & Lopez

30. Schneider MA, Spritzer PM, Soll BMB, et al. Brain maturation, cognition and voice pattern in a gender dysphoria case under pubertal suppression. Front Hum Neurosci 2017;11.
31. Staphorsius AS, Burke SM, Bakker J, et al. Puberty suppression and executive functioning: an fMRI-study in adolescents with gender dysphoria. Psychoneuroendocrinology 2015;56:190–9.
32. Alaa H, Steven W, Ashok A, et al. *Sperm freezing in transsexual women*, . *Archives of Sexual Behavior*41. Springer Science and Business Media LLC; 2012. p. 1069–71.
33. Jarin J, Pine-Twaddell E, Trotman G, et al. Cross-sex hormones and metabolic parameters in adolescents with gender dysphoria. Pediatrics 2017;139(5): e20163173.
34. Swerdloff RS, Wang C, White WB, et al. A new oral testosterone undecanoate formulation restores testosterone to normal concentrations in hypogonadal men. J Clin Endocrinol Metab 2020;105(8):1i.
35. De Sutter P. Gender reassignment and assisted reproduction: present and future reproductive options for transsexual people. Hum Reprod 2001;16(4):612–4.
36. Light AD, Obedin-Maliver J, Sevelius JM, et al. Transgender men who experienced pregnancy after female-to-male gender transitioning. Obstet Gynecol 2014;124(6):1120–7.
37. Valentine A, Nokoff N, Bonny A, et al. Cardiometabolic parameters among transgender adolescent males on testosterone therapy and body mass index-matched cisgender females. Transgender Health 2021;6(6):369–73.
38. Carswell JM, Roberts SA. Induction and maintenance of amenorrhea in transmasculine and nonbinary adolescents. Transgender Health 2017;2(1):195–201.
39. Olson-Kennedy J, Warus J, Okonta V, et al. Chest reconstruction and chest dysphoria in transmasculine minors and young adults. JAMA Pediatr 2018; 172(5):431.
40. Kennis M, Duecker F, T'Sjoen G, et al. Gender affirming medical treatment desire and treatment motives in binary and non-binary transgender individuals. J Sex Med 2022;19(7):1173–84.

Dynamic Gender Identities and Expressions

Detransition and Affirming Non-linear Gender Pathways Among Transgender and Gender Diverse Youth

Brett Dolotina, BS[a], Peter T. Daniolos, MD, DFAACAP[b],*

KEYWORDS

• Transgender youth • Nonbinary youth • Transition • Detransition • Retransition

KEY POINTS

- For some transgender and gender diverse youth (TGD) youth, the exploration of gender identity and expression may be non-linear, encompassing multiple gender embodiments over time.
- Some TGD youth elect to detransition, broadly defined as the cessation or reversal of an already-initiated social and/or medical gender affirmation process.
- Clinicians should support these dynamic gender embodiment goals and facilitate supportive conversations with TGD youth and their families.

INTRODUCTION

Transgender and gender diverse (TGD) youth are those whose gender identity is different from societal expectations associated with their sex assigned at birth.[1] In the United States (U.S.), an estimated 1.4% of adolescents identify as TGD (about 300,000 individuals).[2] Many TGD children and adolescents pursue social gender affirmation, modifying their gender expression to align with their gender identity (eg, changing their name, pronouns, hairstyle, clothing). Some TGD adolescents may meet eligibility criteria for gender-affirming medical interventions, including pubertal suppression and hormone treatments.[3,4] Multiple studies have linked gender-affirming social and medical processes to superior mental

[a] Department of Epidemiology, Mailman School of Public Health, Columbia University, 722 West 168th Street, New York, NY 10032, USA; [b] Member of the Faculty, Harvard Medical School Child and Adolescent Psychiatry, Cambridge Health Alliance/Cambridge Hospital, Macht Building, 1493 Cambridge Street, Cambridge, MA 02139, USA
* Corresponding author.
E-mail address: pdaniolos@challiance.org

Child Adolesc Psychiatric Clin N Am 32 (2023) 803–813
https://doi.org/10.1016/j.chc.2023.05.002
1056-4993/23/© 2023 Elsevier Inc. All rights reserved.

childpsych.theclinics.com

health outcomes among TGD youth.[5–8] To ensure comprehensive support of both medical and social transition pathways, gender-affirming care for TGD youth should be multipronged, consisting of collaborative efforts across psychiatric, social, medical and legal domains.[9,10]

In some cases, TGD youth may elect to *detransition*. While existing research suggests that rates of detransition are quite low among TGD populations, it is essential that clinicians are able to provide comprehensive, individualized support for each patient. The term detransition encompasses a heterogeneous set of experiences that may include a change in gender identity, a myriad of potential shifts in gender expression (eg, change in name, discontinuation of gender-affirming medical interventions, change in pronouns), or a combination of these. Of note, some individuals who have shifts in their gender expression may do so because they have already reached their desired embodiment goals or were forced to stop such gender affirmation processes due to external factors that did not coincide with a change in gender identity (eg, discrimination, undesired reactions to medical treatment, loss of access to care).

It is vital to note that detransition is conceptually distinct from *desistence*, which is another term frequently used in the literature and generally refers to the remission of gender dysphoria, or the psychological distress related to an incongruence between one's sex assigned at birth and their gender identity, as defined by the *Diagnostic and Statistical Manual of Mental Disorders, Fifth Edition, Text Revision (DSM-5-TR)*.[11] Indeed, desistence has been used to describe cases where gender dysphoria subsides with *no initiation of gender affirmation processes*,[12] whereas detransition generally refers to the cessation or reversal of an already-initiated gender affirmation process, or a shift in gender identity. It is possible that some youth may still have gender dysphoria even after they detransition, further demonstrating that detransition and desistence are not synonymous. Moreover, some individuals use the term *retransition*, which refers to the concept of transitioning multiple times between different gender identities and/or expressions, often also mirroring the same discontinuation/reversal processes as those who claim the terms detransition or "detrans."[13] Clinicians must be cognizant of these distinct concepts as they often represent different and unique lived experiences and clinical needs.

Detransition may include a range of evolving gender expressions, including using the name and/or pronouns that a TGD person used prior to their social gender-affirmation process, keeping the name selected during a prior gender-affirmation process, or choosing a new one entirely. Medically, detransition might consist of ceasing pubertal suppression or gender-affirming hormones. It is important to note that detransition is not synonymous with *regret*[14–16]; that is, some TGD youth who discontinue social and/or medical affirmation processes view those processes as fundamentally important for informing their current gender identity and do not experience regret.[17,18] As explicated further in this review, there are a variety of external and internal factors that drive TGD youth to detransition, ranging from external societal pressures to internal gender fluidity.[19,20] As such, it is clear that detransition is a complex process and should not be inherently associated with negative gender-affirmation experiences.[14]

Current research on detransition is limited. In this review, we outline the current state of detransition literature, showcase two clinical composite case studies describing the diverse presentations of patients who elected to detransition, and highlight recommendations for psychiatrists, therapists and other healthcare providers to consider in supporting TGD youth undergoing detransition or shifts in gender expression or identity.

CURRENT LITERATURE ON TRANSITION DISCONTINUATION AND DETRANSITION

The literature regarding detransition includes many definitions of the phenomenon. Among general TGD populations, estimated rates of detransition (broadly defined) appear to range from less than 1% to 13%,[15] with high variability as a result of methodological and conceptual inconsistency. The 13% rate originates from a study of TGD adults who reported diverse histories of detransition, and the vast majority of these individuals cited at least one external factor (eg, social rejection or stigma) as a reason for their detransition. For many of these adults, detransition involved going back in the closet or discontinuing gender-affirming medical care.[21]

Differentiating Detransition and Regret

When studies looked specifically at *regret*, rather than the more variable construct of detransition, rates appear to be quite low. Within one systematic review and meta-analysis of 7928 TGD patients who underwent gender-affirming surgery, 1% experienced regret post-procedure.[22] Some researchers have posited that clinic-based studies may represent an under-estimate of regret rates due to the possibility that individuals would not return to clinics where they received treatments they later regretted. In one study of people who had detransitioned, 24% had informed their doctor or clinic of their detransition.[23] If we assume that clinic-based studies underestimate rates of regret by approximately a factor of four, then rates of regret can be estimated as under 5%. Nevertheless, literature on diverse gender trajectories is woefully lacking. Both patients and providers would clearly benefit from an increased database of methodologically robust studies. For individual mental health providers, it is vital to foster openness and flexibility in clinical spaces in order to support patients regardless of how their gender identities and desires regarding gender expression may evolve.

Prepubertal Youth and Social Transition

Literature on rates of social detransition among TGD children is especially scant. One study following 317 TGD children (mean age 8 years at start of study, with standard deviation of 2 years) found that, over a 5-year follow up period, 7.3% of youth reported changes in their gender identity, with 2.5% of youth reporting that they detransitioned and identified as cisgender thereafter.[24] In a subsequent very small qualitative study inclusive of the youth who had detransitioned (N = 8; 3 children who detransitioned did not participate), none expressed regret at the time of interview.[19] Drivers of detransition or retransition in that study highlighted the impact of social experiences, both positive (eg, meeting a nonbinary person for the first time) and negative (eg, bullying or harassment). To our knowledge, this is the only study that explores social detransition rates among TGD children to date, with only three other studies mentioning cases of children who detransition.[25–27] Other published longitudinal studies of prepubertal youth referred to gender clinics found higher rates of desistence from a *DSM-5-TR* gender-related diagnosis. These studies have been critiqued for including a large number of cisgender youth who were gender non-conforming in their gender expression but had gender identities that aligned with their sex assigned at birth.[28] Of note, prepubertal children are not candidates for any gender-affirming medical interventions under current clinical guidelines.[3,4]

Adolescents and Gender-Affirming Medical Care

TGD adolescents appear to have low rates of discontinuing gender-affirming medical interventions. With respect to pubertal suppression, studies of TGD adolescents at specialized gender clinics demonstrate treatment discontinuation rates of pubertal suppression of 1.9% to 3.5%.[29-32] In a study of 143 adolescents who had started pubertal suppression, five (3.5%) elected to stop gender-affirming medical treatment. Of these, two continued to identify as TGD, and there was no indication that any experienced regret regarding treatment.

Regarding gender-affirming hormonal therapy, one study of 862 TGD individuals receiving gender-affirming hormones through the U.S. Military Health System (MHS) found that individuals who started hormone therapy before age 18 were less likely to discontinue treatment than those who started taking hormones at age 18 or older.[33] This study also found that 25.6% of patients who were younger than 18 year old discontinued hormone treatment within 4 years of initiation. Reasons for discontinuation were unavailable due to the study's methodological design (ie, researchers utilized pharmacy records from the MHS).[33] Indeed, the study authors noted that their data may have over-estimated rates of gender-affirming hormone discontinuation as patients who chose to start obtaining gender-affirming hormones outside of MHS pharmacies (eg, pursued their health care outside of MHS) were incorrectly categorized as having discontinued treatment. In a separate longitudinal study of 55 individuals from a gender clinic in the Netherlands, none discontinued gender-affirming hormones and none expressed regret.[34] As for gender-affirming surgical procedures, one study of 209 patients aged 12 to 17 year old who received a gender-affirming chest surgery demonstrated that 2 (0.95%) expressed post-operative regret, and neither requested nor received a reversal surgery.[35]

Clinical Needs Among Those Who Detransition and Drivers of Detransition

Very few published studies have systematically assessed the needs and experiences of individuals who have detransitioned, including their reasons for detransitioning and regret (if any), as well as what factors may be associated with detransition. Furthermore, most published studies have been primarily of adult samples. The meta-analysis conducted by Bustos and colleagues demonstrated that within the 1% of TGD individuals who expressed regret after gender-affirming surgery, the most pervasive reasons for regret were psychosocial difficulties, particularly low social support and negative reactions from peers and family.[22] Several studies of adults who have detransitioned had similar findings, while also citing additional factors including shifts in gender identity or conceptualizations regarding gender identity, mental health concerns, or coming to believe one's TGD identity was the result of a mental health condition.[23,36] Of note, these latter studies of online convenience samples were not designed to evaluate the rates of detransition or regret, or various drivers of detransition. An additional non-probability study of 17,151 TGD adults in the United States showed that of the 2242 (13.1%) respondents who had reported a history of detransition, 82.5% noted that it was motivated by at least 1 external factor (eg, family pressure, societal stigma), while 15.9% noted at least 1 internal driving factor (eg, psychological challenges, fluidity in gender identity).[21]

CLINICAL CASE EXAMPLES
Case Study 1

Nina is a 9-year-old child who, at the time of first presentation, used she/her pronouns and identified as a transgender girl. She presented to her psychotherapist with symptoms consistent with gender dysphoria. Nina's parents shared that she frequently stated that she is not a boy, insisting that she be called Nina rather than Miles, her name assigned at birth. After a comprehensive clinical assessment, Nina's therapist recommended to her parents that they support her social gender exploration and stated desires to take on aspects of gender expression that matched her gender identity.

Nina chose to undergo multiple forms of social gender affirmation, including wearing more feminine clothes both at home and in public. At school, her teachers and peers were not affirming of her gender. They repeatedly referred to her as Miles and utilized he/him pronouns, despite her request that they use she/her pronouns, and sometimes bullied Nina for her feminine gender expression. Nina became extremely distressed as a result of these constant negative experiences; she decided to detransition (ie, revert to a more masculine gender expression) 3 months later, citing her mistreatment at school as the main reason.

After Nina's family moved towns, Nina began seeing a new psychotherapist with whom she discussed the range of nonbinary gender identities with which some individuals identify. She was interested to learn more about nonbinary identities and felt that she greatly resonated with this, especially the concept of being neither fully a boy nor a girl. After 4 months at her new school, she deduced that her new teachers and peers were affirming TGD people, and subsequently announced that she would like to go by Miles and use they/them pronouns. Miles's teachers, peers, and parents received this information well and quickly affirmed their nonbinary identity and expression (wearing combinations of both masculine and feminine clothes). Their mood greatly improved, and they currently report excitement at the prospect of further exploring their gender. Their parents noted that the more affirming environment has allowed gender to become a less prevalent topic in Miles' life, which allowed them to focus on other interests, including art and spending time with friends. Two years later, Miles still presents to their primary care provider as nonbinary and reports no desire for additional medical intervention. They continue to meet regularly with their therapist for psychosocial support. In particular, they focus on the ways in which Miles sometimes feels anxious or depressed when they read about stories in the news that pathologize TGD people.

Case Study 2

Alanis is an 18-year-old youth who used he/him pronouns, identified as a transgender boy on initial presentation (dating back to when he was 13), and had a history of major depressive disorder and generalized anxiety disorder. At Alanis's request and after a comprehensive clinical evaluation by his psychiatrist, therapist, and primary care provider, his interdisciplinary collaborative care team began gender-affirming hormone therapy with testosterone and closely followed him throughout the course of treatment. For 14 months after initiation, Alanis wore masculine clothing and publicly used he/him pronouns in all social contexts. He was consistently engaged in treatment with his psychotherapist who was well-versed in gender-affirming care.

After deliberate internal reflection, and after 2 years of taking gender-affirming testosterone, Alanis shared with his care team that he began to re-identify as a girl and desired to return to using she/her pronouns as well as discontinue gender-affirming hormone therapy. Alanis expressed that her participation in gender-affirming therapy was pivotal in clarifying her gender and noted that she may seek hormone therapy again sometime in the future. She shared that therapy helped her understand that gender for her is not a binary construct, that only she can know what her gender identity is, and that it might shift for some people. Alanis described this realization as liberating, and her mental health drastically improved. She expressed no decisional regret regarding her social or medical transition and little embodiment unease with respect to more permanent body changes (facial hair growth, fat redistribution). Due to reservations about the permanent deepening of her voice, she elected to seek treatment with a speech and language pathologist to work on voice feminization. Though her physicians noted there is limited literature regarding reversion of voice deepening following gender-affirming testosterone treatment, Alanis read in online forums that some individuals who stopped gender-affirming testosterone treatment after shorter time periods (around 6 months) experienced "vocal lightning" and good results following speech therapy. Her physicians informed her that, if needed in the future, surgeries might be available for voice modification, though this is not a commonly performed procedure. Her lab tests indicate normal hormonal functioning, and she remains in good physical health.

DISCUSSION

Youth are able to explore their gender identities in developmentally appropriate ways via relevant social and/or medical transition processes, which are associated with superior mental health outcomes.[5-8] However, the fact that some TGD youth detransition has been used to argue against social and/or medical transitions during childhood and adolescence.[37,38] Legislators have proposed bills broadly outlawing gender-affirming care for all minors, despite opposition from all major medical organizations.[39] The current literature on detransition showcases that for some individuals, gender trajectories are dynamic and non-linear processes, rather than binary and fixed embodiments. It is critically important for psychiatrists, therapists, and all healthcare providers to support youth with evolving paths regarding their gender identities or expressions.

Multiple studies have noted that, due to detransition being relatively uncommon among TGD people, clinicians may not be well-equipped to provide detransition-related healthcare and guidance, despite a strong need for such information among TGD individuals undergoing detransition.[15,36] Indeed, some individuals will seek additional medical interventions (ie, stopping or changing hormones, surgical reconstruction or reversals) so that they can affirm their evolving gender identity or needs regarding their gender expression. Unfortunately, lack of knowledge among clinicians regarding detransition-related care is to be expected, especially since detransition appears to be a relatively rare occurrence with no ongoing, systematic data collection. To better understand and medically support TGD youth who detransition, we recommend clinicians systematically collect psychological and physiological data, while also recognizing that it will take time to generate sufficiently powered samples to answer key questions around detransition-related care. Additional research studies with robust methodologies are needed to comprehensively understand the diverse goals and needs of TGD youth.

Interpersonally, providers may engage in open, nonjudgmental communication and destigmatize the concept of detransition or dynamic gender identities and expressions with their patients to address individuals' specific social and medical needs more effectively. The overarching goal is to help patients feel comfortable seeking care to promote their mental and physical wellbeing. These topics may be discussed openly within initial evaluations, ongoing care encounters, and/or pre-transition conversations.

For example, to facilitate the exploration of a youth's desired gender trajectory and needs, a psychiatrist may ask: "if your gender identity shifts over time, how will you feel about having a deep voice?" By asking these types of exploratory questions, mental health clinicians can provide the space for patients to express evolving gender identities or desires regarding gender expression. It is vital that we create affirming, safe, and comfortable clinical spaces for *all* patients, including the minority of TGD youth for whom significant shifts or evolution of identities occur over time. Indeed, in the study conducted by MacKinnon et al., some individuals who detransitioned noted that they stopped taking hormones "cold-turkey," or in an abrupt manner without seeking medical follow up, due to anticipated stigma or potential lack of support from their provider.[15] Though this perception from patients may be in part driven by media and societal messaging, rather than on actual interactions with providers themselves, the onus still lies largely on providers to actively combat this notion. Clinicians can communicate to their patients that they will continue to support and guide the patient through any evolving medical and social processes.

Additionally, providers ought to consider the specific needs of a youth's parents, as family support of evolving gender identity or expression desires is crucial for youth wellbeing.[19,40] In light of their TGD child detransitioning, some parents may express confusion or frustration about their child's initial gender transition.[19] Clinicians should approach parents dialectically; that is, clinicians can guide parents to *both* acknowledge challenges with supporting their child's fluid or changing gender trajectory *and* continue to love and support their child however they identify, now and in the future. Providers should also work in tandem with support groups and programs for parents of TGD youth,[41,42] as these programs can cultivate space for parents to better understand and affirm their children's dynamic gender trajectories.

As with all health care options, thorough education and informed consent are critical. Providers should explicitly highlight that all decisions in medicine involve weighing potential risks and side effects of treatment with potential benefits of treatment. For each individual youth and their family, such risks, benefits, and potential side effects ought to be discussed in detail. Part of this discussion should generally include the possibility of gender identity or desires for gender expression evolving in the future, along with a discussion of what is currently known regarding the rates of such experiences (which appear to be low among TGD youth, in the extant literature). In our clinical experience, youth and families are able to process information regarding risks, benefits, and outcome data and integrate them into their decision-making. With support from their interdisciplinary care team, youth and families are better equipped to decide what path forward is most likely to optimize an adolescent's physical and mental health. While a small percentage of individuals may ultimately experience a shift in their gender identity, expression, or medical goals, such shifts do not necessarily indicate that a patient, family, or care team made an uninformed decision or lacked medical competence.[43,44]

Moreover, providers ought to advocate for clinical guidelines that focus on how best to support TGD youth regardless of how their gender identities and hopes regarding gender expression may evolve. One study by Hastings and colleagues outlines a medical framework for pediatric gender-affirming care that centers youth who progress through non-linear gender trajectories.[45] This framework emphasizes an individualized approach to care that highlights a youth's capacity for gender "embodiment," or the fluid process by which one makes their internal gender identity visible, as an alternative to the more linear and static frame of "transition." Furthermore, Turban & Keuroghlian[17] provide a framework of factors for clinicians to consider when working with youth who detransition. This framework includes considering external factors (eg, discrimination) and internal factors (eg, healthy development trajectory), while also noting that external factors can result in internal motivations for detransition (eg, prejudice leading to internalized transphobia). In order to best support and care for youth who detransition, providers can thoughtfully incorporate these specific frameworks into their own practice.

It is of particular importance to note and address external factors that may be causing distress among adolescents. For instance, family therapy may be indicated if a young person is choosing to detransition due to an unsupportive family environment. Additionally, providers may need to prioritize working with school staff if bullying around gender identity or expression is occurring. Structural barriers such as limited access to gender-congruent government identification may also be at play.[21]

The existing detransition literature demonstrates some key insights regarding generally low detransition rates among TGD youth,[24] as well as a qualitative understanding of factors related to TGD youths' detransition.[19] However, review of the current literature also highlights important opportunities for future work. A vast majority of the literature utilizes small samples that are overwhelmingly white and based in the U.S. or Europe. As a result, the current literature is not representative of the experiences, needs, and language conventions of TGD youth of color in the U.S. nor of TGD youth in non-Western countries who detransition. Future studies should aim to recruit larger sample sizes that better represent the diverse experiences of multiply marginalized youth who detransition. Existing literature also often conflates the heterogeneous experiences that may fall broadly under the umbrella of detransition, including shifts in gender identity, regret, stopping treatment due to being satisfied with the changes that have already occurred, or stopping treatment due to harassment or stigma. Future research should be careful to include more specific definitions of reported outcomes and goals. Future studies should also focus on nuanced and comprehensive questions regarding detransition experiences, with the goal of creating more affirming care structures regardless of how gender identities and/or gender expression may evolve. Lastly, little is known about the psychological and physiological effects of certain detransition processes among TGD youth, for example, the precise effects of stopping gender-affirming hormone therapies. Future longitudinal studies should systematically examine psychological and physiological processes to better understand and medically support TGD youth who detransition.

SUMMARY

Although detransition can certainly occur for some TGD youth, rates appear to be quite low, and these experiences appear to be highly heterogeneous. Despite these low rates, clinicians should strive to ensure that clinical services adequately support all patients, regardless of how gender identities and/or expression may evolve. Additionally, providers should create space with youth to explore the nuanced interplay of physical changes induced by gender-affirming interventions and potential future shifts in their goals for gender expression. Efforts should be taken to ensure all TGD youth have positive experiences with care and are able to explore their gender embodiment hopes and express their affirmed identities. Providers can facilitate non-judgmental, open-ended discussions about the possibilities of gender identity and gender expression evolution, with or without regret, with a focus on how clinicians will be available to support young people and their families regardless of how their gender trajectory may evolve.

CLINICS CARE POINTS

- For some TGD youth, gender identities and expressions may be dynamic or non-linear.
- Some youth may decide to detransition, defined as stopping or reversing an already-initiated social and/or medical gender affirmation process.
- Clinicians should provide individualized care to TGD youth with dynamic gender identities and expressions that includes nonjudgmental discussion of embodiment goals and supportive, educational conversations about treatment approaches.

DISCLOSURE

The authors declare no conflicts of interests.

REFERENCES

1. Turban JL, Ehrensaft D. Research review: gender identity in youth: treatment paradigms and controversies. JCPP (J Child Psychol Psychiatry) 2018;59(12):1228–43.
2. Herman J.L., Flores A.R., O'Neill K.K., How Many Adults and Youth Identify as Transgender in the United States? Published online 2022. Available at: https://escholarship.org/content/qt4xs990ws/qt4xs990ws.pdf.
3. Coleman E, Radix A, Bouman W, et al. Standards of care for the health of transgender and gender diverse people, version 8. International Journal of Transgender Health 2022;23(sup1):S1–259.
4. Hembree WC, Cohen-Kettenis PT, Gooren L, et al. Endocrine treatment of gender-dysphoric/gender-incongruent persons: an endocrine society clinical practice guideline. Journal of Clinical Endocrinology & Metabolism 2017;102(11):3869–903.
5. Olson KR, Durwood L, DeMeules M, et al. Mental health of transgender children who are supported in their identities. Pediatrics 2016;137(3):e20153223.
6. Turban JL, King D, Carswell JM, et al. Pubertal suppression for transgender youth and risk of suicidal ideation. Pediatrics 2020;145(2):e20191725.
7. Tordoff DM, Wanta JW, Collin A, et al. Mental health outcomes in transgender and nonbinary youths receiving gender-affirming care. JAMA Netw Open 2022;5(2):e220978.
8. Russell ST, Pollitt AM, Li G, et al. Chosen name use is linked to reduced depressive symptoms, suicidal ideation, and suicidal behavior among transgender youth. Journal of adolescent Health 2018;63(4):503–5.
9. Reisner SL, Radix A, Deutsch MB. Integrated and gender-affirming transgender clinical care and research. J Acquir Immune Defic Syndr 2016;72(Suppl 3):S235.
10. Dolotina B, Turban JL. A multipronged, evidence-based approach to improving mental health among transgender and gender-diverse youth. JAMA Netw Open 2022;5(2):e220926.
11. Diagnostic and statistical manual of mental disorders. In: Text revision. 5th Edition. Washington, DC: American Psychiatric Association; 2022.
12. Steensma TD, Biemond R, de Boer F, et al. Desisting and persisting gender dysphoria after childhood: a qualitative follow-up study. Clin Child Psychol Psychiatr 2011;16(4):499–516.
13. Slothouber V. Narratives of De/Retransition: Disrupting the Boundaries of Gender and Time. Published online 2021. Available at: https://ir.lib.uwo.ca/etd/8070.
14. Hildebrand-Chupp R. More than 'canaries in the gender coal mine': a transfeminist approach to research on detransition. Sociol Rev 2020;68(4):800–16.
15. MacKinnon KR, Kia H, Salway T, et al. Health care experiences of patients discontinuing or reversing prior gender-affirming treatments. JAMA Netw Open 2022;5(7):e2224717.
16. Janssen A. 2.3 Understanding gender "detransition" with and without regret. Journal of the American Academy of Child & Adolescent Psychiatry 2021;60(10):S4.
17. Turban JL, Keuroghlian AS. Dynamic gender presentations: understanding transition and "de-transition" among transgender youth. J Am Acad Child Adolesc Psychiatry 2018;57(7):451–3.

18. Turban JL, Carswell J, Keuroghlian AS. Understanding pediatric patients who discontinue gender-affirming hormonal interventions. JAMA Pediatr 2018;172(10): 903–4.

19. Durwood L, Kuvalanka KA, Kahn-Samuelson S, et al. Retransitioning: the experiences of youth who socially transition genders more than once. International Journal of Transgender Health 2022;23(4):409–27.

20. Pullen Sansfaçon A, Gelly MA, Gravel R, et al. A nuanced look into youth journeys of gender transition and detransition. Infant Child Dev 2023;32(2):e2402.

21. Turban JL, Loo SS, Almazan AN, et al. Factors leading to "detransition" among transgender and gender diverse people in the United States: a mixed-methods analysis. LGBT Health 2021;8(4):273–80.

22. Bustos VP, Bustos SS, Mascaro A, et al. Regret after gender-affirmation surgery: a systematic review and meta-analysis of prevalence. Plastic and Reconstructive Surgery Global open 2021;9(3):e3477.

23. Littman L. Individuals treated for gender dysphoria with medical and/or surgical transition who subsequently detransitioned: a survey of 100 detransitioners. Arch Sex Behav 2021;50(8):3353–69.

24. Olson KR, Durwood L, Horton R, et al. Gender identity 5 years after social transition. Pediatrics 2022;150(2). e2021056082.

25. Edwards-Leeper L, Spack NP. Psychological evaluation and medical treatment of transgender youth in an interdisciplinary "Gender Management Service"(GeMS) in a major pediatric center. J Homosex 2012;59(3):321–36.

26. Menvielle E. A comprehensive program for children with gender variant behaviors and gender identity disorders. J Homosex 2012;59(3):357–68.

27. Steensma TD, McGuire JK, Kreukels BP, et al. Factors associated with desistence and persistence of childhood gender dysphoria: a quantitative follow-up study. Journal of the American Academy of Child & Adolescent Psychiatry 2013; 52(6):582–90.

28. Olson KR. Prepubescent transgender children: what we do and do not know. J Am Acad Child Adolesc Psychiatry 2016;55(3):155–6, e3.

29. De Vries AL, Steensma TD, Doreleijers TA, et al. Puberty suppression in adolescents with gender identity disorder: a prospective follow-up study. J Sex Med 2011;8(8):2276–83.

30. Carmichael P, Butler G, Masic U, et al. Short-term outcomes of pubertal suppression in a selected cohort of 12 to 15 year old young people with persistent gender dysphoria in the UK. PLoS One 2021;16(2):e0243894.

31. Brik T, Vrouenraets LJ, de Vries MC, et al. Trajectories of adolescents treated with gonadotropin-releasing hormone analogues for gender dysphoria. Arch Sex Behav 2020;49(7):2611–8.

32. Wiepjes CM, Nota NM, de Blok CJ, et al. The Amsterdam cohort of gender dysphoria study (1972–2015): trends in prevalence, treatment, and regrets. J Sex Med 2018;15(4):582–90.

33. Roberts CM, Klein DA, Adirim TA, et al. Continuation of gender-affirming hormones among transgender adolescents and adults. Journal of Clinical Endocrinology & Metabolism 2022;107(9):e3937–43.

34. De Vries AL, McGuire JK, Steensma TD, et al. Young adult psychological outcome after puberty suppression and gender reassignment. Pediatrics 2014; 134(4):696–704.

35. Tang A, Hojilla JC, Jackson JE, et al. Gender-affirming mastectomy trends and surgical outcomes in adolescents. Ann Plast Surg 2022;88(4):S325–31.

36. Vandenbussche E. Detransition-related needs and support: a cross-sectional online survey. J Homosex 2021;69(9):1602–20.
37. De Vries AL, Cohen-Kettenis PT. Clinical management of gender dysphoria in children and adolescents: the Dutch approach. J Homosex 2012;59(3):301–20.
38. O'Malley S, Garner M, Withers R, et al. The communication of evidence to inform trans youth health care. Lancet Child & Adolescent Health 2021;5(9):e32–3.
39. Turban JL, Kraschel KL, Cohen IG. Legislation to criminalize gender-affirming medical care for transgender youth. JAMA 2021;325(22):2251–2.
40. Ashley F. Puberty blockers are necessary, but they don't prevent homelessness: caring for transgender youth by supporting unsupportive parents. Am J Bioeth 2019;19(2):87–9.
41. Matsuno E, Israel T. The parent support program: development and acceptability of an online intervention aimed at increasing supportive behaviors among parents of trans youth. J GLBT Fam Stud 2021;17(5):413–31.
42. Kidd KM, Sequeira GM, Thornburgh C, et al. 56."A lifeline for parents and their children": 1: 1 peer mentoring for parents of gender diverse youth. J Adolesc Health 2022;70(4):S30.
43. MacKinnon KR, Ashley F, Kia H, et al. Preventing transition "regret": an institutional ethnography of gender-affirming medical care assessment practices in Canada. Soc Sci Med 2021;291:114477.
44. Ashley F. Adolescent medical transition is ethical: an analogy with reproductive health. Kennedy Inst Ethics J 2022;32(2):127–71.
45. Hastings J, Bobb C, Wolfe M, et al. Medical care for nonbinary youth: individualized gender care beyond a binary framework. Pediatr Ann 2021;50(9). https://doi.org/10.3928/19382359-20210818-03.

Supporting Transgender Youth Across Psychosocial Systems

Brandon Johnson, MD[a],*, Nathalie Szilagyi, MD[b,c,1]

KEYWORDS

- Transgender • Minority stress • Supportive schools • Safe spaces • Religion
- Rural communities

KEY POINTS

- Stigma, marginalization, and victimization contribute to worse health outcomes in transgender youth, consistent with the Minority Stress Model.
- Access to affirming spaces, people, and organizations can bolster resilience and lead to better health outcomes for transgender youth.
- Harnessing supports in environments such as schools, community organizations, religious groups, and rural communities can promote healthy development in transgender youth.

INTRODUCTION

Transgender children and adolescents are at an elevated risk for negative mental health outcomes, as multiple studies have shown higher rates of depression, anxiety, and suicidality in this vulnerable population.[1-3] However, research suggests that diverse gender identities themselves are not pathological and would not be categorized as a mental illness. While incongruence between one's gender identity (a person's own internal sense of their gender) and external, physical characteristics can cause distress, external factors such as stigma and discrimination appear to have more significant negative effects.[4,5]

One framework through which to understand this is the Minority Stress Model, which posits that social factors that create a chronically hostile and stressful social environment can lead to elevated rates of psychological distress as well as poor mental and physical health outcomes for individuals in oppressed minority groups. For example,

[a] Department of Psychiatry, Icahn School of Medicine at Mount Sinai, 1090 Amsterdam Avenue 16th Floor, New York, NY 10025, USA; [b] Yale Child Study Center, Yale School of Medicine, New Haven, CT, USA; [c] Aurora Psychiatric Associates, Greenwich, CT, USA
[1] Present address: 120 Greenwich Avenue, Greenwich, CT 06830.
* Corresponding author.
E-mail address: Brandon.johnson2@mountsinai.org

Child Adolesc Psychiatric Clin N Am 32 (2023) 815–837
https://doi.org/10.1016/j.chc.2023.05.003
1056-4993/23/© 2023 Elsevier Inc. All rights reserved.

exposure to stigma in religious beliefs or political policies that are non-affirming or even frankly rejecting transgender identities would be considered *distal* stress factors for transgender individuals. These factors could contribute to and amplify the additional external stressors of gender-based discrimination and victimization.

Such external stressors may then increase subjectively processed, internally experienced stresses such as internalized transphobia, negative expectations, and the belief in the need to conceal transgender identities (*proximal* factors). Combined, these stress factors can have detrimental effects on the mental and physical health of transgender people, with increased risk for depression, suicidality, and substance abuse, among other negative outcomes.[6–8] Notably, the Gender Minority Stress and Resilience Model proposed by Testa, Hendricks, and others also include *resilience* factors, which are external supports that can mitigate the negative effects of stress factors and have powerful positive effects on mental and physical health outcomes. They highlighted community connectedness and pride (in one's gender identity) as significant resilience factors.

In this article, we will briefly review some stressors commonly faced by transgender children and adolescents. More importantly, we will provide an overview of supports across domains that can help increase resilience and promote positive outcomes. While the data specifically focusing on transgender youth is expanding, many studies combine sexual and gender minorities together by looking at the LGBTQ community as a whole. This article will specify which populations various studies refer to, including when they are specific to transgender youth.

SUPPORTING TRANSGENDER YOUTH IN SCHOOLS
School Vulnerabilities for Transgender Youth

Schools play a vital role in the development of children and adolescents. The amount of time that youth spend in school settings can provide both significant threats as well as opportunities to the healthy development and well-being of transgender youth. Negative school climates have been shown to contribute to both academic and health disparities among LGBTQ youth.[9] Victimization in schools can even have lasting effects on gender-diverse youth through poorer psychosocial adjustment into young adulthood.[10]

Threats to health and academic progress can come from adults and peers alike in the school setting. Stigmatizing school policies such as limiting gender expression, lack of access to gender-affirming facilities or activities, and lack of protection against bullying and harassment contribute to negative school climates for transgender youth. School staff may act on conscious or unconscious bias, censor classroom content related to gender identity, or even participate directly in the harassment of transgender youth. Indeed, many schools and communities are actively trying to limit transgender youths' access to affirming spaces in schools, school sports, or even health care by supporting discriminatory legislation. Disturbingly, transgender youth with a lack of access to gender-affirming restrooms and locker rooms report a higher incidence of experiencing sexual assault.[11]

Transgender youth experience higher rates of victimization by peers in school settings compared with their cisgender peers.[9,12] Bullying of LGBTQ youth can take on many forms: verbal, relational, physical, cyber, and destruction of property. There are many negative implications of peer victimization based on gender identity, such as school truancy, risky sexual behaviors, and poor physical and mental health outcomes.[13] Absence from school due to mistreatment can have a ripple effect as transgender students lose access to a safe educational space. The mistreatment itself as well as its sequelae can perpetuate school absence. For example, in a large sample of adolescents from California, transgender youth reported school truancy for multiple reasons: safety concerns, symptoms of depression, and substance use.[14] Transgender youth experiencing bullying and school absenteeism also report a negative view of school connectedness, thereby diminishing the positive impact that educational settings can have on youth and potentially impacting future educational trajectories.[15]

Characteristics of Supportive Schools

Despite the existence of significant vulnerability factors for transgender youth in schools, there are many initiatives in schools designed to protect and support transgender youth. School connectedness is defined as a meaningful engagement in school activities and the development of caring relationships at school.[16] It is associated with higher academic achievement[17] as well as decreased suicidal ideation in LGBT youth.[18] In this section, we discuss qualities of supportive schools that can promote school connectedness in transgender youth and thereby promote improved outcomes.

Gender and Sexuality Alliances

Gender and Sexuality Alliances (GSAs) are extracurricular clubs in schools meant to provide a safe space for LGBTQ youth. They are made up of staff or teachers as advisors and a contingent of LGBTQ youth and allies. GSAs engage in various affirming activities such as creating an LGBTQ social network, educating on LGBTQ-related topics, providing emotional support, and working to create a more affirming school environment. GSAs have grown in prevalence over the last decades, with nearly 62% of schools having a GSA in 2019 compared to only about a third in 2001.[19] Data consistently shows that GSAs positively impact the school experience of LGBTQ youth and can mitigate some of the risks of a hostile school climate.[20] Notably, rates of victimization of LGBTQ youth were found to be lower in schools with a GSA.[21]

Additionally, participation in a GSA is associated with higher connectedness to the school community among LGBTQ students.[19] The benefits of GSAs may even continue beyond high school, as one study found LGBTQ young adults who had participated in GSAs were more likely to obtain a college education.[22] The 1984 Federal Equal Access Act prevents schools that accept federal funding from discriminating against student groups. As a result, the right to assemble a GSA has been upheld in multiple court cases where GSA assembly was initially denied by various school districts in the United States.[23,24]

Inclusive School Curricula

The presence of school curricula that address transgender students' identities and needs also contributes to a supportive school environment. For instance, inclusive sexual education curricula were associated with decreased suicidal ideation in LGBTQ youth.[25] Conversely, inaccurate or non-inclusive sexual education programs in schools can have negative consequences for transgender youth, given their unique experiences and needs that are not generally covered in traditional sexual education programs. Several content areas are important for transgender-inclusive sex education: puberty-related gender dysphoria, non-medical gender-affirming interventions, medical gender-affirming interventions, consent and relationships, sex and desire, sexually transmitted infection prevention, fertility and contraception, and health care access.[26] The inclusion of these topics promotes safety as well as improved mental and physical health in transgender youth.

Beyond the sexual health curriculum, the mere visibility of gender-diverse identities as early as the elementary school may provide an opportunity for children to normalize transgender identities. The absence of such a curriculum can reinforce gender stereotypes that have been linked to gender-related harassment and bullying. Some organizations have proposed and cultivated gender-inclusive classroom curricula targeted at different ages and developmental levels.[27] Qualitative studies have shown that exposing children to gender diversity in elementary school allows them to challenge gender norms and develop a more flexible framework for gender in general.[28] Supportive educators and inclusive curricula were associated with decreased victimization in schools in a national study of transgender students in the United States.[29] Furthermore, transgender students from schools with inclusive curricula were found to have higher grade point averages and were more likely to pursue higher education.[30]

Inclusive School Policies

Creating a safe school environment for transgender youth protects against school-related traumas and absenteeism. There are many ways schools can create this safe environment for their gender-diverse students. Official transgender and gender-diverse student policies decrease the rates of gender-based discrimination against transgender students. Comprehensive policies are noted to be more effective in enhancing transgender students' sense of safety and school connectedness.[20] Such school policies include the use of affirmed names and pronouns, access to gender-affirming or gender-neutral bathrooms, the ability to change one's name on official school documents, and participation in affirming gendered extracurricular activities.[30] Referring to students by their "chosen" name in as many contexts as possible, including school, is associated with decreased rates of depression, suicidal ideation, and suicidal behavior.[31] Generally speaking, sports participation in schools is associated with higher self-esteem, lower depression, and greater school belonging. The lack of inclusive and comfortable environments has been identified as a barrier to transgender youth participation in school sports.[32] Notably, less than 5% of schools have specific inclusive policies that allow transgender students to participate in sports teams that align with their gender identity. Protective policies, approachable teachers and coaches, and safe locker rooms are associated with higher participation in school sports for transgender students, thereby providing them access to the potential benefits of such participation.[33]

Policies aimed to protect transgender youth against bullying and harassment have proliferated across the United States. Enumerated protection against bullying based on sexual orientation and gender identity has been found to protect these students more effectively than anti-bullying policies without such enumeration. Teachers need to be equipped to help support transgender youth when they observe these behaviors in schools. GLSEN found that teachers who received in-service education on LGBT student issues reported intervening more when they heard biased remarks and were more likely to engage in LGBT-supportive practices. In this research, it was found that inclusive policies that enumerate protection against sexual and gender-based harassment allowed teachers to identify and intervene in supporting LGBT students more readily. Importantly, rates of victimization and absenteeism were found to be lower for transgender students in schools with comprehensive policies against bullying and harassment based on gender identity.[29]

Role of School Mental Health Professionals

School mental health professionals (SMHPs) can play a vital role in supporting transgender students. SMHPs with LGBTQ-specific training in graduate school, along with professional development in working with LGBTQ youth, expressed greater comfort in working with and advocating for transgender youth. These SMHPs supported LGBTQ youth in diverse ways, including providing individual and group counseling, advocating for inclusive school policy, training staff on LGBTQ issues, and promoting inclusion in the curriculum. An SMHP may also be the best-equipped adult in the school to provide referrals to community health resources applicable to transgender youth. Linking these students to appropriate sexual and reproductive health care, mental health care, and gender specialists can further meet their needs and bridge the gap between supports available inside and outside the school setting.[34]

Advocating in School Settings

It is imperative that clinicians and parents understand the resources available to transgender youth in schools. Helping these students connect to affirming adults and spaces in their schools can reduce risk and promote school connectedness. While not all schools are equal in their support, protection, and affirmation of transgender youth, knowing what resources have been shown to be effective can help clinicians and parents advocate for these resources if they do not exist in a particular school setting. Federal, state, and local laws may impact what affirming supports and resources are available in local schools, so understanding the legal landscape is often a useful first step. While all schools have some version of anti-bullying policies, they may not be effective in protecting transgender youth specifically. Clinicians and parents may need to advocate with school leadership when policies are not effectively protecting transgender youth from bullying and harassment. Utilization of resources from many of the organizations discussed above[35-37] may help this advocacy by highlighting the negative outcomes associated with school victimization as well as describing policies that can create a safer and more affirming school environment for all students.

SUPPORTING TRANSGENDER YOUTH IN COMMUNITIES

Community supports for transgender youth form an important scaffold that provides safe spaces, access to resources, and opportunities to commune with other transgender youth and allies. The resources available in individual communities vary widely and are often influenced by community demographics such as region, size, political climate, degree and type of religious affiliations, and visibility of LGBT individuals and families, among others. Due to the heterogeneity of available resources among communities, various organizations have collated national, state, and local resources available to transgender youth and their families.[35-37] Lack of resources and a discriminatory environment can conversely have a deleterious effect on transgender youth. Data suggests that campaigns supporting discriminatory laws against sexual and gender minority individuals may lead to increased rates of harassment for these minorities in addition to the psychological burden of being in an openly marginalized group.[38]

Safe Spaces and Events

Affirming spaces where transgender youth are able to congregate can have a positive impact on their mental health and identity development. Community centers for sexual and gender minority youth exist in cities across the United States and provide a vast array of needed support. In a survey of transgender youth, community centers were noted to meet their needs in many domains. For instance, community centers can provide services such as lists of medical providers, shelters, transitional living programs, and employment support to meet the basic needs of transgender youth. They often promote mental health through the delivery of individual, group, and family counseling. School advocacy is another service that these centers may provide to promote safety in schools and equitable access to facilities. Conferences, workshops, and social spaces were also found to be valuable contributions to community centers, according to transgender youth.[39]

Pride festivals across the world offer opportunities for LGBTQ individuals to come together to foster community, resilience, and visibility. While many pride activities are tailored to LGBTQ adults, pride events that are geared toward youth can provide a safe space for transgender youth to build community. Specific youth-targeted pride festivals have been shown to reduce barriers to attendance at pride activities for LGBTQ youth.[40] Other targeted opportunities to commune can fill in the gaps when community resources, in general, are sparse. For instance, a transgender youth who attended an LGBTQ camp in the Midwest shared that the camp provided a vital social opportunity that they could not find elsewhere, thereby promoting resilience and a positive outlook toward the future.[41]

Symbols of support in the community can contribute to feelings of connectedness and safety among transgender youth. Depictions of the rainbow pride flag, for instance, have been shown to foster a sense of identity and community among transgender youth. Neighborhoods, businesses, or schools that display these symbols can signify that transgender youth are welcome and can express themselves authentically in those spaces. These symbols have also been associated with positive feelings and memories, which can promote individual well-being. Rainbows and other affirming symbols may also direct youth to resources and safe people in the community.[42]

Online Supports

Transgender youth often turn to online spaces in order to research their identity, seek out transgender health care, and find other transgender individuals. Social support online may be especially useful to transgender youth who lack those support in their physical communities. In a survey conducted by GLSEN, LGBT youth spent 45 minutes more per day online than their non-LGBT peers. LGBT youth identified as having more online friends and feeling more supported by those friends than non-LGBT respondents. At least half of the youth reported using online resources in the absence of support in their own community, like close LGBT friends or GSAs. Online spaces can also provide a safe space for transgender youth to come out, highlighted by the fact that many LGBT youth identified as being more out online than in person.[43]

Online communities also offer a space for transgender youth to participate in civic engagement. Two-thirds of LGBT youth reported participating in an online community that supports a cause or issue. These youth are also more likely to utilize online forums to plan and recruit for in-person civic events. LGBT youth participation in such online civic activities was found to be twice that of their non-LGBT peers, highlighting that minority youth value these online communities as a way of connecting with other like-minded individuals to promote change.[43]

Family Supports

The data are clear that having a supportive family member protects against negative mental health outcomes associated with stigma and oppression.[12,44] Parents of transgender youth may look for community resources to help them understand and support their transgender child. One study found that parents of transgender youth show a strong interest in joining support groups as they can help parents navigate school systems and learn about local resources.[45] Organizations such as PFLAG provide support groups and resources for parents and families of transgender youth. The needs of these families can be somewhat different than those of families with LGB children.[46] Having groups specifically designed for families of transgender children to come together may provide additional benefits compared to broader LGBT groups.

The Family Acceptance Project (FAP) has created educational materials for the parents and families of LGBTQ youth, emphasizing the important role of families in helping sexual and gender minority youth to thrive. The FAP approach focuses on shared values such as love, family connections, and wanting their offspring to live a healthy, happy life. Educational materials list simple actions families can take, such as using preferred names and pronouns, which can have measurable effects on the mental and physical health of transgender youth.[44]

Access to Affirming Health Care

Access to affirming medical care is paramount for transgender youth. Lack of competent professionals and uncoordinated care have been identified by transgender youth and their caregivers as two of the barriers to accessing gender-affirming medical treatment.[47] Additionally, data suggest that transgender youth report poorer health and access health care at lower rates than their cisgender peers. Past negative experiences with the health care system often drive this population's lower utilization of resources.[48] Transgender adolescents have suggested that better LGBTQ training for health care professionals and the use of correct pronouns in the office would increase their use of these services.[49] There are many interventions to make health care spaces and experiences more affirming, such as displaying affirming symbols in the space, providing training on working with LGBTQ youth, and utilizing registration forms that are gender inclusive. Together with expanding the number of health care professionals competent in working with transgender youth, these interventions may support better health care utilization and outcomes in this population.

SUPPORTING TRANSGENDER YOUTH IN RELIGIOUS INSTITUTIONS
Role of Religion and Spirituality

Religion and spirituality hold an important role in human experience across time, geography, ethnicity, and culture. For many people, religious or spiritual beliefs can provide a framework to find meaning and purpose, a means to cope with stressors, and a source of hope for the future.[50–52] Across the United States, religion is an integral component in individual and community life: in a 2021 Pew Research Center survey, approximately 70% of Americans reported religious affiliation, with those identifying as Christian making up the largest group at 63% of survey respondents.[53] Of note, more than 45% of LGBT adults also identified as Christian.[54] Finally, many Americans who don't participate in religious institutions still endorse spiritual beliefs and practices: in a separate survey of American adults in 2017, 27% of respondents reported that they think of themselves as spiritual but not religious.[55]

For the general population, multiple studies have suggested that religion, spirituality, and engagement in religious activities can protect mental and physical health. And for many marginalized groups, such as people of color, those from lower socioeconomic status, or those living in rural areas, religious beliefs, and affiliation can serve as a source of identity and resilience, as well as provide opportunities for support and community.[50,51,56,57]

Unfortunately, for LGBT individuals, the evidence suggests that religious affiliation can have variable effects, with both positive and negative mental and physical health outcomes reported.[50,52,56,58,59] Many religious institutions and traditions have a history of heteronormative and cisnormative beliefs, with some going as far as teaching that LGB sexuality and transgender identities are "unnatural," immoral, or pathological.[56,60–63] Although there has been some moderation of such beliefs among more liberal or progressive branches of Christianity, Judaism, and Islam over the past 50 years, many contemporary religious institutions continue to teach theological beliefs condemning sexualities and gender identities outside of heterosexual and cisgender norms.

Religious rejection of LGB sexuality and transgender identities is widely discussed in public media and discourse, familiar to the point of being considered common knowledge in the general population and among sexual and gender minorities.[50,56] Large percentages of LGBT adults surveyed described experiencing some religious traditions as non-affirming (or "unfriendly") to LGBT people, ranging from 44% who found mainline Protestant denominations non-affirming to 84% who reported finding Muslim religious traditions non-affirming.[64]

Research around the specific effects of religious affiliation and engagement in transgender children and adolescents is unfortunately limited. However, research about the experiences of LGBT individuals across age groups appears to support these models: rejecting or non-affirming religious experiences were generally associated with negative outcomes. Dahl and Galliher found that transgender adolescents and young adults who were raised in conservative Christian religious traditions reported experiencing religious-related guilt and feelings of inadequacy suggestive of internalized transphobia, as well as depressive symptoms and suicidal ideation.[50] In a 2006 study exploring the mental health experiences of transgender adolescents and young adults, Grossman and D'Augelli reported that some transgender youth themselves made a connection between being raised in conservative Christian religious environments with rigid gender roles and expectations and increased risk for self-harm or even suicide.[65,66] Multiple studies on efforts to change a youth's gender identity or sexual orientation - sometimes called "conversion therapy" - have shown such efforts to be both ineffective and harmful. Adolescents exposed to "conversion" attempts often experience increased psychological distress and other negative mental health outcomes, including increased suicidal ideation. Of note, many religious institutions describe gender identity as a behavioral or lifestyle choice and actively attempt to persuade transgender youth to change it, though they may not use the term "conversion therapy."[67,68]

In contrast, affiliation or engagement with affirming religious institutions has been linked to decreased internalized transphobia and negative expectations, with resultant improvement in mental and physical health outcomes. Grossman and colleagues found that among transgender and gender-diverse youth who reported having a religion themselves - that is, of their own choosing - religious service attendance was associated with lower suicidal ideation and fewer suicide attempts, which was consistent across racial and ethnic groups.[66] Additional studies of transgender and gender-diverse youth and adults found that many reported experiencing religion and spirituality to be sources of resilience in the context of discrimination, adversity, and trauma. And even some transgender adolescents and young adults who reported leaving the conservative, non-affirming religious institutions in which they had been raised spoke positively of some of the general values learned there, such as a commitment to justice or service to others.[50]

In summary, religious institutions can serve as powerful influences for transgender children and adolescents, with both the risk of increasing external stress factors such as gender-related discrimination, rejection, and non-affirmation and the opportunity to strengthen resilience by providing identity affirmation and a sense of community connectedness.

Increasing Affirmation Within Religious Institutions

Finding affirming faith communities

Fortunately, there are many opportunities for transgender youth to establish religious affiliations in institutions where diverse sexualities, gender identities, and expressions are embraced, and leaders intentionally support the spiritual and psychological needs of LGBTQ congregants.[56,69] In spite of the fact that many conservative religious institutions continue to espouse non-affirming beliefs and policies, there are others that are openly affirming LGBT people. Many progressive Christian denominations, such as the United Church of Christ, the Episcopal Church in America, and Metropolitan Community Churches, have moved away from heteronormative and cis-normative theologies in favor of more affirming teachings about gender and sexuality.[56,61,70] LGBT people are officially welcomed as members and invited equally to serve in leadership roles in these churches, though, in practice, local congregations can vary substantially.

In addition, separate gender- and sexuality-affirming organizations have been created in almost every faith tradition, though often unsanctioned by formal religious bodies. These include *Dignity* for Catholics, *Eshel* for people from Orthodox Jewish traditions, and *Affirmation* for Mormons (Latter Day Saints), among many others. Extensive lists of these affirming groups, as well as summaries of formal, institutional teachings on LGBTQ issues by different religions and denominations, can be found online at the Human Rights Campaign (HRC) website (Appendix 1).[71] Of note, membership in a church or other religious institution does not always mean that an individual's personal beliefs uniformly align with the teachings of their church or religious institution. For example, while Catholic Church tradition and teaching prohibit gay or lesbian sexual relationships, 67% of Catholics surveyed personally supported same-sex marriage.[72] The beliefs and attitudes of local congregations may vary considerably from national church dogma and policy. Additionally, there is evidence that some Christians in churches that don't identify as liberal or progressive theologically may be open to more accepting or inclusive beliefs around LGBTQ individuals within the context of their current religious beliefs.[61] Such variations may make individual houses of worship more or less affirming and could perhaps help explain the ongoing affiliation of many LGBT people with officially non-affirming religious institutions.

For many people, religious affiliation can provide emotional and spiritual support and a sense of community and belonging, which may explain some of its established benefits for psychological well-being. And as above, religious institutions often play prominent roles for otherwise marginalized populations, such as those in Black, immigrant, or rural communities. It would be too facile - and culturally insensitive - to simply advise transgender youth and their families to switch houses of worship or stop engaging with religious practice entirely. Additionally, some research suggests that the abrupt severing of religious affiliation carries a risk of deleterious effects on psychological well-being.[50,56,73]

Mental health providers working with transgender youth can provide a safe, therapeutic space and opportunities to explore complex issues around identity, religious and spiritual beliefs, and the role of their religious affiliation in their lives. For some youth, the impact of gender-based rejection by their congregation may outweigh the resilience factors it provides, making a move out of the congregation appropriate and protective. For those youth, providers can offer emotional support, information about more affirming religious communities, and referrals to other faith-based organizations, such as those listed above (see Appendix 1).

However, some transgender youth may find moving away from long-established religious affiliations infeasible or overwhelming in the context of family and community relationships. For example, many people living in small towns or rural areas lack access to more affirming congregations or many other religious institutions at all. Parents already struggling to accept an adolescent's transgender identity or gender-diverse gender expression may experience a youth's wish to leave their religious congregation as a broader rejection of the family's beliefs and culture. Because religious institutions can serve as important sources of support for parents during a child or adolescent's social transition, parents may experience the move to a different institution as a significant source of stress and loss.[74,75]

In such cases, it would make sense to explore other options. For example, it might be possible to find affirming adults or groups within an otherwise rejecting congregation, such as by joining a religious education class, specific service activity, or youth group for adolescents. Likewise, avoiding or minimizing participation in some aspects of congregational life may decrease a transgender youth's exposure to transphobic comments and discrimination, much like avoiding participation on sports teams led by biased and hostile coaches. Joining activities such as religious youth groups or community service projects at *other,* more affirming, local religious institutions while still maintaining affiliation at the original congregation could also help transgender youth optimize resilience factors in a challenging situation. Similarly, if transportation and other family resources permit, traveling to affirming religious institutions or activities outside the youth and family's community, such as attending Pride events or LGBTQ-focused religious youth groups, could introduce additional community connections and pride. If there's a nearby article of PFLAG, an organization for the parents and families of LGBTQ individuals, local members may be able to share information about trans-friendly organizations and activities in the area.

Online resources can supplement local or in-person religious engagement with other gender-affirming resources or provide information about alternatives. In addition to the resources mentioned above, many other organizations maintain lists of faith-based resources for affirming interfaith or nondenominational organizations, which may be helpful for trans youth and families.

Educating individuals, families, and congregations
As noted above, many religiously affiliated people may be open to learning more about gender and sexuality and would be willing to consider more inclusive and affirming ideas within the context of their current religious beliefs. Educating members of religious congregations can have a real impact on their attitudes and behaviors toward transgender youth. Unfortunately, people belonging to very conservative or fundamentalist Christian congregations appear less likely to be open to new ideas around gender and sexuality than those belonging to more progressive congregations.[61]

The FAP model described above promotes values consistent with the belief systems of most religious institutions. Of note, the FAP approach does NOT include trying to change religious beliefs or moral values, making it likely to be more palatable for even adherents to conservative religious traditions.[44] In addition, FAP information created by and for members of the Latter Day Saints (Mormon) church uses language reflecting the emphasis the LDS church places on families and eternity.[44] Similar approaches to helping members of other religious groups reframe their understanding of issues around gender and sexuality within the context of their own religious beliefs have been proposed, and a variety of resources focusing on different religious traditions is available in print and online. Simply providing a list of reliable resources to religious leaders and communities may be a helpful start. However, cautious evaluation of websites or organizations listed online is essential, as many anti-transgender groups and otherwise harmful information sources exist, and some may superficially masquerade as affirming.

Responsibility for educating others should not be placed on transgender youth and families. Surveys of Christian congregants and pastors have suggested an openness to learning more about transgender issues and an interest in better serving transgender congregants, with pastors especially interested in in-person programs involving knowledgeable speakers.[61] Many LGBTQ-friendly organizations have volunteer speakers willing to address community and religious groups, including those listed above. In addition, child and adolescent psychiatrists and other mental health and medical providers who work with gender-diverse youth can serve as an important source of information.

SUPPORTING TRANSGENDER YOUTH IN RURAL SETTINGS

According to U.S. Census Bureau data, approximately 20% of the U.S. population resides in rural areas, accounting for about 61 million people nationwide.[76,77] While many stereotypes persist about rural communities and their residents in popular culture, the reality is far more complex and heterogeneous, reflecting unique combinations of community strengths and challenges. However, there are some characteristics common to many rural areas which can have an impact on the lived experience of transgender youth and their families.

Rural areas are more likely to be majority politically conservative, with fewer anti-discrimination laws and policies protecting the rights of LGBTQ individuals. Unfortunately, politically conservative states are more likely to enact blatant anti-trans laws. For example, most of the 25 U.S. states currently considering or have recently enacted legislation to ban gender-affirming care for transgender youth have maintained predominantly conservative voting patterns over the past two decades.[78,79] Surveys of people living in rural areas also reveal high rates of Christian religious affiliation and religiosity, with conservative Christian denominations representing a larger presence, especially in the South.[64,78] Perhaps not surprisingly, affiliation with more conservative religious traditions has been associated with decreased support for diverse gender identities and anti-discrimination laws.[61,80]

In multiple studies, transgender people residing in rural settings have described feeling isolated within heteronormative and cis-normative communities and experiencing significant social stigma and discrimination, with low perceived levels of community support.[81-84] Some studies suggest that transgender youth and adults in rural regions of the U.S. and Canada have higher rates of concealment of their gender identity, with some citing concerns about the risks of standing out as gender diverse in small, tight-knit communities.[78,84,85] These concerns appear to be well-founded, as research revealed that in a Midwestern state, transgender adolescents in rural high schools experienced significantly higher levels of gender-based physical bullying victimization and harassment than their urban or suburban peers. Additionally, transgender students in rural schools across the U.S. described school as an unsafe environment due to not blending in with traditional (cisgender) norms expected in the community.[84,86,87] Perhaps most dire is the increased rates of physical aggression and assault experienced by transgender youth and adults in rural areas: multiple nationwide studies confirm that transgender people in rural areas are exposed to physical aggression and sexual assault at much higher rates than cisgender peers, with transgender people of color at highest risk.[78,81,84]

As mentioned above, schools and religious institutions often play a central role in rural community life, made all the more important by the relative dearth of other community resources. There is a lower prevalence of LGBT-focused or gender-affirming programs for transgender children and adolescents in rural areas than in urban or suburban settings. Geographic isolation and transportation issues can be especially impactful in rural areas: younger children and adolescents depend on adults for transportation, and although older adolescents may be able to drive, they often lack access to vehicles or the financial means to pay for fuel.[78,87–89]

This combination of factors is entirely consistent with the Minority Stress Model: rural areas' social and cultural environment can be anti-transgender, hostile, and rejecting. Transgender children and adolescents internalize transphobia, with self-loathing, belief in the need for concealment, and low expectations for the future. Isolation and the lack of transgender visibility or role models can prevent the development of gender-related community connection and pride. These, unfortunately, could be expected to lead to worse mental and physical health outcomes for transgender youth - which is exactly what the research shows. Transgender adolescents in rural areas have markedly elevated rates of depression and anxiety, as well as non-suicidal self-directed violence and suicide attempts.[81,84,86,89]

People living in rural areas often cite the strong sense of community and interconnectedness with neighbors as an important strength. In communities with small populations, overlap between contexts may be inevitable. For example, youth may encounter peers, family, and other community members at school, sports leagues, church, jobs, and public settings such as gas stations or grocery stores. Thus confidentiality is a real concern. Revealing one's transgender identity to others ("coming out") in rural areas often does not occur in isolation and can have what some sources describe as a "ripple effect."[78,82,86,90]

Some of the most striking challenges for transgender youth in rural settings occur in health care. Unfortunately, people living in rural communities experience significant health disparities compared to those living in other geographic locations, including higher rates of tobacco use, obesity, diabetes, substance abuse, and suicide.[77,91] Longstanding health care provider shortages in rural areas have led to inadequate medical and mental health care access, with psychiatric services for children and adolescents especially hard hit. Per 2022 data from the American Medical Association and AACAP, forty-two of fifty states were considered to have a severe shortage of child and adolescent psychiatrists, and many rural counties lack child and adolescent psychiatrists entirely.[92,93]

For transgender children and adolescents, access to health care is crucially important. In addition to the routine care all children and adolescents need, transgender youth have a higher risk for mental health issues, as previously described. It is important to remember that transgender children and adolescents also need access to Gender-Affirming Care (GAC), which is the evidence-based standard of care for the treatment of Gender Dysphoria. Strong and consistent evidence shows that GAC improves mental health outcomes for transgender children and adolescents - and that denial of care for transgender youth with intense and persistent Gender Dysphoria leads to increased psychological distress and worse mental health outcomes.[67,94–96] Although the number of specialty gender clinics providing GAC in the U.S. has increased substantially over the past two decades, that increase has largely been limited to urban or suburban locations; there are few specialty gender clinics in rural areas.[97]

The ongoing shortage of health care providers in rural areas thus includes primary care physicians, psychiatrists and other mental health providers, and other medical specialists. Practically speaking, this creates barriers to access, such as having to travel farther for even primary care and having fewer choices, even when providers are available.[78,81,88] Multiple studies suggest that rural providers don't always have sufficient training and education, familiarity, or comfort with sexual and gender minorities. Many transgender youth and adults have reported experiencing bias, discrimination, mistreatment, and even refusal of care from medical providers.[90] In rural settings especially, this can lead to the expectation of future discrimination and negative treatment, avoidance of care, and suboptimal health outcomes. Likewise, confidentiality is a major concern for sexual and gender minority youth and adults in rural settings, and many have described reluctance to disclose information about their sexuality or gender identity to providers who may see multiple family and community members and overlap across settings within a small community. Rural transgender youth have expressed discomfort with other aspects of the rural health care setting, such as hetero- and cis-normative intake forms, educational brochures, and non-affirming office staff. Finally, many rural transgender individuals have reported religion-based rejection and discrimination from providers - again, not unreasonably, given studies that show an inverse relationship between health care providers' level of (conservative) religiosity and acceptance of transgender people and identities.[65,81,84]

Using Strengths and Resources in Rural Communities

Although there may be fewer community resources in rural settings, the resources that are available may have the potential to make a bigger impact. The same interconnectedness of rural residents and overlap of relationships across contexts - the "ripple effect" - that can make coming out challenging for transgender youth can also have positive effects. For example, a supportive and affirming teacher at school may also be a neighbor, the parent of classmates at school, the coach of a community sports team, and a member of a local church - with the potential to extend individual support across contexts and influence others to follow their example. And in the absence of bureaucratic structures more common in urban or suburban areas, leaders of small, locally-run institutions may have the flexibility to enact affirming changes relatively quickly.

In some small school districts, teachers, administrators, and staff get to know their students well and have the opportunity and flexibility to make adjustments to improve school climate and safety for transgender students. Family members of transgender children and adolescents who accept and affirm their offspring in communities that include multiple extended family members can likewise have a big impact that extends far beyond their immediate family.

Rural communities with predominantly conservative religious or political populations often include individuals and groups with diverse beliefs or perspectives. For example, many predominantly Republican rural counties still have a local Democratic Party organization, though it may be much smaller. Surveys of rural residents suggest that rural people of color, women, and younger rural residents support LGB and trans-affirming policies more than others. And it is important to remember that many transgender adults reside in rural areas; in fact, CDC data suggests that more than 50% of transgender adults reside in majority-rural states - though, as above, not all may have revealed their gender identity to other members of their communities.[12,78,98]

Within rural communities, finding LGBT role models and openly affirming allies can have an enormous impact on the resilience of transgender children and adolescents by countering some of the anti-trans bias they may encounter otherwise and helping them to develop stronger community connections. Creating LGBT-affirming programs and groups within existing community institutions, such as libraries, schools, churches, and community organizations such as YMCA or 4H clubs, can also foster resilience via an improved sense of belonging and pride in identity.

Mental health and medical providers are often respected and influential figures in rural communities, so providing better education and training to providers about gender and sexuality issues, as well as the medical and mental health needs of transgender youth and their families, could have an enormous impact. Surveys of primary care providers have shown an interest and willingness to learn more and provide better care for transgender patients.[49,85] Studies have shown that actions that health care providers could easily do, such as simply using a transgender youth's preferred name and pronouns, can improve mental health outcomes, including decreasing the risk of suicide attempts.[31] Likewise, a 2019 survey by The Trevor Project found that youth with at least one accepting adult were 40% less likely to report a suicide attempt in the past year.[99] Even in the absence of other supportive adults, rural health care providers often have distinct opportunities to positively impact transgender children and adolescents. Likewise, by educating medical office staff and creating visibly affirming and inclusive office spaces, health care providers can convey strong messages of support to transgender youth and the entire community. Rural health care providers can also help transgender youth and their families by becoming educated about gender-affirming care and regional specialty gender clinics and making appropriate referrals.[49,81,90]

Both rural providers and urban/suburban specialty clinics can help improve support for transgender youth by offering education to community organizations about issues around diverse sexualities and gender identities, as well as what the evidence shows about the appropriate uses and benefits of gender-affirming care. This can be crucial for families living in states with anti-transgender laws or proposed gender-affirming care bans, often based on erroneous information.[67]

Finally, online or remote resources can serve as important links to affirmation and support for transgender children, adolescents, and their families. Telehealth, or remote video sessions with mental health providers, have been effective across many contexts, including therapy sessions with gender-diverse adolescents with other psychiatric diagnoses, such as depression and anxiety. Similarly, patients and families have found remote visits with endocrinologists from specialty gender clinics to be generally useful and effective.[100–103] Unfortunately, remote video sessions from the patient's home may not always be possible because many rural areas lack reliable, high-speed internet access. In those cases, alternate sites, such as in a private room in a school or library with internet access or the use of a medium less favored by patients and providers, such as an audio-only telephone, may be necessary.

SUMMARY

Transgender youth are developing in a complex landscape of conflicting messages about the validity of their identities. In many instances, they face stigma, marginalization, and victimization that predisposes them to worse physical and mental health outcomes via the Minority Stress Model. While it is important to understand these risk factors and associated negative outcomes, it is just as imperative to grasp factors that contribute to resilience in transgender youth. Generally speaking, access to affirming spaces, people, and organizations can buffer some of the minority stress faced by transgender youth and lead to better outcomes.

The work with transgender youth should be approached from the same framework as with any youth. Clinicians must use a developmental lens that takes into account both strengths and vulnerabilities and work with the youth and family to tip the balance toward spaces and experiences that will support their development and build resilience. The resources available to individual youth depend highly on the systems around them. Opportunities for support exist within schools, broader communities, religious organizations, and with medical professionals who practice gender-affirming care. Clinicians who are familiar with resources in their communities can effectively guide transgender youth and their families to these affirming spaces.

Based on the continued high rates of negative health outcomes in transgender youth, it is clear that not enough resources are accessible to these kids and their families. It is paramount that clinicians, especially in underserved communities, are knowledgeable about resources within their communities and how to connect transgender youth to broader resources (online spaces, telehealth visits with competent providers, and advocacy groups). Additionally, adults across all domains of children's lives (parents, teachers, religious leaders, politicians, medical providers) must further educate themselves about gender-diverse youth and their needs to broaden the supportive scaffold that protects them from negative outcomes. Only then might we turn the tide toward a safe and affirming world for transgender youth to develop into their authentic selves.

CLINICS CARE POINTS

- Accessing supportive people and spaces in schools improves educational and mental health outcomes for transgender youth.
- The presence of GSAs decreases rates of victimization of LGBTQ youth in schools.
- Various organizations have developed inclusive school curricula that can decrease victimization and improve educational outcomes for transgender youth.
- Understanding federal, state, and local laws can help parents and providers advocate more effectively for gender affirming resources in schools.
- Supporting families helps them be more affirming to their transgender children, thereby protecting against negative mental health outcomes.
- Access to affirming care improves medical and mental health outcomes in transgender youth.
- Religion, spirituality, and engagement in religious activities play a significant role in the lives of many people, including transgender youth and their families, and can provide many opportunities to help support and affirm transgender youth.
- Religious institutions vary widely in their beliefs and practices about diverse gender identities, and even within organizations, there can be significant heterogeneity among adherent congregations and individuals.
- Gender affirming religious institutions can help mitigate negative effects of external stressors such as discrimination and stigma, and increase resilience, leading to improved mental health outcomes among transgender youth.
- While rural areas often lack more visible LGBTQ-affirming resources, the personal interconnectedness, strong local institutions and flexibility often found in rural communities can provide significant sources of support for transgender youth.

DISCLOSURE

Authors have nothing to disclose.

REFERENCES

1. Spack NP, Edwards-Leeper L, Feldman HA, et al. Children and adolescents with gender identity disorders referred to a pediatric medical center. Pediatrics 2012; 129(3):418–25.
2. Olson J, Schrager SM, Belzer M, et al. Baseline physiologic and psychosocial characteristics of transgender youth seeking care for gender dysphoria. J Adolesc Health 2015;57(4):374–80.
3. Becerra-Culqui TA, Liu Y, Nash R, et al. Mental health of transgender and gender nonconforming youth compared with their peers. Pediatrics 2018; 141(5):e20173845.
4. Adelson SL. Practice parameter on gay, lesbian, or bisexual sexual orientation, gender nonconformity, and gender discordance in children and adolescents. J Am Acad Child Adolesc Psychiatry 2012;51(9):957–74.
5. Rafferty J, Yogman M, Baum R, et al. Ensuring comprehensive care and support for transgender and gender diverse children and adolescents. Pediatrics 2018; 142(4). https://doi.org/10.1542/peds.2018-2162.
6. Meyer IH. Prejudice, social stress, and mental health in lesbian, gay, and bisexual populations: conceptual issues and research evidence. Psychol Bull 2003;129(5):674–97.
7. Hendricks ML, Testa RJ. A conceptual framework for clinical work with transgender and gender nonconforming clients: an adaptation of the Minority Stress Model. Prof Psychol Res Pract 2012;43(5):460–7.
8. Testa RJ, Habarth J, Peta J, et al. Development of the gender minority stress and resilience measure. Psychol Sex Orientat Gend Divers 2015;2(1):65–77.
9. Greytak EA, Kosciw JG, Villenas C, et al. From teasing to torment: school climate revisited, A survey of U.S. Secondary school students and teachers. New York: GLSEN; 2016.
10. Toomey RB, Russell ST. Gay-straight alliances, social justice involvement, and school victimization of lesbian, gay, bisexual, and queer youth: implications for school well-being and plans to vote. Youth Soc 2011;45(4):500–22.
11. Murchison GR, Agénor M, Reisner SL, et al. School restroom and locker room restrictions and sexual assault risk among transgender youth. Pediatrics 2019;143(6):e20182902.
12. James SE, Herman JL, Rankin S, et al. The report of the 2015 U.S. Transgender survey. Washington, DC: National Center for Transgender Equality; 2016.
13. Earnshaw VA, Bogart LM, Poteat VP, et al. Bullying among lesbian, gay, bisexual, and transgender youth. Pediatr Clin 2016;63(Issue 6):P999–1010.
14. Day JK, Perez-Brumer A, Russell ST. Safe schools? Transgender youth's school experiences and perceptions of school climate. J Youth Adolesc 2018 Aug; 47(8):1731–42.
15. Pampati S, Andrzejewski J, Sheremenko G, et al. School climate among transgender high school students: an exploration of school connectedness, perceived safety, bullying, and absenteeism. J Sch Nurs 2020;36(4):293–303.
16. Greytak EA, Kosciw JG, Diaz EM. Harsh realities: the experiences of transgender youth in our nation's schools. New York: GLSEN; 2009.
17. Blum RW. A case for school connectedness. Educ Leader 2005;62(7):16–20.

18. Whitaker K, Shapiro VB, Shields JP. School-based protective factors related to suicide for lesbian, gay, and bisexual adolescents. J Adolesc Health 2016; 58(1):63–8.
19. Truong NL, Clark CM, Rosenbach S, et al. The GSA study: results of national surveys about students' and advisors' experiences in gender and sexuality alliance clubs. New York: GLSEN; 2021.
20. Kosciw JG, Clark CM, Truong NL, et al. The 2019 National School Climate Survey: the experiences of lesbian, gay, bisexual, transgender, and queer youth in our nation's schools. New York: GLSEN; 2020.
21. Marx RA, Kettrey HH. Gay-Straight alliances are associated with lower levels of school-based victimization of LGBTQ+ youth: a systematic review and meta-analysis. J Youth Adolesc 2016;45(7):1269–82.
22. Toomey RB, Ryan C, Diaz RM, et al. High school gay-straight alliances (GSAs) and young adult well-being: an examination of GSA presence, participation, and perceived effectiveness. Appl Dev Sci 2011;15(4):175–85.
23. American Civil Liberties Union (ACLU) Okeechobee, FL high school gay-straight alliance wins groundbreaking federal lawsuit. 2008 July 30; Available at: http://www.aclu.org/lgbt-rights_hiv-aids/okeechobee-fl-high-school-gay-straight-alliance-wins-groundbreaking-federal-law. Accessed July 15, 2022.
24. American Civil Liberties Union (ACLU) ACLU settles Yulee high school gay-straight alliance lawsuit; students to meet on campus. 2009 August 10; Available at: http://www.aclufl.org/news_events/?action=viewRelease&emailAlertID=3768. Accessed July 15, 2022.
25. Proulx CN, Coulter RWS, Egan JE, et al. Associations of lesbian, gay, bisexual, transgender, and questioning-inclusive sex education with mental health outcomes and school-based victimization in U.S. High school students. J Adolesc Health 2019;64(5):608–14.
26. Haley SG, Tordoff DM, Kantor AZ, et al. Sex education for transgender and nonbinary youth: previous experiences and recommended content. J Sex Med 2019;16(11):1834–48.
27. GLSEN. "Inclusive Curriculum Guide." Available at: https://www.glsen.org/activity/inclusive-curriculum-guide.
28. Ryan CL, Patraw JM, Bednar M. Discussing princess boys and pregnant men: teaching about gender diversity and transgender experiences within an elementary school curriculum. J LGBT Youth 2013;10(1–2):83–105.
29. Greytak EA, Kosciw JG, Boesen MJ. Putting the "T" in 'Resource': the benefits of LGBT-related school resources for transgender youth. J LGBT Youth 2013; 10(1–2):45–63.
30. GLSEN. Improving school climate for transgender and nonbinary youth (research brief). New York: GLSEN; 2021.
31. Russell ST, Pollitt AM, Li G, et al. Chosen name use is linked to reduced depressive symptoms, suicidal ideation, and suicidal behavior among transgender youth. J Adolesc Health 2018;63(4):503–5.
32. Jones BA, Arcelus J, Bouman WP, et al. Sport and transgender people: a systematic review of the literature relating to sport participation and competitive sport policies. Sports Med 2017;47(4):701–16.
33. Clark CM, Kosciw JG, Chin J. LGBTQ students and school sports participation (research brief). New York: GLSEN; 2021.
34. GLSEN, ASCA, ACSSW, & SSWAA. Supporting safe and healthy schools for lesbian, gay, bisexual, transgender, and queer students: a national survey of school counselors, social workers, and psychologists. New York: GLSEN; 2019.

35. GLAAD resource list. Available at: https://www.glaad.org/resourcelist. Accessed July 16, 2022.
36. Lambda Legal Resource List. Available at: https://www.lambdalegal.org/know-your-rights/article/youth-resources#:~:text=Legal%20Help%20Desk%20866-542-8336%20Lambda%20Legal%20is%20a,through%20impact%20litigation%2C%20education%20and%20public%20policy%20work. Accessed July 16, 2022.
37. National Center for Transgender Equality Resource List. Available at: https://transequality.org/additional-help. Accessed July 16, 2022.
38. Hatzenbuehler ML, Shen Y, Vandewater EA, et al. Proposition 8 and homophobic bullying in California. Pediatrics 2019;143(6).
39. McGuire JK, Conover-Williams M. Creating spaces to support transgender youth. Prev Res 2010;17(4):17–20.
40. Taylor J. Queerious youth: an empirical study of a queer youth cultural festival and its participants. J Sociol 2014;50(3):283–98.
41. Weinhardt LS, Wesp LM, Xie H, et al. Pride Camp: pilot study of an intervention to develop resilience and self-esteem among LGBTQ youth. Int J Equity Health 2021;20(1):150.
42. Wolowic JM, Heston LV, Saewyc EM, et al. Chasing the rainbow: lesbian, gay, bisexual, transgender and queer youth and pride semiotics. Cult Health Sex 2017;19(5):557–71.
43. GLSEN, CiPHR, & CCRC. Out online: the experiences of lesbian, gay, bisexual and transgender youth on the Internet. New York: GLSEN; 2013.
44. Ryan C, Russell ST, Huebner D, et al. Family acceptance in adolescence and the health of LGBT young adults. J Child Adolesc Psychiatr Nurs 2010;23(4):205–13.
45. Lawlis SM, Butler P, Middleman A. Evaluating transgender youth and parent interest and preferences regarding support groups. Glob Pediatr Health 2020;7. 2333794X20954680.
46. Field TL, Mattson G. Parenting transgender children in PFLAG. J GLBT Fam Stud 2016;12(5):413–29.
47. Gridley SJ, Crouch JM, Evans Y, et al. Youth and caregiver perspectives on barriers to gender-affirming health care for transgender youth. J Adolesc Health 2016;59(3):254–61.
48. Rider GN, McMorris BJ, Gower AL, et al. Health and care utilization of transgender and gender nonconforming youth: a population-based study. Pediatrics 2018;141(3).
49. Eisenberg ME, McMorris BJ, Rider GN, et al. "It's kind of hard to go to the doctor's office if you're hated there." A call for gender-affirming care from transgender and gender diverse adolescents in the United States. Health Soc Care Community 2020;28(3):1082–9.
50. Dahl AL, Galliher RV. LGBTQ adolescents and young adults raised within a Christian religious context: positive and negative outcomes. J Adolesc 2012;35(6):1611–8.
51. Ano GG, Vasconcelles EB. Religious coping and psychological adjustment to stress: a meta- analysis. J Clin Psychol 2005a;61(4):461–80.
52. Brandt PY. Religious and spiritual aspects in the construction of identity modelized as a constellation. Integr Psychol Behav Sci 2018;53(1):138–57.
53. Pew Research Center, Dec 14, 2021, "About Three-in-Ten U.S. Adults Are Now Religiously Unaffiliated".

54. Conron, KJ; Goldberg, SK; O'Neill, K. (2020). Religiosity Among LGBT Adults in the U.S. Williams Institute, UCLA School of Law. Retrieved Jul 31, 2022 Available at: https://williamsinstitute.law.ucla.edu/publications/lgbt-religiosity-us/. Accessed July 31, 2022.
55. Lipka, M & Gecewicz, C. More Americans now say they're spiritual but not religious. Pew Research Center. Retrieved Jul 23, 2022 Available at: https://www.pew.research.org/fact-tank/2017/09/06/more-Americans-now-say-they're-spiritual-but-not-religious/. Accessed July 23, 2022.
56. Raedel DB, Wolff JR, Davis EB, et al. Clergy attitudes about ways to support the mental health of sexual and gender minorities. J Relig Health 2020;59(6): 3227–46.
57. Wong YJ, Rew L, Slaikeu KD. A systematic review of recent research on adolescent religiosity/spirituality and mental health. Issues Ment Health Nurs 2006; 27(2):161–83.
58. Lease SH, Horne SG, Noffsinger-Frazier N. Affirming faith experiences and psychological health for caucasian lesbian, gay, and bisexual individuals. J Counsel Psychol 2005;52(3):378–88.
59. Yakushko O. Influence of social support, existential well-being, and stress over sexual orientation on self esteem of gay, lesbian, and bisexual individuals. Int J Adv Counsell 2005;27(1):131–43.
60. Drescher J. Queer diagnoses: parallels and contrasts in the history of homosexuality, gender variance, and the diagnostic and statistical manual. Arch Sex Behav 2009;39(2):427–60.
61. Wilkins CL, Wellman JD, Toosi NR, et al. Is LGBT progress seen as an attack on Christians?: examining Christian/sexual orientation zero-sum beliefs. J Pers Soc Psychol 2022;122(1):73–101.
62. Hornsby TJ, Guest D. Transgender, intersex, and biblical interpretation (Semeia studies). 1st edition. SBL Press; 2016.
63. Canales AD. Ministry to transgender teenagers (Part One): pursuing awareness and understanding about trans youth. J Pastor Care Counsel 2018;72(3): 195–201.
64. Murphy, C. (2015). Lesbian, gay and bisexual Americans differ from general public in their religious affiliations. Pew Research Center. Retrieved Jul 28, 2022 Available at: http://www.pewresearch.org/fact-tank/2015/05/26/lesbian-gay-and-bisexual-americans-differ-from-general-public-in-their religious-affiliations/. Accessed July 28, 2022.
65. Grossman AH, D'augelli AR. Transgender youth. J Homosex 2006;51(1):111–28.
66. Grossman AH, D'Augelli AR. Transgender youth and life-threatening behaviors. Suicide Life-Threatening Behav 2007;37(5):527–37.
67. Boulware S.Kamody R.Kuper,L., Olezeski, C., Szilagyi, N., Alstott, A. (2022). Biased science: The Texas and Alabama Measures criminalizing medical treatment for transgender children and adolescents rely on Inaccurate and Misleading scientific claims. Retrieved on Jul 19, 2022 Available at: https://medicine.yale.edu/childstudy/policy/lgbtq-youth/. Accessed July 19, 2022.
68. American Academy of Child & Adolescent Psychiatry. (2018). Conversion Therapy. Retrieved on Jul 23, 2022 Available at: https://www.aacap.org/aacap/Policy_Statements/2018/Conversion_Therapy.aspx. Accessed July 23, 2022.
69. Fontenot E. Unlikely congregation: gay and lesbian persons of faith in contemporary U.S. culture. In: Pargament KI, editor. APA handbook of psychology, religion and spirituality, vol. 1. Washington, DC: AmericanPsychological Association DC; 2013. p. 617–33.

70. Chaves M, Roso J, Holleman A, et al. Congregations in 21st Century America. Durham, NC: Duke University Department of Sociology; 2021.
71. HRC Foundation. Faith Positions. Retrieved Jul 19, 2022 Available at: https://www.hrc.org/resources/faith-positions. Accessed July 19, 2022.
72. Pew Research Center. (2017). Support for same-sex marriage grows, even among groups that had been skeptical. Retrieved Jul 23, 2022 Available at: https://www.pewresearch.org/politics/2017/06/26/support-for-same-sex-marriage-grows-even-among-groups-that-had-been-skeptical/. Accessed July 23, 2022.
73. Canales AD. Ministry to transgender teenagers (Part Two): providing pastoral care, support, and advocacy to trans youth. J Pastor Care Counsel 2018; 72(4):251–6.
74. Aramburu Alegría C. Supporting families of transgender children/youth: parents speak on their experiences, identity, and views. Int J Transgenderism 2018; 19(2):132–43.
75. Abreu RL, Rosenkrantz DE, Ryser-Oatman JT, et al. Parental reactions to transgender and gender diverse children: a literature review. J GLBT Fam Stud 2019; 15(5):461–85.
76. Ratcliffe M, Burd C, Holder K, et al. Defining rural at the U.S. Census Bureau. Washington, DC: U.S. Census Bureau; 2016.
77. Grundy SA, Brown RC, Jenkins WD. Health and health care of sexual minority individuals in the rural United States: a systematic review. J Health Care Poor Underserved 2021;32(4):1639–52.
78. Movement Advancement Project. November 2019. Where We Call Home: Transgender People in Rural America. Retrieved on Jul 19, 2022 Available at: www.lgbtmap.org/rural-trans. Accessed July 19, 2022.
79. Daily Kos Elections. (2021). Statewide election results by congressional and legislative districts. Retrieved Jul 30, 2022 Available at: https://www.dailykos.com/stories/2013/07/09/1220127/-Daily-Kos-Elections-2012-election-results-by-congressional-and-legislative-districts. Accessed July 30, 2022.
80. Lipka,M & Tevington, P. (2022). Attitudes about transgender issues vary widely among Christians, religious 'nones' in U.S. Pew Research Center. Retrieved Jul 24, 2022 Available at: https://www.pewresearch.org/fact-tank/2022/07/07/attitudes-about-transgender-issues-vary-widely-among-christians-religious-nones-in-u-s/. Accessed July 24, 2022.
81. Rosenkrantz DE, Black WW, Abreu RL, et al. Health and health care of rural sexual and gender minorities: a systematic review. Stigma and Health 2017;2(3): 229–43.
82. Paceley MS, Sattler P, Goffnett J, et al. "It feels like home": transgender youth in the Midwest and conceptualizations of community climate. J Community Psychol 2020;48(6):1863–81.
83. Bowman S, Nic Giolla Easpaig B, Fox R. Virtually caring: a qualitative study of internet-based mental health services for LGBT young adults in rural Australia. Rural Rem Health 2020. https://doi.org/10.22605/rrh5448.
84. Renner J, Blaszcyk W, Täuber L, et al. Barriers to accessing health care in rural regions by transgender, non-binary, and gender diverse people: a case-based scoping review. Front Endocrinol 2021;12. https://doi.org/10.3389/fendo.2021.717821.
85. Kano M, Silva-Banuelos AR, Sturm R, et al. Stakeholders' recommendations to improve patient-centered "LGBTQ" primary care in rural and multicultural practices. J Am Board Fam Med 2016;29(1):156–60.

86. Eisenberg ME, Gower AL, McMorris BJ, et al. Emotional distress, bullying victimization, and protective factors among transgender and gender diverse adolescents in city, suburban, town, and rural locations. J Rural Health 2018;35(2): 270–81.

87. Palmer NA, Kosciw JG, Bartkiewicz MJ. Strengths & Silences: the experiences of lesbian, gay, bisexual and transgender students in rural and small town schools. New York: GLSEN; 2012.

88. Toliver, Z. (2016). LGBTQ Healthcare: Building Inclusive Rural Practices. Rural Health Information Hub/Rural Health Monitor. Retrieved Jul 22, 2022 Available at: https://www.rural.health.info.org/rural-monitor/lgbtq-healthcare/. Accessed July 22, 2022.

89. Paceley MS, Okrey-Anderson S, Heumann M. Transgender youth in small towns: perceptions of community size, climate, and support. J Youth Stud 2017;20(7): 822–40.

90. Paceley MS, Ananda J, Thomas MMC, et al. "I have nowhere to go": a multiple-case study of transgender and gender diverse youth, their families, and healthcare experiences. Int J Environ Res Publ Health 2021;18(17):9219.

91. Ivey-Stephenson AZ, Crosby AE, Jack SPD, et al. Suicide trends among and within urbanization levels by sex, race/ethnicity, age group, and mechanism of death - United States, 2001-2015. MMWR Surveill Summ 2017;66(18):1–16.

92. National Rural Health Association. (2022). Workforce Shortage Problems. Retrieved Jul 19, 2022 Available at: https://ruralhealth.us/about-nrha/about-rural-health-care.

93. American Academy of Child & Adolescent Psychiatry. (2022). Severe Shortage of Child & Adolescent Psychiatrists Illustrated in AACAP Workforce Maps. Retrieved on Jul 29, 2022 Available at: https://www.aacap.org/aacap/Advocacy/Federal_and_State_Initiatives/Workforce_Maps/Home.aspx. Accessed July 29, 2022.

94. World Professional Association for Transgender Health. (2022). Standards of Care for the Health of Transgender and Gender Diverse People Version 8. Available at: https://www.wpath.org/publications/soc. Accessed July 22, 2022.

95. Hembree WC, Cohen-Kettenis PT, Gooren L, et al. Endocrine treatment of gender-dysphoric/gender-incongruent persons: an endocrine society clinical practice guideline. Endocr Pract 2017;23(12):1.

96. McNamara M, Lepore C, Alstott A, et al. Scientific misinformation and gender affirming care: tools for providers on the front lines. J Adolesc Health 2022. https://doi.org/10.1016/j.jadohealth.2022.06.008.

97. Bazelon, E. (2022, June 15). The Battle Over Gender Therapy. New York Times. Retrieved Jul 20, 2022, Available at: https://www.nytimes.com/2022/06/15/magazine/gender-therapy.html. Accessed July 20, 2022.

98. Badgett, MV Lee; Choi, SK; Wilson, BDM. (2019). LGBT Poverty in the United States: A Study of Differences Between Sexual Orientation and Gender Identity Groups. Williams Institute, UCLA School of Law. Retrieved Jul 31, 2022. Available at: https://williamsinstitute.law.ucla.edu/publications/lgbt-poverty-us/. Accessed July 31, 2022.

99. The Trevor Project. (2019). The Trevor Project Research Brief: Accepting Adults Reduce Suicide Attempts among LGBTQ Youth. Retrieved Jul 26, 2022. Available at: https://www.thetrevorproject.org/research-briefs/accepting-adults-reduce-suicide-attempts-among-lgbtq-youth/. Accessed July 26, 2022.

100. Simpson SG, Reid CL. Therapeutic alliance in videoconferencing psychotherapy: a review. Aust J Rural Health 2014;22(6):280–99.

101. Smith K, Ostinelli E, Macdonald O, et al. COVID-19 and telepsychiatry: development of evidence-based guidance for clinicians. JMIR Mental Health 2020;7(8): e21108.

102. Lee JY, Eimicke T, Rehm JL, et al. Providing gender-affirmative care during the severe acute respiratory syndrome coronavirus 2 pandemic era: experiences and perspectives from pediatric endocrinologists in the United States. Transgender Health 2022;7(2):170–4.

103. Sequeira GM, Kidd KM, Rankine J, et al. Gender diverse youth's experiences and satisfaction with telemedicine for gender-affirming care during the COVID-19 pandemic. Transgender Health 2022;7(2):127–34.

APPENDIX 1: RESOURCES TO SUPPORT TRANSGENDER YOUTH

One-to-One Support/Hotlines:
From The Trevor Project:
Trevor LifeLine: 1-866-488-7386
Trevor Text: Text START to 678678
TrevorChat - helpline for young people: www.thetrevorproject.org/get-help-now
TrevorSpace: www.trevorspace.org
Other Youth Resources:
LGBT National Youth Talkline: 1-800-246-PRIDE
LGBTQ Teens Online Talk Group: https://www.lgbthotline.org/youthchatrooms
Trans Youth Online Talk Group: https://www.lgbthotline.org/lgbtteens
Trans Teens Online Talk Group: https://www.lgbthotline.org/transteens
General:
LGBT National Hotline: 1-888-843-4564
Trans Lifeline: 877-565-8860
School Resources:
GLSEN
Educator Resources: https://www.glsen.org/resources/educator-resources
Student Resources: https://www.glsen.org/resources/student-and-gsa-resources
Human Rights Campaign (HRC)
School Resources: https://www.hrc.org/resources/schools
Educator Resources: https://www.thehrcfoundation.org/professional-resources/education-professionals
National Center for Transgender Equality
School Rights: https://transequality.org/know-your-rights/schools
Youth & Student Resources: https://transequality.org/issues/youth-students
Gender Spectrum
Educator Resources: https://www.genderspectrum.org/audiences/educators-and-education-professionals
Community Resources:
CenterLink - list of LGBT community centers by state: http://www.lgbtcenters.org/LGBTCenters
Trans in the South: A Directory of Trans-Affirming Health & Legal Providers: https://southernequality.org/resources/transinthesouth/
Information about Gender-Affirming Religious Institutions and Faith-Based Organizations:
HRC: https://www.hrc.org/resources/faith-positions

Strong Family Alliance: http://www.strongfamilyalliance.org

PFLAG: https://pflag.org/nondenominational

TransFaith: http://www.transfaithonline.org

Gender Spectrum: http://www.genderspectrum.org

Transmission Ministry Collective: http://www.transmissionministry.com

Freed Hearts: http://www.freedhearts.org

Q Christian Fellowship: www.qchristian.org/for-you

Many Voices - a Black Church Movement for Gay and Transgender Justice: www.manyvoices.org

Additional Religion-Based Resources:

Family Acceptance Project: https://familyproject.sfsu.edu

United Church of Christ and Unitarian Universalist Church - "Our Whole Lives" is a theologically-based, developmentally-appropriate, affirming and inclusive curriculum about gender and sexuality for ages ranging from kindergarten to adult: http://www.ucc.org/owl

HRC - "Coming Home" is a program curriculum to educate religious congregants and communities of color about the lives and experience of transgender and gender-diverse individuals through an exploration of gender through a theological and culturally aware lens: https://www.hrc.org/resources/religion-faith

Systems-Involved Transgender and Gender-Diverse Youth

Homelessness, Juvenile Legal Systems, and Child Welfare and Foster Care

Jonathon W. Wanta, MD[a],*, George Gianakakos, MD[a],
Austin Nguy, BA[b], Dalia N. Balsamo, MD[c]

KEYWORDS

- Transgender • Gender diverse • Juvenile justice • Foster care • Child welfare
- Homelessness

KEY POINTS

- Transgender and gender-diverse youth are overrepresented among youth experiencing homelessness as well as those in the juvenile legal, child welfare, and foster care systems.
- Systems-involved transgender and gender-diverse youth face unique challenges navigating their day-to-day lives that may increase the risk for adverse mental health outcomes.
- Working with systems-involved transgender and gender-diverse youth requires a compassionate, curious, and nonjudgmental approach in addition to a steadfastness for advocacy and social justice.

INTRODUCTION

There can be no keener revelations of a society's soul than the way in which they treat its children.
—Nelson Mandela, May 8th 1995 in a speech for the Launch of the Nelson Mandela's South African Children's Fund[1]

[a] Pritzker Department of Psychiatry and Behavioral Health, Ann and Robert H. Lurie Children's Hospital of Chicago, 225 East Chicago Avenue, Box 10, Chicago, IL 60611, USA; [b] University of California, Riverside, School of Medicine, 900 University Avenue, Riverside, CA 92521, USA; [c] Department of Psychiatry and Neuroscience, University of California, Riverside, School of Medicine, 900 University Avenue, Riverside, CA 92521, USA
* Corresponding author. 225 East Chicago Avenue, Box 10, Chicago, IL 60611.
E-mail address: jwanta@luriechildrens.org

Child Adolesc Psychiatric Clin N Am 32 (2023) 839–848
https://doi.org/10.1016/j.chc.2023.04.003
1056-4993/23/© 2023 Elsevier Inc. All rights reserved.

To maintain function and order, a society forms systems through its policies and services. Social services may be nonspecific and for the benefit of all, such as public education, or targeted to vulnerable populations like the elderly. Collective attitudes and values may change drastically over time and vary widely among countries, states, or even cities, resulting in dramatically different support for implementing or adapting services. In the United States (U.S.), various systems have been put in place to address housing, social services, and the mental and physical health needs of our youth. Because children lack a direct role in public government or planning, it is up to adults to create and implement systems that support and protect youth. It is of utmost importance to advocate for and uphold children's rights and safety nets.

Systems in place for youth must serve and nurture those who are most disenfranchised. We focus exclusively on the experience and treatment of systems-involved transgender and gender-diverse (TGD) youth. A 2021 Gallup Poll found that about 1.8% of American youths identified as transgender, although less is known about youth with other diverse gender identities.[2] Understanding the complexity of systems-involved TGD youth starts with understanding the systems in place that address, or fail to address, their needs. We explore the experiences of TGD youth within some of society's most complex systems, highlighting those who are experiencing homelessness, those involved in the juvenile legal system, and those involved in child welfare and/or foster care systems. We explore the unique needs of TGD youth and disparities in their outcomes, in the setting of collective societal shortcomings. Our aim is to equip providers to advocate for a kinder version of "society's soul" for all youth, even our most vulnerable.

TRANSGENDER AND GENDER-DIVERSE YOUTH EXPERIENCING HOMELESSNESS

Hope clung to her purple backpack as she hurried under the city's streetlights, each casting an orange glow onto the pools of half-melted snow left by her boots. She dusted off a park bench before throwing herself onto it, rummaging through her backpack to find something with which to wipe her runny nose. Her heaving breaths formed a smoky wreath over her head, mirroring the tangle of thoughts twisting in her mind. She was sure her family was different, that her family would understand. If she had any doubts, she never would have said anything. The looks on their faces as she told them she was transgender, however, made it clear that they didn't understand. This was only confirmed by the hurtful words that followed, although Hope was barely able to hear much through the fog of her disbelief. As she shivered on the bench, the only thing she knew now was that she couldn't go back; she couldn't return home.

Children and adolescents experiencing homelessness are a dynamic and heterogenous population. Homelessness, in and of itself, can take various forms. According to the U.S. Department of Education, homelessness encompasses all individuals who lack a "fixed, regular, and adequate nighttime residence."[3] While this notion may bring to mind images of individuals sleeping on the streets or in parks, homelessness includes those who sleep in cars, motels, or homeless shelters. Not uncommonly, youth with unstable housing may "couch surf," spending a few nights at a time with different family or friends without a permanent homebase.[4] Naturally, these different living arrangements confer very different risks regarding stability and safety.[5]

As with all youth, it is important to consider the family system for youth who are experiencing homelessness. Youths may be accompanied by a parent or caregiver or entirely on their own ("unaccompanied"). Youth who experience homelessness with their family unit face a greater risk of unaccompanied homelessness later in life, for example, if a family member passes away.

Many mental health providers feel ill-prepared to care for youth experiencing homelessness. They may have implicit bias about those who are experiencing homelessness and/or knowledge gaps about their patients' lived experiences. Homeless youth may also not "seem" homeless when initially presenting in health care settings and may be otherwise overlooked, resulting in a disconnect between needs and services provided.[6]

In a nationally representative sample, 1 in 30 youth aged 13 to 17 and 1 in 10 young adults aged 18 to 25 experienced some form of homelessness over the previous 12 months. Black/African-American and Hispanic non-White youth had an 83% and 33% higher risk of reporting homelessness than white peers, respectively. Lesbian, gay, bisexual, transgender, and/or queer (LGBTQ) youth exhibit over twice the rate of homelessness as their cisgender heterosexual peers, with LGBTQ youth of color experiencing the highest rates of homelessness.[5] TGD youth face more discrimination than cisgender LGB youth and are thus further overrepresented in the population of those experiencing homelessness. Despite making up less than 2% of the total population,[7] 7% to 9% of the homeless population may identify as transgender or gender diverse.[8] Among youth homelessness human service agency providers, almost 80% reported TGD youth having longer periods of homelessness compared to cisgender and heterosexual peers.[9]

Transgender youth may come to experience homelessness through 2 general pathways. "Runaway youth" are those who have left the home without consent, whereas "throwaway youth" are those who are forced out by a parent. Those who run away may experience a more episodic course, for example, returning home after some period of time, whereas those who are forced out are more likely to face a chronic course.[3] For transgender youth, issues around their gender identity are often the main driver for either running away or being forced out. In one study, two-thirds of providers identified issues around sexual orientation and/or gender identity as the primary driver for homelessness for their transgender youth population.[9]

Navigating homelessness comes with inherent risks and challenges, especially around safety and securing one's basic needs. Youth experiencing homelessness have high rates of victimization at baseline, and this risk is disproportionate for transgender youth experiencing homelessness. Agency providers estimate that 90% of transgender youth experiencing homelessness have experienced harassment or bullying; 75% having experienced physical, emotional, or sexual abuse; and 25% having experienced intimate partner violence.[7] Rates of sexual exploitation and trafficking vary by study but are estimated to be between 20% and 65%.[9,10] Youth may be denied access to shelters consistent with their gender identity or may face discrimination, aggression, or assault therein.[11] Some transgender youth experiencing homelessness may resort to survival sex in order to get their basic needs met.[12]

TGD youth experiencing homelessness are at an increased risk of worse physical and mental health outcomes than cisgender youth experiencing homelessness.[13] About 75% of TGD youth experiencing homelessness were identified as having a mental health condition.[9] Several theoretic models have been proposed to explain these extreme disproportionalities. First, the Minority Stress Model explains how chronic internal and external stressors related to one's minoritized status accumulate over time and increase the risk for adverse mental health outcomes.[14] The Risk Amplification Model was specifically created with homeless youth in mind. In it, Whitbeck and Hoyt explain that existing psychosocial problems are exacerbated once homeless and that extended homelessness results in increased psychosocial problems.[15] Together, the Minority Stress Model and Risk Amplification Model help inform providers as they work to conceptualize and assist their TGD youth experiencing homelessness.

TRANSGENDER AND GENDER-DIVERSE YOUTH AND THE JUVENILE LEGAL SYSTEM

"You can't be here young man!" Hope turned her head toward the voice, locking eyes with an officer craning his head through the passenger-side window of his car. "It's 'young lady,'" Hope replied, as the policeman's head cocked to the side in confusion. Then suddenly, knowingly, the officer closed his eyes and nodded, opening the car door and stepping onto the sidewalk. "Ok 'Miss,' why don't you come with us? It's cold out here. We can try to get you help back at the station." "Really, I'm fine," shot Hope, "but thanks." As she pivoted to start heading in the other direction, she felt a hand rest on her shoulder: "Come on, let's go."

Historically, data on the experience and treatment of transgender and gender-diverse youth in the juvenile legal system have been limited. Many jurisdictions do not collect data on sexual orientation or gender identity by practice.[16] Some youth fear further victimization by authority figures for whistleblowing.[17] And transphobic practices may be overlooked to avoid public critique. Without proper transparency, data collection and evaluation remain stymied.

Transgender and gender-diverse youth may face unique challenges that increase the risk for and perpetuate involvement with the juvenile legal system. Family rejection may prompt TGD youths to run away from or be kicked out of their homes. Unaccompanied TGD minors face the slew of stressors and challenges described in the previous section, and they can also face legal ramifications upon interfacing with the law. For example, runaway TGD youths may be unable to attend school safely and end up facing offense changes for truancy. Ultimately, many TGD youths fall into a vicious cycle of family rejection, trauma, and detention that can be difficult to escape.

While navigating the legal system, TGD youth face stigmatization and additional barriers compared to their cisgender peers. Many TGD youth have reported being misgendered by their attorneys and being held in contempt by the judge for wearing clothing consistent with their gender identity. TGD youth are more likely to be sent to detention for offenses that may not warrant such a highly restrictive level of control and confinement. They may not be considered for less restrictive alternatives due to prevailing beliefs that more mainstream placements are ill-equipped to provide the care they need.[18] Unfortunately, these risks are further compounded for TGD youth of color.

Youth detention centers present additional challenges for TGD youth. They may be housed inappropriately or even face segregation from the general population. Legal experts have weighed in to oppose this practice as it can cause undue trauma to the youth.[19] Additionally, TGD youth may be denied gender-affirming medical interventions that have been shown to potentially protect against negative mental health outcomes.[20,21]

Federal law provides guidance for the treatment of transgender youth in juvenile settings. The Prison Rape Elimination Act (PREA) was signed into law in 2003 to address sexual assault in correctional settings.[22] A PREA-compliant policy requires that housing and programming assignment be done on a case-by-case basis while placing great emphasis on the youth's own view regarding their safety. It also limits the use of solitary confinement and mandates staff to receive training in effective communication with TGD youth.[16] However, juvenile justice policies and procedures can differ greatly from one jurisdiction to another, depending on state, county, and municipality legislatures.[23] **Fig. 1** demonstrates the heterogeneity of protections and policies by state within the juvenile legal system.

The American Academy of Child and Adolescent Psychiatry (AACAP) has a clear policy statement regarding the treatment of juvenile justice-involved TGD youth.[24]

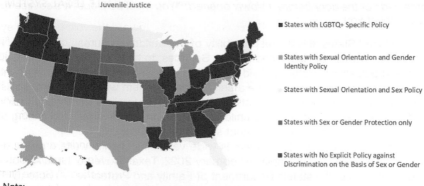

Note:
Purple: Juvenile Justice (JJ) policy includes specific protections for LGBTQ+ groups.
Green: Protections for sexual orientation and gender identity (self-identified gender labels)
Yellow: Protections in place for the basis of sexual orientation and sex/gender (sex assigned at birth male vs. female). However, do not mention any protections for gender identity.
Green: Protections for only sex/gender. No sexual orientation protections or gender identity protection.
Red: These states have no protections for sex/gender, sexual orientation, or gender identity.

Trans-inclusive/ Gender Diverse-inclusive policies: Purple and Green
Trans-exclusive/ Gender Diverse-exclusive policies: Yellow, Blue and Red

Fig. 1. State-by-state protections for juvenile justice-involved TGD youth. (*Adapted from Lambda Legal, currently in correspondence for permissions.*)

AACAP recommends that the names and pronouns of TGD youth be respected and that TGD youth not be segregated or isolated in the absence of serious safety concerns. In addition, AACAP advocates for TGD youth to receive psychiatric and medical care consistent with current standards and guidelines. The National Commission on Correctional Health Care (NCCHC) also has a position statement recommending the creation of a safe environment for TGD youth, staff training, and individualized gender-affirming care, when applicable.[25]

TRANSGENDER AND GENDER-DIVERSE YOUTH AND THE CHILD WELFARE AND FOSTER CARE SYSTEMS

The Child Welfare Agent took off her coat and hung it on the back of her chair, brushing snow off the sleeves. She plopped into the seat and heaved a briefcase onto her lap, rummaging through it before pulling out a sheet of paper. She returned the bag to the floor, her eyes darting across the document. Suddenly, her eyes peeked over the paper: "So you're Daniel. My name's Alice. It's nice to meet you." "It's Hope. Please call me Hope." Alice's eyes returned to the paper before she placed it on the desk beside her. "Of course, I'm sorry. It's really nice to meet you, Hope." Her eyes softened as a warm smile spread across her face: "I understand your folks haven't been picking up the phone. Let me make some calls and see what I can do."

"Third time's a charm" chirped Alice, her voice full of sincerity. Hope wasn't so sure. Her parents wanted nothing to do with her, and any family members they had reached out to didn't feel comfortable housing her for longer than a few weeks. Alice's footsteps slowed in front of a small yellow house, the walkway to the front door lined with tulips peeking through the soil. The pair made their way to the front door. Alice glanced at Hope before gingerly pushing the doorbell, hearing it ring throughout the home. Footsteps and voices could be heard on the

other side of the door before it slowly opened: "You must be Hope. It's so nice to finally meet you."

In the United States, it is the responsibility of the Children's Bureau, a subsidiary of the U.S. Department of Health and Human Services, to help develop federal requirements and guidelines related to child protection and welfare throughout the country. Each state must create and operate a child welfare system with the general goals of "preventing child abuse and neglect by strengthening families, protecting children from further maltreatment, reuniting children safely with their families, and finding permanent families for children who cannot safely return home."[26]

As with juvenile legal systems, there is wide variability in child welfare policy on a state-by-state basis. For example, in February 2022, Texas Governor Greg Abbott ordered all officers of the state's Department of Family and Protective Services (DFPS) to begin investigations of parents and healthcare providers delivering evidence-based gender-affirming care for TGD youth and their families. Investigations were initially mired in legal challenges with the future of gender-affirming care uncertain in the state of Texas.[27] In other states, such restrictions are not legal. **Fig. 2** provides a visual representation of protections offered in each state within the child welfare system.

A large part of the child welfare system run by any state is their foster care program, with "foster care" defined as "24-h substitute care for children placed away from their parents or guardians and for whom the [State] agency has placement and care responsibility." This can include placement with foster families, group homes, residential treatment centers, and others. Of the estimated 73 million children under the age of 18 living in the United States in 2018, approximately 437,000 interfaced with the foster care system. Among these children, roughly 25% (100,000) were awaiting were awaiting adoption, with an additional quarter of these (about 23,000) aging out each year without permanent families.[28] There has been limited research within the child welfare system related to the experiences of TGD youth specifically, but there is evidence to

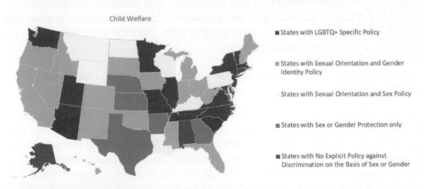

Child Welfare

■ States with LGBTQ+ Specific Policy

■ States with Sexual Orientation and Gender Identity Policy

States with Sexual Orientation and Sex Policy

■ States with Sex or Gender Protection only

■ States with No Explicit Policy against Discrimination on the Basis of Sex or Gender

Note:
Purple: Child Welfare (CW) policy includes specific protections for LGBTQ+ groups.
Green: Protections for sexual orientation and gender identity (self-identified gender labels)
Yellow: Protections in place for the basis of sexual orientation and sex/gender (sex assigned at birth male vs. female). However, do not mention any protections for gender identity.
Green: Protections for only sex/gender. No sexual orientation protections or gender identity protection.
Red: These states have no protections for sex/gender, sexual orientation, or gender identity.

Trans-inclusive/ Gender Diverse-inclusive policies: Purple and Green
Trans-exclusive/ Gender Diverse-exclusive policies: Yellow, Blue and Red

Fig. 2. State-by-state protections for child welfare-involved TGD youth. (*Adapted from Lambda Legal, currently in correspondence for permissions.*)

suggest that TGD youth are overrepresented in the foster care system. For example, 5.6% of foster youth in Los Angeles identified as transgender, compared to approximately 2% in the general population.[29]

Despite TGD youth often entering the foster care system for many of the same reasons as cisgender youth—including abuse, neglect, and parental substance abuse—many TGD youth face additional unique challenges related to their identities. LGBTQ youth have a higher average number of foster care placements and a higher likelihood of living in a group home setting than their cisgender heterosexual peers. These disparities are likely related to the non-affirming nature of foster placements for LGBTQ youth and the high level of bias and discrimination LGBTQ youth face, regardless of where they end up.[30,31] Additionally, TGD youth may experience verbal or physical abuse in group homes or foster homes owing to their gender identity and/or their outward gender expression. Establishing and identifying supportive and affirming group homes and foster families can help mitigate discrimination within the child welfare system.[32]

SUMMARY

Systems-involved TGD youth often navigate harsh and stigmatizing conditions. Inherently, they bridge the intersection of at least two marginalized identities, but they may additionally experience compounding discrimination on the basis of intersecting identities. Systems-involved TGD youth include racial/ethnic minorities, people living with disabilities, undocumented immigrants, and people living with HIV. We recommend a clinician explore each patient's multifaceted identities and how these may interact with their different systems and supports.[33]

Given the marked heterogeneity of TGD youth populations, there is no "single way" to best support systems-involved TGD youth, although there are general guiding principles that are useful to consider. First and foremost, it is important to keep systems-involved TGD at the center of our discourse and work to uplift their voices.[34] So-called photovoice projects, in which participants select their own photographs to engage in conversation on their lived experiences, have been successfully utilized with LGBTQ youth experiencing homelessness. In one photovoice study, youth reported feeling more empowered to self-advocate, and researchers found the method to be helpful in highlighting the many strengths and resilience factors often overlooked in this group.[35]

Second, the clinician should be mindful of supporting systems-involved TGD youth transitioning into adulthood. While this is certainly important with any youth population, it is particularly relevant in working with systems-involved TGD youth who may face additional barriers such as terminating high school before completion or having a criminal record. These youth may benefit from a higher level of support, including streamlined access opportunities for pursuing a GED or job training programs.[34]

Lastly, working with systems-involved TGD youth necessitates compassion, curiosity, and tenacity. Many systems-involved youth perceive a dearth of resources when it comes to their wellbeing. TGD youth face a higher risk of victimization and discrimination than their cisgender peers in all legal and social systems. Further, for TGD youth, there may be discriminatory policies in place that compound risk for adverse mental health outcomes. Though federal guidelines do exist, implementation and protections vary state-by-state. Advocacy work at the state and local levels therefore can bring about palpable change to better support the health and well-being of systems-involved TGD youth.

In closing, the policies in place to support systems-involved youth often fail to meet the needs of the TGD community across the country. Mental health providers are likely to interface with currently or previously systems-involved TGD youth during their career. If the ways in which a society treats children truly reflect its soul, then mental health providers are at the forefront of ensuring a kinder soul over time through compassionate care, curiosity about their patients' lived experiences, equitable care, and advocacy for some of society's most vulnerable members.

CLINICS CARE POINTS

- Health care providers can screen for common risk factors experienced by TGD youth experiencing homelessness in order to provide the highest level of care and resources.
- Within the juvenile legal system, health care providers can advocate for alternatives to detention or placement that respect the youth's gender identity if safe to do so.
- Health care providers working with TGD youth in the foster care system can support affirming foster families and group homes when necessary.
- Health care providers who care for systems-involved TGD youth should strive to uplift their voices, assist TGD youth as they transition into adulthood, and advocate for improved access and more equitable care.

DISCLOSURE

Authors do not have any financial disclosures or conflicts of interests to disclose.

REFERENCES

1. Mandela, N. Speech by President Nelson Mandela at the launch of the Nelson Mandela Children's Fund. Nelson Mandela Foundation. Available at: http://db.nelsonmandela.org/speeches/pub_view.asp?pg=item&ItemID=NMS250&txtstr=Mahla). Accessed July 25, 2022.
2. Jones, J. LGBT Identification Rises to 5.6% in Latest U.S. Estimate. Gallup. Available at: https://news.gallup.com/poll/329708/lgbt-identification-rises-latest-estimate.aspx. Accessed July 25, 2022.
3. Federal Definitions. Youth.gov. Available at: https://youth.gov/youth-topics/runaway-and-homeless-youth/federal-definitions. Accessed July 25, 2022.
4. Amore K. Severe housing deprivation in Aotearoa/New Zealand 2001-2013. Wellington NZ: He Kainga Oranga/Housing Health Ressearch Programme University of Otago; 2016.
5. Morton Samuels GM, Dworsky A, Patel SMH. Missed opportunities: LGBTQ youth homelessness in America. Voices of the Youth Count 2018;1–15.
6. Seip, N. New Study Reveals the Scope of Youth Homelessness. True Colors United. Available at: https://truecolorsunited.org/2017/11/15/new-study-reveals-scope-youth-homelessness/. Accessed July 25, 2022.
7. Johns MM, Lowry R, Andrzejewski J, et al. Transgender identity and experiences of violence victimization, substance use, suicide risk, and sexual risk behaviors among high school students — 19 states and large urban school districts, 2017. Morb Mortal Wkly Rep 2019;68(3):67.
8. Seip N. At the intersections: a collaborative resource on LGBTQ youth homelessness 2019. True Colors United 2019;13–90.

9. Choi SK, Wilson BDM, Shelton J, et al. Serving our youth 2015: the needs and experiences of Lesbian, gay, bisexual, transgender, and Questioning youth experiencing homelessness. Los Angeles: The Williams Institute with True Colors Fund; 2015.

10. Wright CD, Tiani AG, Billingsley AL, et al. A Framework for understanding the role of Psychological Processes in Disease development, Maintenance, and treatment: the 3P-Disease model. Front Psychol 2019;10:2498.

11. Fraser B, Pierse N, Chisholm E, et al. LGBTIQ+ homelessness: a Review of the Literature. Int J Environ Res Public Heal 2019;16(15):2677.

12. Greenfield B, Alessi EJ, Manning D, et al. Learning to endure: a qualitative examination of the protective factors of homeless transgender and gender expansive youth engaged in survival sex. Int J Transgend Health 2020;22(3):316–29.

13. Durso L.E. and Gates G.J., *Serving Our Youth: Findings from a National Survey of Services Providers Working with Lesbian, Gay, Bisexual and Transgender Youth Who are Homeless or At Risk of Becoming Homeless*, Available at: https://escholarship.org/uc/item/80x75033?. 2010.

14. Meyer IH. Prejudice, social stress, and mental health in Lesbian, gay, and bisexual populations: Conceptual issues and research evidence. Psychol Bull 2003;129(5):674.

15. Whitbeck LB, Hoyt DR, Yoder KA. A risk-amplification model of victimization and depressive symptoms among runaway and homeless adolescents. Am J Community Psychol 1999;27(2):273–96.

16. Owen MC, Wallace SB. Advocacy and collaborative health care for Justice-involved youth. Pediatrics 2020;146(1).

17. Irvine A. We've had three of them: addressing the invisibility of lesbian, gay, bisexual, and gender nonconforming youths in the juvenile justice system. Columbia J Gend Law 2010;19(3). https://doi.org/10.7916/CJGL.V19I3.2603.

18. Benson K. What's in a pronoun?: the ungovernability and misgendering of trans native kids in juvenile justice in Washington state. J Homosex 2020;67(12): 1691–712.

19. Marrett S. Beyond rehabilitation: constitutional violations associated with the isolation and discrimination of transgender youth in the juvenile justice system. Bost Coll Law Rev 2017;58(1).

20. Tordoff DM, Wanta JW, Collin A, et al. Mental health outcomes in transgender and Nonbinary youths receiving gender-affirming care. JAMA Netw Open 2022;5(2). https://doi.org/10.1001/jamanetworkopen.2022.0978.

21. Turban JL, King D, Carswell JM, et al. Pubertal Suppression for transgender youth and risk of Suicidal Ideation. Pediatrics. Feb 2020;145(2). https://doi.org/10.1542/peds.2019-1725.

22. Prison Rape Elimination Act in Juvenile Facilities. Office of Juvenile Justice and Delinquency Prevention. Available at:https://ojjdp.ojp.gov/programs/prea. Accessed July 25, 2022.

23. Cook, A. State-by-State Analysis of Juvenile Justice Systems. Lambda Legal. Available at:https://www.lambdalegal.org/juvenile-justice. Accessed July 25, 2022.

24. Transgender Youth in Juvenile Justice and other Correctional Systems. American Academy of Child & Adolescent Psychiatry. Available at:https://www.aacap.org/aacap/Policy_Statements/2016/Policy_Statement_on_Transgender_Youth_in_Juvenile_Justice_and_other_Correctional_Systems.aspx. Accessed July 25, 2022.

25. Transgender and Gender Diverse Health Care in Correctional Settings. National Commission on Correctional Health Care. Available at:https://www.ncchc.org/transgender-and-gender-diverse-health-care-in-correctional-settings-2020/. Accessed July 25, 2022.
26. Child Welfare Information Gateway. (2020). How the child welfare system works. Washington, DC: U.S. Department of Health and Human Services, Administration for Children and Families, Children's Bureau.
27. Abbot, G. Letter to The Honorable Jaime Masters Commissioner. Texas Governor's Office. Available at: https://gov.texas.gov/uploads/files/press/O-MastersJaime202202221358.pdf. 2022. Accessed November 9, 2022.
28. Child welfare outcomes 2018: Report to Congress. Children's Bureau 2021; 91(156):214, 208.
29. Wilson BDM, Cooper K, Kastanis A, Nezhad S. Sexual and Gender Minority Youth in Foster Care. Williams Institute. Available at: https://williamsinstitute.law.ucla.edu/publications/sgm-youth-la-foster-care/. Published October 21, 2021. Accessed August 3, 2022.
30. Baams L, Wilson BDM, Russell ST. LGBTQ youth in unstable housing and foster care. Pediatrics 2019;143(3). https://doi.org/10.1542/PEDS.2017-4211.
31. Wilson BDM, Kastanis AA. Sexual and gender minority disproportionality and disparities in child welfare: a population-based study. Child Youth Serv Rev 2015. https://doi.org/10.1016/j.childyouth.2015.08.016.
32. Love A. A room of one's own: safe placement for transgender youth in foster care. N Y Univ Law Rev 2014;89(6):2268–300.
33. Golden RL, Oransky M. An intersectional approach to therapy with transgender adolescents and their families. Arch Sex Behav 2019;48(7):2011–25.
34. Supporting Pathways to Long-Term Success for Systems-Involved Youth: Lessons Learned. American Youth Policy Forum. 2017.
35. Forge N, Lewinson T, Garner BM, et al. "Humbling experiences": a photovoice project with sexual and gender-expansive youth experiencing homelessness. J Community Psychol 2018;46(6):806–22.

Transgender and Gender Diverse Youth in Inpatient and Other Residential Care

Jaime Stevens, MD, MPH

KEYWORDS

- Gender • Transgender • Gender diverse • Youth • Inpatient • Residential
- Psychiatry • Mental health

KEY POINTS

- TGD youth are at higher risk of more serious mental health concerns that require intensive psychiatric care.
- Inpatient and other residential care environments require special considerations for safety and can also provide unique opportunities to provide affirming care.
- Gender-positive policies, staff training, communication, placement, and programming are imperative in these settings.
- Mindful discharge planning is essential for maintaining progress achieved and supporting the positive development of TGD youth.

BACKGROUND

It is well established that transgender and gender diverse (TGD) youth experience more trauma, bullying, abuse, sexual assault and rape, home and dating violence, survival sex work, placement in juvenile confinement, negative social determinants of health (poverty, homelessness, school exclusion, and violence), higher risk of STIs and obesity, and lower family connectedness than their non-TGD peers. Many of these factors have been shown to be connected to increased depression, anxiety, suicidal ideation and attempt, and substance use rates seen in this population.[1–18]

DISCUSSION
Safety

Discrimination, verbal and physical abuse, and being recognized as transgender are all risk factors for suicidal behavior in TGD individuals,[18] and attempts to transition gender are associated with more suicidal ideation and attempts if patients are exposed to such risk factors at a young age.[19] Gender-related harassment at school

Affirming Psychiatry LLC, University of Hawai'i, PO Box 22148, Honolulu, HI 96823, USA
E-mail address: jaimestevensmd@gmail.com

Child Adolesc Psychiatric Clin N Am 32 (2023) 849–866
https://doi.org/10.1016/j.chc.2023.05.004
1056-4993/23/© 2023 Elsevier Inc. All rights reserved.

is associated with high levels of suicide attempt, worsened when teachers are the perpetrators of harassment or physical or sexual assault.[20]

This mistreatment leads to TGD youth being more likely to be placed in group care, dependency, and delinquency systems,[21] and they are more than twice as likely to access inpatient mental health care as their non TGD peers.[12]

For TGD youth in the inpatient psychiatric setting, "it is important to ensure that additional psychosocial stress is not encountered during hospitalization."[22]

Health Care Experience of Transgender and Gender Diverse Individuals

Large surveys of the United States TGD population have revealed high rates of.

- Refusal of healthcare due to gender
- Mistreatment from healthcare providers
- Harassment and violent treatment in medical settings
- Avoidance of care due to fear of disrespect, mistreatment, and discrimination related to gender identity all of which lead to poor general and mental health outcomes.[20,23–25]

These experiences have been reported not only in general medical care but also in mental health-specific treatment.[26,27] TGD youth, in particular, avoid health care due to negative experiences, fear of stigma and discrimination, concerns regarding confidentiality, and providers' inability to provide affirming care.[28]

Position of Medical Associations

Multiple medical societies support access to affirming the treatment of TGD youth,[29–34] and many oppose discrimination in accommodations, facilities, and programming.[35–39] Clinicians caring for TGD youth in these environments "have a responsibility to provide medical care that is non-judgmental and comprehensive."[33]

Scope and Limitations

Given the paucity of data regarding institutional approaches to gendered programming and facilities for TGD youth, particularly in the inpatient setting,[40] this chapter draws from published research regarding affirming care of TGD, intersex, and sexual and gender minority (SGM) youth in other clinical settings (such as primary care), best practices for the care of TGD adults, and supportive approaches to TGD youth in other environments (such as schools and detention homes). It offers clinical guidance for an organization's clinicians, administrators, educators, and advocates to provide safer care for TGD youth in facilities, to support their mental and physical health.

While these recommendations focus on facilities in which youth receive round-the-clock mental healthcare, affirming practices can be applied to other environments that affect the youth's development and community engagement, such as in intensive outpatient, partial hospitalization, group homes, shelters, extracurricular activities, and other youth programming.

Transgender and Gender Diverse Youth and Mental Health Settings

TGD children and their families are increasingly turning to mental health professionals to help explore gender.[41] However, TGD youths' first encounters with mental health services tend to be for psychosocial concerns as opposed to gender issues and typically occur prior to receiving services for gender transition.[42,43]

Regardless of chief complaint, it is the role of mental health clinicians to provide a safe and welcoming space for TGD youth to discuss, explore, and live in their gender without restriction and with support. Recognition of an individual's gender identity is "critical for the health and wellbeing of transgender people"[44] as restriction increases risk for negative psychosocial outcomes,[41] and social acceptance is associated with better mental health.[45]

What Patients Need

TGD youth report needing the following from their providers.

- Private time
- Patience and being heard
- Flexibility to appreciate their individual identity, and
- Validation that they know who they are.[46]

Recommendations from TGD youth and caregivers to health systems include mandatory training for providers/staff, protocols for the care of TGD youth, roadmaps for families, asking and recording of chosen name/pronoun, and designating a navigator for TGD patients.[47]

Multiple sources[17,43,48–56] recommend the following affirmative practices for the general healthcare of patients with TGD.

- Nondiscrimination policies and leadership commitment
- Relevant staff training
- Use of appropriate language and inclusive forms and data collection
- A welcoming physical environment and inclusive marketing
- Specific considerations for confidentiality
- Awareness of local needs and partnerships with resources
- Inclusive community outreach

These practices may be especially important in the residential or inpatient setting where interpersonal interactions with staff and other providers are extended and more intimate than in outpatient care.[57] In the inpatient psychiatric environment in particular, TGD youth recommend staff members proactively ask for a patient's preferred identifiers (instead of waiting to be told), acknowledge mistakes in identifier use, and have formal training in transgender cultural competency.[58]

Policies

Staff members in inpatient and residential care settings have a fiduciary responsibility to protect youth given limitations on patients' rights and freedoms due to their age, compounded by dependency on professionals in this restricted environment. In the United States, the absence of policies and staff training, inadequate staffing and supervision, failure to impose discipline for violating rules, using isolation as protection from abuse, and lack of functioning grievance and classification systems to protect vulnerable youth have been interpreted as deliberate indifference and failure to protect the health and safety of SGM youth and are a violation of institutional legal obligations.[59]

Non-discrimination policies protect a patient's ability to participate fully in their treatment; however governmental policy protections are subject to change and have not been shown to ameliorate the history of healthcare mistreatment and resultant avoidance by gender minority individuals.[25] Therefore, healthcare institutions must establish their own policies, practice guidance, training requirements, and accountability for the care of patients with TGD.[52]

Similar to how supportive school policies "have been shown to lower odds of bullying not only for gender diverse students but for the entire student body,"[60] supportive healthcare institutional policies may benefit not only individual patients but the entire program.

Policies should explicitly state:[14,17,48,49,51,52,55]

- A prohibition of discrimination, harassment, and bullying based on actual or perceived gender identity and expression by employees, volunteers, contract providers, youth, and visitors
- Specifics as to what types of behaviors are prohibited
- An expectation that staff models respectful language and behavior to individuals of all genders
- The requirement of staff to immediately and adequately respond to all gender-based harassment and abuse - including from patients, visitors, and colleagues
- Instructions to access a confidential system to report violations of the policy
- The requirement for any staff member to accept reports of violations from a patient or a third party on the patient's behalf
- How complaints will be investigated, resolved, and responded to in writing
- Consequences for the violation of the policy
- Prompt discipline of any staff violating the policy, including perpetrating or failing to respond to reported or witnessed harassment
- The inclusion of policy adherence in the employment evaluation process
- Protection from retaliation for reports of non-adherence to policy
- Placement, rooming, and bathroom guidelines as outlined later in discussion.
- Access to assessment and care from sex and gender specialists as outlined later in discussion.

Policies should be reviewed with staff at orientation, youth and guardians at admission, and visitors upon arrival; posted in reception and on every unit; publicized in written and digital form; and reviewed in periodic training for employees.[49,51,52,55]

Although only 1/4 of respondents in an inpatient pediatric mental health facilities survey report this, the TGD non-discrimination policy should be posted on every unit as patients may be in distress on arrival and not prepared to read or thoroughly consider policy details at the time.[40]

System-Wide Considerations

System-wide navigation and support networks may lead to positive patient outcomes. As in any health care environment, TGD youth in intensive mental health care may benefit from:[14,17,48,49,53,55,61]

- Compensated youth/family/community advisory committees to reflect on demographics and needs and make recommendations
- A staff committee, employee resource group, and/or dedicated resource professional raising awareness; supporting initiatives for affirming TGD youth care including education, advocacy, and community outreach and referrals; and providing a safe space for open dialogue
- Recruitment and hiring of gender diverse staff
- A TGD-confident provider list
- Patient navigators (including staff and/or community providers) to literally or figuratively walk patients through the logistics of their care episode
- Visits from TGD mentors and other supportive adults, in addition to affirming family members
- TGD-specific questions on patient and staff surveys

Community awareness of an organization's affirming practices may help to decrease the expectation of discrimination that contributes to minority stress. Because inpatient and residential facilities often have a larger catchment area than outpatient providers, communications - including digital and print materials - should include TGD-inclusive images and language. Inclusion of pronouns in one's introductions, e-mail signature, and webinar username should be normalized and encouraged.[49,55]

Training

Healthcare providers often lack clinical training in the care of patients with TGD [62,63] and those that are trained may be more likely to be so in the care of adults than in the care of children. In particular, mental health providers typically have not received adequate training to support younger TGD children and their families.[41] As with policy development, healthcare organizations are left to determine their own training protocols. Despite this, a study of child and adolescent inpatient psychiatric units in the United States showed only about half required education about gender diversity.[40]

Recommendations include training on the care of TGD youth with the following attributes.

Who:[43,52,57,64]
- Required of all staff (including mental and physical health care providers, nursing staff, therapists, case managers/care coordinators, volunteers, lab and x-ray staff, front desk and clerical staff, administration, health information technology, housekeeping, dietary, and maintenance staff, security, as well as all consultants and contractors), as staff members with the least clinical training often have the most direct patient contact
- Advanced training for direct care staff
- Taught by professional trainers with expertise in TGD youth

What (Content):[17,43,48,49,52,55,65]
- Agency policies
- Cultural humility
- Sex and gender diversity including intersex traits and identities; nonbinary, fluid, genderqueer, agender, and other gender identities; cultural concepts of gender such as Two Spirit, māhū, and so forth.
- Intersectional identities, experiences, challenges, and strengths including but not limited to: socioeconomic status, rural communities, structural oppression and privilege, religion and spirituality, family history (ex. historical trauma, migration, dislocation), preferred language, diverse intellectual and physical abilities, neurodiversity, body size, youth of color
- Power differential and institutional barriers
- Adolescent development and skills to meet the needs of patients at all ages and developmental levels
- Specific needs of TGD youth
- Updated/current best practices
- Culturally affirming communication with, and respectful care of, patients with TGD
- Apologizing for a mistake and/or correcting a mistake of another staff member or patient
- What constitutes discrimination and harassment
- Practice responding to unacceptable gender-based language and behaviors, including intervention with the perpetrator and reporting

- Identifying and mitigating one's internal/implicit biases, prejudices, privilege, and identifying areas for personal growth

When:[55,66]

- Prior to interacting with patients
- On a regular basis, but at least annually

Where/How:[52,55]

- Incorporated into general training for staff members
- Multi-method (for example, staff meetings and other communication can be used as reminders for appropriate behavior)

Approach and Communication

Because youth may travel to regions outside of their home communities for intensive psychiatric care and may have never been offered a safe opportunity to share their authentic identity, it may be particularly important for these environments to provide safe environments in which to do so. Staff should appreciate that some patients may have an expectation of mistreatment, a history of which is particularly prevalent in patients with TGD, and approach all from a trauma-informed perspective.

All staff should approach patients with cultural humility and the awareness that others' experiences and identities may vary from their own. Recognition of an individual's gender identity should not depend on any social or medical preconditions.[44] Staff should be aware that a patient's identity may not align with their perceived gender expression for a variety of reasons, including, but not limited to safety, resources, and fluidity. A patient's gender identity should not be assumed from their appearance, mannerisms, or other personal expressions; sexual orientation; family, community, or religious background; or other demographic factor.[55] A patient whose appearance is consistent with the societal or regional expectations of their sex assigned at birth should not be presumed to be cisgender, and conversely, one whose presentation is expansive should not be presumed to identify as TGD.[67,68]

Gender neutral pronouns should be used both with the patient and with colleagues until the patient makes their pronouns known.[53,69] Introductions should demonstrate a welcoming environment by routinely asking all patients for the appropriate use of their current name and pronouns.[43,48] Current name and pronouns should be shared among all staff and used consistently regardless of identity documents or court records.[17,48] In fact, research has demonstrated the use of chosen name "has the potential to reduce depressive symptoms, suicidal ideation, and suicidal behavior" in TGD youth.[70]

All patients should be asked about any needs regarding their gender identity or expression. This should include ascertaining the patient's wishes regarding the use of name and pronouns in communications with those outside the facility, including parents and guardians, regardless of others' opinions of the patient's gender.[17,51] Finally, staff should refrain from asking a patient about their physical characteristics, anatomy, or surgical history, except as medically necessary.[17]

Registration, medical records, and data

Registration
Registration should include a routine, but voluntary, opportunity for all patients to identify their gender identity.[51,55,57] Patients may feel more comfortable sharing personal identification information on forms as opposed to verbally to staff.[43] This may be especially true for youth who are accompanied by an adult to whom they have not disclosed their gender; thus all forms should contain inclusive, gender-neutral language.[55]

Name and gender marker on insurance and legal documents should be noted in a private process. While true for all TGD individuals, as minors, TGD youth may have had fewer resources and opportunities to update these to reflect their true identity.[48,51,52]

Medical Records

TGD youth in inpatient settings have noted the importance of the integration of current name and pronouns into all hospital information systems, for example, on wristbands, medication administration records, census, and kitchen and dietary services, to ensure consistency in affirming care.[51,55,58]

Data

"The authentic experiences, strengths, and needs of transgender and nonbinary youth have been essentially erased from science and from the health research evidence base."[71]

Providing opportunities to share gender information benefits not only the individual patient, but can aid in program development, quality improvement, and ultimately identify and address disparities in the health of TGD youth.[43,55]

Confidentiality

Differences between a patient's assigned name, pronouns, and gender and those in use should be kept confidential, as failure to do so deprives youth of their autonomy and may expose them to harassment.[72] Since patients may identify differently in different settings, patients with TGD should be asked which name and pronouns should be used in communications with those outside the milieu.[17,49,57,73]

It is essential for the provider and institutional billing department to know and share with patients local laws related to disclosure, including parental or guardian access to medical records.[17]

ENVIRONMENT

The Transgender Law Center suggests decreasing the risk of violence by "providing a multigendered environment in which transgender and gender non-conforming people do not automatically stand out simply because of their gender expression or presentation."[74]

Recommendations for a welcoming physical space in outpatient clinics apply to residential and inpatient care settings as well and may lower stress and anxiety for patients. These include:[43,49,52,53,55,57]

- Waiting rooms, reception, and units with Safe Zone and Hate Free Space signs
- Gender diverse posters, artwork, pamphlets, magazines, and health information materials
- Gender neutral bathrooms with a policy that patients, staff, and visitors can use restrooms that reflect their gender identity
- Gender neutral and gender-affirming rewards and recreational and creative activities
- Opportunities for staff to demonstrate support of gender diversity in their workspace (for example with a safe space sticker) and attire (such as on a pin)

Placement

Residential and inpatient services are more likely than outpatient settings to be segregated by sex or gender. These often include only binary options, which may cause extra stress for those who are fluid or nonbinary.[57] TGD youth should ideally be offered treatment in a mixed-gender program to decrease the risk of the harassment and violence associated with gender-segregated placements.[52]

If unavailable, a TGD youth should be offered facilities and programming consistent with their gender identity as opposed to their anatomy or identity documents.[17,43,51,68] Failure to do so may compromise confidentiality, compound stigma and discrimination associated with negative mental and physical health problems, and is contrary to appropriate medical treatment.[15,35,39,75]

Units and rooming

When units, floors, or rooms are segregated by gender, youth should be offered assignment consistent with their gender identity,[51,56] and involved in determining where they would be safest and best supported.[17]

Twenty four percent of staff respondents to a United States survey on inpatient psychiatric care reported their institution required TGD youth patients to room with another TGD patient or use a private room when others had roommates.[40] TGD youth should not be automatically assigned to or pressured to choose a private room as this contributes to stigma and discrimination associated with negative health consequences.[17,75]

Conversely, if a TGD patient requests a private room, this should be granted. If unavailable, the patient should be placed in an empty multiple-bed room. This may involve the movement of other patients, which is acceptable as long as this does not compromise the health or safety of the patient(s) being relocated.[51,52]

Bath, toilet, dressing, and locker rooms

TGD individuals experience high rates of harassment and physical assault in gender-segregated bathrooms,[76] and many TGD youth are prevented access to school bathrooms and locker rooms consistent with their gender identity.[77] One study showed restroom/dressing room use to be one of the top five concerns for both TGD youth and their parents.[9]

Multiple healthcare organizations and hospital recommendations suggest TGD youth should have access to bathrooms and locker rooms consistent with their gender identity.[51,75] As with room assignments, forcing TGD youth to use separate or private restrooms is stigmatizing and detrimental to their health, but this should be an option if the patient chooses for their safety and privacy.[52,56,75] If single user facilities are desired but not available, TGD youth may be offered alternate times to use multiple user facilities in private.[17]

Safety

When contraband searches are indicated, staff should take into consideration that TGD youth may have more discomfort with undressing than non-TGD youth and are at high risk of exploitation during these procedures.[52]

Patient rights

Sharing the non-discrimination policy with all patients and guardians prior to admission "lets all patients know that the program will expect them to be tolerant of diversity."[57] Patients and/or guardians concerned about the presence of a fellow patient with different anatomy or other sex characteristics may be counseled on patient rights, standards of care, and expectations of appropriate dress and behavior on the unit.[52,78,79] If needed, the patient with concerns or concerned guardians may be moved. Concerns from others do not constitute grounds for changing a TGD patient's rooming or facility use.[51]

Facilities have an obligation to stop any bullying or harassment, including gender-based harassment by staff, visitors, or another patient. The offender should be segregated or moved as opposed to the targeted patient.[52] If unsafe to do so, the targeted patient may be moved.[51]

Psychiatric and Medical Assessments

TGD patients admitted to a psychiatric unit may not yet have had a safe opportunity to disclose their gender identity or express their true gender. A mental healthcare facility in which they are separated from their environment of origin may be the first chance for them to do so.

Conversely, other TGD youth may be open about and supported in their identities and simply require continued affirming care.

Psychiatric assessment

In conducting an initial psychiatric evaluation, it is important to recognize that a TGD patient's current mental health concerns may be primarily, partially, or entirely unrelated to their gender. A patient's gender should be neither ignored nor a forced topic of focus.[80] Care for TGD adolescents should take a holistic approach that includes cultural, economic, psychosocial, sexual, and spiritual influences on health.[42]

As in the outpatient setting, psychiatrists should consider the possibility of TGD patient's internalization of harmful views of TGD individuals, as well as marginalization, isolation, potential stressors of concealing one's identity, or exposure to harmful policies or inadequate resources.[25,42]

In the trauma assessment, history of medical trauma and gender change efforts should be ascertained, as these are associated with psychiatric symptoms.[81–83]

TGD youth have a high incidence of safety concerns at home and in school, and because intolerance leads to negative determinants of health, the inpatient or residential setting offers a unique and important opportunity to assess these environments separately from unaffirming individuals. If there is a concern, providers should be prepared to advocate for TGD youth prior to their discharge and offer this advocacy to patients.[18,56,77]

Medical assessment

Whether the medical history and physical examination are performed by the psychiatrist or a primary care consultant, patients should receive gender-informed care. The presence or absence of certain organs or physiologic processes should not be assumed and medical history forms should not include a "female only" or "male only" designation on questions.

For patients with pre-pubertal TGD, anticipatory guidance around natal puberty may be indicated, especially if patients have not yet discussed these with their primary care provider.

Providers should be aware of the possibility of pain or rash related to binding or tucking and be prepared with resources to support physical health if patients are using specific undergarments for this.

Patients requiring screening or care of the chest or genitourinary system during their stay should be asked their preferred terms for this anatomy[84] and about comfort around examinations. Preferred terms should be used, and providers should advocate for patient preferences if possible (eg, self-sampling of cervical cells).

For patients at risk of undesired pregnancy (in themselves or their partner[s]) or menses, providers should be prepared to discuss options for prophylaxis or suppression, respectively, and aid in facilitating access to these before discharge. For those who have not previously had a safe space to ask questions regarding puberty blockers and/or hormone therapies, providers should be prepared to discuss these and make appropriate referrals.[43]

Clinicians should be aware of potential side effects and specific monitoring requirements of any hormonal interventions for patients on gender-affirming medical treatment prior to admission.[7]

Programming

"Programs are more effective and sustainable when young people are partners in the programs' design, development, operations, and evaluation."[49]

Healthcare associations support gender-affirming access not only to facilities but also to activities and programming.[75] As in schools,[77,85] it is important to avoid.

- Needlessly separating youth by gender
- Holding those of different genders to different rules or standards
- Enforcing "traditional" gender norms

Gender-segregated activities should be limited to activities in which this is essential for health and wellbeing. In those situations, patients should participate consistent with their gender identity.

Dress codes, rules regarding grooming, makeup, and haircut, styling, and removal, and access to grooming and personal items should be universal and consistent for all genders.[17,49,51,52] Patients should be allowed to use personal items that assist gender expression, such as those used in binding, padding, and tucking, as much as this can be safely arranged on the unit.[17,51,52] Youth, who may have fewer financial freedoms to purchase these items, may require assistance in obtaining them.

TGD youth are at risk for feelings of fear and isolation, and care in an inpatient or residential facility may compound this. Unit programming may include education about intersectional identities and understanding the harms of harassment and bias.[52] Organizational acknowledgment and events for Transgender Day of Remembrance, Pride, and National Coming Out Day may help patients to feel supported while unable to participate in their home communities.[49,55]

Gender-Related Medical Care

Living fully in one's gender "is often a critically important part of treatment" for TGD youth. Those who do not experience higher levels of anxiety and depression than non-TGD youth, whereas those who have transitioned experience similar levels of these mental health concerns.[45,75] To avoid iatrogenic harm, all aspects of gender-affirming treatment started prior to admission should be continued in an inpatient or residential setting.[17,43,52]

For patients whose gender identity is still in development, the inpatient or residential care environment can and should provide an opportunity to explore gender identity and expression in a supportive and safe environment.

TGD youth requiring access to gender-related care should be provided with such treatment regardless of the care environment, including foster, group, detention, or other facility type.[86] This includes assessment for any indicated medical treatment and arrangements to receive this care.[51,52] Accordingly, facilities should have procedures for youth to confidentially request and receive care from medical providers competent in gender-affirming treatment.[17]

Health care providers are often legally obligated to obtain informed consent from a parent or guardian before the medical treatment of a youth; however, jurisdictions vary as to who has the right to consent, when, under what circumstances, and how to proceed should multiple guardians disagree.[87] Therefore, all medical providers on the care team should be aware of the region's legal requirements regarding guardianship and consent and have a relationship with the organization's legal counsel to ensure appropriate treatment. When necessary, the care team should assist a youth in obtaining consent for recommended treatment from a guardian or the court.[17,52,88]

Disposition

Acute residential care has been shown to significantly improve psychiatric symptoms in TGD youth but has not been shown to be sufficient enough to decrease symptom severity to the level of their non-TGD peers, highlighting the importance of discharge care planning for these patients.[89]

Often dependent on others for basic needs, some youth will be discharged to a supportive environment of origin, while others may be expected to return to an unaffirming situation or one altogether unknown.[42] As lack of support or safety issues in a patient's home or community may have been a major factor in a TGD youth requiring an intensive level of care in the first place, discharge planning should include ascertaining any concerns from the patient and determining a safe living and social environment.[42,56,58] With patient consent, team members can offer to meet with families, schools, outpatient providers, and community members to provide education on gender, ways to affirm and support a TGD youth after discharge, and peer and professional resources related to their respective role.[7,28,51]

Patients with TGD are at risk of discontinuation of mental health treatment if that care exposes them to negative experiences around gender identity,[80] so it is essential the patient's mental health follow-up is with safe and informed providers. Prior to discharge providers should work with the team to ensure:[17,42,49]

- Follow-up care is scheduled with affirming health care providers, therapists, agencies, and community organizations
- Gender-affirming health insurance/coverage is established (see transhealthproject. org)
- An adequate supply of all medications, including hormones or GnRH agonists, if indicated

When a youth is compelled to be discharged to a rejecting or unsafe environment despite the advocacy of the treatment team, planning should explicitly address harm reduction options. TGD youth disproportionately find themselves homeless due to a rejecting or unsafe living environment.[52] Shelters with inappropriate policies around gender-segregated placement increase risk for violence against TGD individuals, leaving many TGD youth at risk for living on the street without food or health care and can result in survival sex work, exploitation, and arrest.[20,90] Discussion of controlled disclosure is particularly important for youth whose gender expression may be considered incongruent with their anatomy, as they have limited access to affirming surgery and may be at risk of harm if discovered.[42]

Mindful discharge planning for TGD youth is imperative to prevent the development or recurrence of a serious psychiatric or safety concern and readmission.

SUMMARY

TGD youth are disproportionately exposed to stressors that may contribute to the more severe mental health symptoms and higher rate of safety concerns seen in this population. These circumstances require higher levels of psychiatric care and TGD youth are overrepresented in inpatient psychiatric treatment.

In the absence of standards of care for TGD youth in intensive psychiatric facilities, the recommendations above draw from guidelines in the care of adjacent populations to minimize harm and maximize the benefits of treatment in this unique environment.

CLINICS CARE POINTS

- TGD youth are at higher risk of more serious mental health concerns that require intensive psychiatric care.
- Inpatient and other intensive residential care environments require special considerations for safety and unique opportunities to provide affirming care.
- Gender-positive policies, staff training, communication, placement, and programming are imperative in these settings.
- Mindful discharge planning is essential for maintaining progress achieved and supporting the positive development of TGD youth.

DISCLOSURE

Dr J. Stevens has no commercial or financial conflicts of interest or any funding sources related to this chapter.

REFERENCES

1. 2018 Gender-Expansive Youth Report. Human Rights Campaign. Available at: https://www.hrc.org/resources/2018-gender-expansive-youth-report.
2. Baams L. Disparities for LGBTQ and gender nonconforming adolescents. Pediatrics 2018;141(5):e20173004.
3. Becerra-Culqui TA. Mental health of transgender and gender nonconforming youth Compared with their peers. J Adolesc Health 2017;61(5):642–8.
4. de Vries AL, Doreleijers TA, Steensma TD, et al. Psychiatric comorbidity in gender dysphoric adolescents. J Child Psychol Psychiatry 2011;52(11):1195–202.
5. Eisenberg ME, Gower AL, McMorris BJ, et al. Risk and protective factors in the lives of transgender/gender nonconforming adolescents. J Adolesc Health 2017;61:521–6.
6. Grossman AH, D'Augelli AR. Transgender youth and life-threatening behaviors. Suicide Life Threat Behav 2007;37(5):527–37.
7. Guss C, Shumer D, Katz-Wise SL. Transgender and gender nonconforming adolescent care: psychosocial and medical considerations. Curr Opin Pediatr 2015;26(4):421–6.
8. Kimberly LL, Folkers KM, Friesen P, et al. Ethical issues in gender-affirming care for youth. Pediatrics 2018;142(6):e20181537.
9. Lawlis SM, Donkin HR, Bates JR, et al. Health concerns of transgender and gender nonconforming youth and their parents upon presentation to a transgender clinic. J Adolesc Health 2017;61(5):642–8. https://doi.org/10.1016/j.jadohealth.2017.05.025.
10. National Survey on LGBTQ Youth Mental Health. The Trevor Project. Available at: https://www.thetrevorproject.org/wp-content/uploads/2021/05/The-Trevor-Project-National-Survey-Results-2021.pdf.

11. Perry JR, Frazer S. On all sides: how Race & gender influence health risk for transgender students of color. Advocates for Youth; 2020. Available at: https://actionnetwork.org/forms/on-all-sides.

12. Reisner SL, Vetters R, Leclerc M, et al. Mental health of transgender youth in care at an adolescent urban community health center: a matched retrospective cohort study. J Adolesc Health 2015;56(3):274–9.

13. Swaner R, Labriola M, Rempel M, et al. Youth Involvement in the sex trade: a National study. Center for Court Innovation; 2016. Available at: https://www.ojp.gov/pdffiles1/ojjdp/grants/249952.pdf.

14. Tobin V, Bockting WO, Hughes TL. Mental health Promotion for gender minority adolescents. J Psychosoc Nurs Ment Health Serv 2018;56(12):22–30.

15. Toomey RB, Ryan C, Diaz RM, et al. Gender-nonconforming lesbian, gay, bisexual, and transgender youth: school victimization and young adult psychosocial adjustment. Dev Psychol 2010;46(6):1580–9.

16. Turban JL, Ehrensaft D. Research Review: gender identity in youth: treatment paradigms and controversies. J Child Psychol Psychiatry 2018;59(12):1228–43.

17. Wilber S, Szanyi J. Model policy: transgender, gender Nonconforming and intersex youth in confinement facilities. National Center for Lesbian Rights and Center for Children's Law and Policy; 2019. Available at: https://www.nclrights.org/wp-content/uploads/2019/05/TGNCI-Model-Policy.pdf.

18. Winter S., Diamond M., Green J., et al., Transgender people: health at the margins of society, Lancet, 388 (10042), 2016, 390–400. Available at: https://www.thelancet.com/journals/lancet/article/PIIS0140-6736(16)00683-8/fulltext#.

19. Turban JL, Beckwith N, Reisner SL, et al. Association between Recalled exposure to gender identity conversion efforts and Psychological distress and suicide attempts among transgender adults. JAMA Psychiatr 2020;77(1):68–76.

20. Grant J.M., Mottet L.A., Tannis J., et al., Injustice at every Turn: a report of the National transgender discrimination survey. National Center for Transgender Equality and National Gay and Lesbian Task Force. 2011. Available at: https://www.thetaskforce.org/injustice-every-turn-report-national-transgender-discrimination-survey/.

21. Majd K, Marksamer J, Reyes C. Hidden Injustice: lesbian, gay, bisexual, and transgender youth in juvenile courts. Legal services for children. National Juvenile Defender Center, and National Center for Lesbian Rights; 2014. Available at: https://www.nclrights.org/wp-content/uploads/2014/06/hidden_injustice.pdf.

22. Alastanos JN, Mullen S. Psychiatric admission in adolescent transgender patients: a case series. Ment Health Clin 2018;7(4):172–5.

23. James S., Herman J., Rankin S., et al., The report of the 2015 US transgender survey. 2016. Available at: https://transequality.org/sites/default/files/docs/usts/USTS-Full-Report-Dec17.pdf.

24. Cruz TM. Assessing access to care for transgender and gender nonconforming people: a consideration of diversity in combating discrimination. Soc Sci Med 2014;110:65–73. Available at: http://www.sciencedirect.com/science/article/pii/S0277953614002111.

25. Clark KD, Luong S, Lunn MR, et al. Healthcare mistreatment, state level policy protections, and healthcare avoidance among gender minority people. Sex Res Soc Policy 2022. https://doi.org/10.1007/s13178-022-00748-1.

26. White BP, Fontenot HB. Transgender and non-conforming persons' mental healthcare experiences: an integrative review. Arch Psychiatr Nurs 2019;33:203–10.

27. Panchal A, Piper C, Whitmore C, et al. Providing supportive transgender mental health care: a systemized narrative review of patient experiences, presferences, and outcomes. J Gay Lesbian Mental Health 2002;26(3):228–64.

28. Call DC, Challa M, Telingator CJ. Providing affirmative care to transgender and gender diverse youth: disparities, interventions, and outcomes. Curr Psychiatry Rep 2021;23(6):33. https://doi.org/10.1007/s11920-021-01245-9.

29. AACAP Statement Responding to Efforts to ban Evidence-Based Care for Transgender and Gender Diverse Youth. 2019. Available at: https://www.aacap.org/AACAP/Latest_News/AACAP_Statement_Responding_to_Efforts-to_ban_Evidence-Based_Care_for_Transgender_and_Gender_Diverse.aspx.

30. Position Statement on treatment of transgender (Trans) and gender diverse youth. American Psychiatric Association; 2020. Available at: https://www.psychiatry.org/File%20Library/About-APA/Organization-Documents-Policies/Policies/Position-Transgender-Gender-Diverse-Youth.pdf.

31. Frontline Physicians Oppose Legislation That Interferes in or Penalizes Patient Care. American Academy of Family Physicians, American Academy of Pediatrics, American College of Physicians, American College of Obstetricians and Gynecologists, American Osteopathic Association. 2021. Available at: https://www.aap.org/en/news-room/news-releases/aap/2021/frontline-physicians-oppose-legislation-that-interferes-in-or-penalizes-patient-care/.

32. Madara JL. Letter from the CEO and Executive Vice President of the American medical association to Bill McBride, Executive director. National Governors Association; 2021. https://www.ama-assn.org/press-center/press-releases/ama-states-stop-interfering-health-care-transgender-children.

33. Recommendations for promoting the health and well-being of lesbian, gay, bisexual, and transgender adolescents: a position paper of the Society for Adolescent Health and Medicine. J Adolesc Health 2013;52(4):506–10. https://doi.org/10.1016/j.jadohealth.2013.01.015.

34. The Pediatric Endocrine Society Opposes Bills that Harm Transgender Youth. 2021. Available at: https://pedsendo.org/news-announcements/the-pediatric-endocrine-society-opposes-bills-that-harm-transgender-youth-2/.

35. Access to basic human services for transgender individuals H-65.964. American Medical Association; 2017.

36. APA Resolution on opposing discriminatory laws, policies, and practices Aimed at LGBTQ+ Persons. American Psychological Association; 2020. https://www.apa.org/about/policy/resolution-opposing-discriminatory-laws.pdf.

37. Rafferty J. Ensuring comprehensive care and support for transgender and gender-diverse children and adolescents. Pediatrics 2018;142(4):e20182162.

38. WPATH/USPATH Statement on the Bills Barring Trans Girls from Sports. 2021. Available at: https://www.wpath.org/media/cms/Documents/Public%20Policies/2021/WPATH%20_%20USPATH%20Statement%20on%20the%20Bills%20Barring%20Trans%20Girls%20from%20Sports.pdf?_t=1617217300.

39. Yarbrough E. Position Statement on discrimination against transgender and gender diverse individuals. APA Caucus of LGBTQ Psychiatrists and the Council on Minority Mental Health and Health Disparities; 2018.

40. Halloran J, Szilagyi N, Stevens J, et al. Assessment of transgender/gender-expansive Accessibility in inpatient pediatric mental health facilities. Transgender Health 2022. https://doi.org/10.1089/trgh.2021.0124.

41. Keo-Meier CE, Ehrensaft DE. Introduction to the gender affirmative model. In: The gender affirmative model: an interdisciplinary approach to supporting

transgender and gender expansive children. Washington DC: American Psychological Association; 2018. p. 3–19.

42. de Vries ALC, Cohen-Kettenis PT, Delemarre-Van de Waal H, et al. Caring for transgender adolescents in BC: Suggested guidelines. Vancouver Coastal health. Transcend Transgender Support & Education Society, and the Canadian Rainbow Health Coalition; 2006. Available at: http://www.vch.ca/transhealth.

43. UCSF Gender Affirming Health Program, Department of Family and Community Medicine, University of California San Francisco. Guidelines for the primary and gender-affirming care of transgender and gender nonbinary people. 2nd edition. Deutsch MB; 2016. transcare.ucsf.edu/guidelines.

44. Winter S, Settle E, Wylie K, et al. Synergies in health and human rights: a call to action to improve transgender health. Lancet 2016;388(10042):318–21.

45. Olson KR, Durwood L, DeMeules M, et al. Mental health of transgender children who are supported in their identities. Pediatrics 2016;137(3):e20153223.

46. Hawkins LA. Gender identity development among transgender youth: a qualitative analysis of contributing factors. Dev Psychol 2010;71(2–A):666.

47. Gridley SJ, Crouch JM, Evans Y, et al. Youth and caregiver perspectives on barriers to gender-affirming health care for transgender youth. J Adolesc Health 2016;59(3):254–61.

48. Affirmative services for transgender and gender diverse people: best practices for Frontline health care staff. National LGBT Health Education Center, Fenway Institute; 2020. Available at: https://www.lgbtqiahealtheducation.org/publication/affirmative-services-for-transgender-and-gender-diverse-people-best-practices-for-frontline-health-care-staff/.

49. Butler A. Creating safer spaces for LGBTQ youth: a Toolkit for education, Healthcare,and community-based organizations. Advocates for youth; 2020. Available at: https://www.advocatesforyouth.org/resources/curricula-education/creating-safer-spaces-for-lgbtq-youth/.

50. Community Standards of Practice For Provision of Quality Health Care Services For Gay, Lesbian, Bisexual And Transgendered Clients. GLBT Health Access Project. Available at: http://www.glbthealth.org/CommunityStandardsofPractice.htm.

51. Creating Equal access to quality health care for transgender patients: transgender affirming hospital policies. Lambda Legal; 2016. Available at: https://www.lambdalegal.org/publications/fs_transgender-affirming-hospital-policies?gclid=EAlaIQobChMI1uO3vY2k-QIVZsLCBB0_NgEQEAAYASAAEgLw_fD_BwE.

52. Marksamer J, Spade D, Arkles G. A place of Respect: a Guide for group care facilities serving transgender and gender non-conforming youth. National Center for Lesbian Rights, Sylvia Rivera Law Project; 2011. Available at: https://www.nclrights.org/wp-content/uploads/2013/07/A_Place_Of_Respect.pdf.

53. McClain Z, Hawkins LA, Yehia BR. Creating welcoming spaces for lesbian, gay, bisexual, and transgender (LGBT) patients: an evaluation of the health care environment. J Homosex 2016;63(3):387–93.

54. Redfern JS, Sinclair B. Improving health care encounters and communication with transgender patients. J Commun Healthc 2014;7(1):25–40.

55. Advancing effective communication, cultural competence, and patient- and family-Centered care for the lesbian, gay, bisexual, and transgender (LGBT) community: a Field Guide. Oak Brook, IL: The Joint Commission; 2011. LGBTFieldGuide.pdf.

56. Wilber S, Ryan C, Marksamer J. Best practice guidelines: Serving LGBT youth in out-of-home care. Child Welfare League of America; 2006. Available at: https://www.nclrights.org/get-help/resource/child-welfare-league-of-america-cwla-best-practice-guidelines-serving-lgbt-youth-in-out-of-home-care/.

57. Walton HM, Baker SL. Treating transgender individuals in inpatient and residential mental health settings. Cognit Behav Pract 2019;26(4):592–602.

58. Acosta W, Qayyum Z, Turban JL, et al. Identify, engage, Understand: supporting transgender youth in an inpatient psychiatric hospital. Psychiatr Q 2019;90(3): 601–12.

59. RG et al v. Koller et al. United States District Court for the District of Hawai'i. Civil No. 05-566 JMS/LEK. June 15, 2006.

60. Gower AL, Forster M, Gloppen K, et al. School practices to foster LGBT-supportive Climate: associations with adolescent bullying Involvement. Prev Sci 2018;19: 813–21.

61. Madrigal C. Improving LGBTQ+ patient outcomes Utilizing navigation and support networks across hospital systems. New Orleans, LA: GLMA Health Professionals Advancing LGBTQ Equality; 2020.

62. Vance SR, Halpern-Felsher BL, Rosenthal SM. Health care providers' comfort with and barriers to care of transgender youth. J Adolesc Health 2015;56:251–3.

63. LGBT Health Readiness Assessments in Health Centers. Key Findings. National LGBT health education Center. Fenway Institute; 2017. Available at: https://www.lgbtqiahealtheducation.org/wp-content/uploads/2017/11/LGBT-Health-Readiness-Assessment-Key-Findings.pdf.

64. Reisner S. Meeting the Health Care Needs of Transgender People. Available at: https://www.lgbtqiahealtheducation.org/wp-content/uploads/Sari-slides_final1.pdf.

65. Hollenbach AD, Eckstrand KL, Dreger A, editors. Implementing curricular and institutional climate changes to improve health care for individuals who are LGBT, gender nonconforming, or born with DSD: a resource for medical educators. Association of American Medical Colleges; 2014.

66. Kidd JD, Bockting W, Cabaniss DL, et al. Special-"T" training: extended follow-up results from a Residency-wide professionalism Workshop on transgender health. Acad Psychiatry 2016;40(5):802–6.

67. Cicero EC, Wesp LM. Supporting the health and well-being of transgender students. J Sch Nurs 2017;33(2):95–108.

68. World Professional Association for Transgender Health. Standards of Care for the Health of Transsexual, Transgender, and Gender Nonconforming People 7th Version. 2012. Available at: https://www.wpath.org/publications/soc.

69. Providing Affirmative Care for Patients with Non-Binary Gender Identities. National LGBT Health Education Center, Fenway Institute. Available at: https://www.lgbtqiahealtheducation.org/wp-content/uploads/2017/02/Providing-Affirmative-Care-for-People-with-Non-Binary-Gender-Identities.pdf.

70. Russell ST, Pollitt AM, Li G, et al. Chosen name Use is Linked to reduced depressive symptoms, suicidal ideation, and suicidal behavior among transgender youth. J Adolesc Health Off Publ Soc Adolesc Med 2018;63(4):503–5.

71. Dixon M., Hawke L.D., Relihan J., et al., Let's Talk gender: Ten Things transgender and nonbinary youth want all Researchers to know, JAACAP, 61 (8), 2022, 963.

72. American Academy of pediatrics opposes Legislation that Discriminates against transgender children. American Academy of Pediatrics 2016. Available at: https://www.aap.org/en-us/about-the-aap/aap-pressroom/Pages/AAPOpposes LegislationAgainstTransgenderChildren.aspx.

73. Practice Parameter on gay, lesbian, or bisexual sexual orientation, gender Nonconformity, and gender Discordance in children and adolescents. JAACAP 2012;51(9):957–74.

74. Peeing in Peace: a resource Guide for transgender Activists and Allies. Transgender Law Center; 2005. Available at: http://transgenderlawcenter.org/wp-content/uploads/2012/05/94930982-PIP-Resource-Guide.pdf.

75. Brief of Amici Curiae American Academy of Pediatrics, American Medical Association, American Psychiatric Association, and 10 Other Medical, Nursing, Mental Health, and Other Health Care Organizations in support of defendants-appellees. Joel Doe, a minor, et al v. Boyertown area school district, et al. US court of appeals for the 3rd circuit. No. 17-3113. 2018.

76. Herman JL. Gendered restrooms and minority stress: the public Regulation of gender and its Impact on transgender People's lives. J Public Management & Social Policy 2013;19(1):65.

77. Kosciw JG, Clark CM, Truong NL, et al. The 2019 National School Climate Survey: the experiences of lesbian, gay, bisexual, transgender, and queer youth in our nation's schools. GLSEN; 2020. Available at: https://www.glsen.org/research/2019-national-school-climate-survey.

78. Maza C, Brinker L. 15 Experts Debunk Right-Wing Transgender Bathroom Myth. Media Matters for America. March 19, 2014. Available at: https://www.mediamatters.org/sexual-harassment-sexual-assault/15-experts-debunk-right-wing-transgender-bathroom-myth.

79. Samar VJ. The right to privacy and the right to Use the bathroom consistent with one's gender identity. Duke J Gender Law and Policy 2016;24:33. https://scholarship.law.duke.edu/cgi/viewcontent.cgi?article=1312&context=djglp.

80. Simeonov D, Steele LS, Anderson S, et al. Perceived sarisfaction with mental health services in the lesbian, gay, bisexual, transgender, and traanssexual communities in Ontario, Canada: an internet-based survey. Canadian J Community Mental Health 2015;34(1):31–44.

81. APA Resolution on gender identity change efforts. American Psychological Association; 2021. Available at: https://www.apa.org/about/policy/resolution-gender-identity-change-efforts.pdf.

82. Substance Abuse and Mental Health Services Administration, Ending Conversion Therapy: Supporting and Affirming LGBTQ Youth. HHS Publication No. (SMA) 15-4928. Rockville, MD: Substance Abuse and Mental Health Services Administration, 2015. Available at: http://store.samhsa.gov/shin/content/SMA15-4928/SMA15-4928.pdf.

83. Fish JN, Russel ST. Sexual orientation and gender identity change efforts are Unethical and harmful. Am J Public Health 2020;110(8):1113–4.

84. Ragosta S., Obedin-Maliver J., Fix L., et al., From 'Shark-Week' to 'Mangina': an analysis of Words used by people of marginalized sexual orientations and/or gender identities to Replace Common sexual and Reproductive health terms, Health Equity, 5 (1), 2021, 707–717.

85. Model school District policy on transgender and gender Nonconforming students: Model language, Commentary, & resources. GLSEN, National Center for Transgender Equality; 2018. Available at: https://transequality.org/sites/default/files/images/resources/trans_school_district_model_policy_FINAL.pdf.

86. Anton BS. Proceedings of the American Psychological association for the legislative year 2008: Minutes of the annual meeting of the Council of Representatives. Am Psychol 2009;64:372–453. Available at: https://www.apa.org/about/policy/transgender.pdf.

87. Stiff M. Breaking Down barriers: an Administrator's Guide to state law & best policy practice for LGBT healthcare access. HRC Foundation; 2010. Available at:

https://lavenderhealth.files.wordpress.com/2013/12/administrators-guide-for-lgbt-healthcare-access.pdf.

88. Ikuta E. Overcoming the parental veto: how transgender adolescents can access puberty-Suppressing hormone treatment in the absence of parental consent under the mature minor Doctrine. South Calif Interdiscipl Law J 2016;25:179–228.

89. Silveri MM, Schuttenberg EM, Schmandt K, et al. Clinical outcomes following Acute residential psychiatric treatment in transgender and gender diverse adolescents. JAMA Netw Open 2021;4(6):e2113637.

90. Rooney C, Durso LE, Gruberg S. Discrimination against transgender Women Seeking access to homeless shelters. DC: Center for American Progress; 2016. Available at: https://www.americanprogress.org/issues/lgbt/report/2016/01/07/128323/discriminationagainst-transgender-women-seeking-access-to-homelessshelters/.

Puberty for Transgender Kids and Their Parents
Impressions from a Mom

Justine Larson, MD, MPH

KEYWORDS

• Gender • Lived experience • Family

KEY POINTS

• Decision making around medical interventions for families of transgender adolescents can be challenging.
• Puberty is a difficult time for adolescents, and uniquely so for transgender adolescents.
• Listening to the perspectives of family members and youth can help a child and adolescent psychiatrist gain insights into the patients they serve.

I am a parent of a transgender adolescent boy who transitioned at the age of 11 years. As I've written previously,[1] I've felt many emotions over the past 5 years: denial, grief, confusion, resolution, and pride. Throughout this article, I will refer to my son as "he," even though before he transitioned at the age of 11 years, we had referred to him as "she." In addition, for the purposes of this article, I have changed his name for privacy purposes. It should be noted that he is supportive of my writing about our experiences.

Puberty is an awkward word for many parents and adolescents. From my work as a child and adolescent psychiatrist, I know that for many adolescents, growing breasts, hair popping out in different places, having your voice crack—all of that can be stressful and embarrassing at the best of times. But what about for parents and kids when the child is transgender? Most children hope that going through puberty will be a private enterprise. Most tweens cringe at the idea of their parent talking to them about getting a bra, for example, or the logistics of their periods. For transgender kids and their families, puberty can be even more complicated.

PUBERTY WAS A CRISIS

Before puberty began, my son, Ian, seemed relatively happy being a girl that people commonly saw as a boy, at least from my limited perspective. He dressed in boys' clothes, and people frequently accidentally referred to him as "he" when he was still known as "she." If you had asked me then, I would probably have described him as

Sheppard Pratt, 4915 Aspen Hill Road, Rockville, MD 20852, USA

Child Adolesc Psychiatric Clin N Am 32 (2023) 867–871
https://doi.org/10.1016/j.chc.2023.05.005
1056-4993/23/© 2023 Elsevier Inc. All rights reserved.

a girl who was kind of a tom boy and who sometimes dressed like a boy and was interested in typically boy-ish things like running around, climbing trees, and jumping off tree stumps.

When puberty hit, however, he became despondent. He told me later that before puberty, he "didn't realize he was that different" from boys. He actually liked it when people mistook him for a boy.

"I'm a boy," he insisted, at the age of 11.

At first, I did not fully understand what he was saying or how to respond, despite my training as a child and adolescent psychiatrist. Was he transgender? Was this something that would be sustained? I was scared and confused.

Thinking back on it, I see that part of what was driving his sense of urgency at that time was the aversive experience of his changing body. Later, he admitted to me that he'd been using duct tape to tape his breasts, causing his skin to break down. As I struggled to understand, he put it this way: "If I get my period, that will be the end for me." As we were learning about our options, Ian told my husband that he would rather "live on the streets" than have to get his period.

One hears from transgender youth that having their body develop in a way that is not consistent with their sense of their own gender is simply horrible to the point of being unbearable. I have not experienced it myself, but when one considers the ends to which kids will go to "correct" and avoid these bodily changes, one can get a sense of how awful it must be.

Have you wanted to escape something so badly that you'd rather die than experience it? Have you ever chosen to be homeless instead of living in a place where you must live with your body being a certain way?

For transgender youth, additional factors contribute to negative outcomes like suicidal ideation and homelessness. They face outright rejection for simply existing, as evidenced by the recent legislative activities in Texas, Alabama, and Florida, among other states. They experience microaggressions and macroaggressions in day-to-day interactions, like the time my son was called a "pervert" for using the girls' bathroom—this was before he had transitioned, but he still was read as looking like a boy.

External factors aside, living in a body that doesn't fit with one's sense of self is a powerful contributing factor to low mood and suicidality.

In the midst of what felt like the biggest crisis I had faced as a parent, I was trying to figure out what to do, so I did what medical training advises: consult an "expert." I made some desperate calls to a gender clinic. A blasé staff person informed me that the waiting time for an initial evaluation was 8 months. I explained that it was "kind of an emergency." The staff person was unmoved.

Through professional connections and with the help of supportive grandparents, we were able to pay privately for a sooner clinical evaluation. I did wonder during this process what it would be like for families without either financial or professional resources. Once again, the unfairness hits some folks harder than others.

HORMONE BLOCKERS OR NO?

Hormone blockers were not a decision that we made lightly. Before I learned about medical interventions for transgender youth, and before I became educated about gender dysphoria, I was mildly opposed to the idea of interfering with the natural process of adolescent development. My general philosophy is that "nature" holds many secrets that are still unknown to us; therefore, one should generally not meddle with natural processes unless one must, because you might mess something up.

When it came to hormone blockers, we weighed the pros and cons. On the one hand, the pubertal delay itself could have unintended consequences. First, the physical consequences could include changes in bone growth. There are also, potentially, social or cognitive consequences that we do not yet understand as well. Would hormone blockers impact my son's social and cognitive development? What else do we not understand about long term effects?

We were scared and confused but agreed to the hormone blockers because of my son's forceful and compelling description of the emotional pain he was experiencing. He looked exhausted and sad. After a lot of deliberating and some arguing, my husband and I agreed to hormone blockers to put a "pause" on puberty. This decision was somewhat eased by it being temporary and reversible: if we discontinued the blockers, puberty would resume its natural course.

Ian received the hormone blockers for about 6 months until he one day said to me, "I don't want to get the shots anymore."

My husband and I, and our son's pediatrician, were all a little befuddled by this turn of events after all of Ian's advocacy to start the hormone blockers and the mental health crisis we'd experienced leading up to it.

When I asked for clarification, my son told me the shots were "super painful," and he no longer minded having some female characteristics because he felt supported and understood by the people in his life. Both the pediatrician and I tried to push him on this question: "How come," I asked, "Are you fine with it now?"

He just shrugged and said, "I just am." For Ian at that time, not being understood by us, his parents, and by other people in his life was contributing to the terrible feeling he was having about going through female puberty. In other words, he was saying he didn't mind having female secondary sex characteristics now that the people in his life understood that he identified as male.

Initially, I wondered if this was a sign that he was having some ambivalence about transitioning to male.

"You can change your mind," I said.

"Mama," he said, rolling his eyes, "I'll always be a boy. I might be a more feminine boy, but always a boy." I hear comments from other parents and in the media that kids are "too young to decide what gender they are." Ian, though, has been unwavering on his feeling that he is male.

For a time, right after Ian came out to us, I felt hurt about the idea of him rejecting "being a girl." I wondered if I'd done something wrong in the way that I'd messaged what it is to be female. But Ian has since explained it to me very well: "I think women are great. In fact," he said to me earnestly, "Maybe even better than men. The thing is—I'm not a girl, I'm a boy. It doesn't have anything to do with what I think about how women are."

I have heard other parents trying to talk their child out of being transgender by saying, "You can be any kind of girl (or boy) you want!" I have realized that these parents, like I was, are under the mistaken belief that their child simply does not understand the full spectrum of what a girl or boy can be. I'm grateful to my son for helping me understand that it's not about understanding *how girls can be*, but rather just *who he is* inside, plain and simple.

NEXT STOP: TESTOSTERONE

After Ian was off the hormone blockers for about a year and his progression toward puberty resumed, my husband and I fretted about when The Dreaded Period would drop. I purchased some special transmale boxers that could accommodate sanitary napkins and set up a "go kit" for him so that he would not have tell me right away when it happened. Occasionally, I would ask him if he was still feeling good about not being on the blockers. He was annoyed by my questions, saying, "Why do you keep bugging me about it?"

One spring a year ago, in the midst of this waiting, he said, "So, when am I going on testosterone?"

If we were nervous about puberty blockers, we were even more nervous about the idea of going on testosterone. There were several reasons for our nervousness. First of all, the concept of "irreversible" changes—such as the voice lowering, or the shape of his body changing—was scary. Second, the idea of my child growing facial hair or having a low voice gave me the shivers. Lastly, I was particularly concerned about any impact on fertility and had concerns about him making potentially irrevocable decisions now when he could change his mind later.

Even among parents of cisgender children, it is normal for parents to feel uncomfortable with watching their child go through puberty and acquire secondary sex characteristics. Many parents experience a sense of "weirdness" about seeing their little child develop adult characteristics. I recall a friend of mine seeing her adolescent cisgender son's legs—"They're all … hairy!" She said with dismay, "Whose legs *are* those?!"

Similarly, a transgender patient of mine described to me his mother's conversation with him as his voiced changed, when he had recently started on testosterone. "She doesn't like to hear my voice change," he said.

So, there is an element of this discomfort for parents of transgender children that is simply part of the normal experience of seeing their child become an adult. Part of what makes parents uncomfortable, I think, is the discordance of who we think our child is—how we understand our child—with who they are becoming. In a way, puberty is part of the separation-individuation process of adolescence. In actual corporeal terms, the body is saying, "Who was I before, and what am I becoming?"

In addition to the "normal" discomfort of my child going through puberty, I was concerned about the impact of testosterone on fertility. We were told that in order for a person to have fertile eggs, they need to fully go through female puberty; it's not generally known how long-term exposure to testosterone may impact a person's ova. In other words, if my son decides later he wants to have biological children, it's not clear if having been on testosterone would enable him to go through "female" puberty at a later time and have fertile eggs. For his part, Ian was clear that he envisioned himself, at least right now, marrying a woman and either adopting or having a sperm donor. Egg harvesting is an option for many individuals, but it involves surgery, hormone treatments, and other uncomfortable and expensive procedures. Putting him through all those interventions for something he says he does not want did not seem like a reasonable plan.

For individuals transitioning from male to female, sperm banking sounds a lot easier than egg harvesting, right? But for some youth, producing viable sperm is not a simple endeavor either. First, there is the problem of having to experience male puberty. Second, for some people, like one of my transgender patients, interacting with their penis in that way—perhaps a reminder of their masculine characteristics—is extremely upsetting and disturbing. Although this patient will potentially have to deal with that in the future in order to have a healthy sex life, it is not fair that she should have to deal with it before she feels ready. Third, both of these processes are costly, with ongoing costs for cryopreservation that are not covered by health insurance.

In regard to the question of testosterone for Ian, the whole idea of having to "agree" to have my child go through male puberty felt like an odd position. Under cisgender circumstances, kids go through puberty without their parent having to "agree" to it.

If all parents did have to "agree" for their child to start going through puberty, I am willing to bet that there are some parents out there who would choose to delay it.

After much deliberation and research, we agreed to have him start the testosterone about 1 year ago. His voice has started to lower, and people who meet him for the first time "read" him as entirely male. I get the sense that he enjoys the changes that testosterone is bringing. He seems more at ease with himself, more relaxed.

What's next?

Experiencing the changes that Ian has gone through—from seeming fairly comfortable in a girl body, to feeling urgently averse to the changes that puberty brought, to feeling more comfortable with female characteristics, to seeking a male body again—I realize that this is just the middle of the journey. I'm ready and interested to hear what my son has to say next.

CLINICS CARE POINTS

- Psychiatry providers have an important role in supporting parents and their children as they go through puberty.
- Transgender patients and their families have both common as well as distinct experiences in relation to puberty when compared to cisgender patients.
- Psychiatrists should be familiar with key decision-points required of transgender patients, including decisions around hormones and fertility preservation considerations.

DISCLOSURE

Dr J. Larson has received honoraria from the Center of Excellence for LBGTQ + Behavioral Health. No other conflict of interests.

REFERENCE

1. Larson J. Parenting my transgender child: from loss to acceptance. Ann Fam Med 2021;19(6):556–9.

UNITED STATES POSTAL SERVICE®
Statement of Ownership, Management, and Circulation
(All Periodicals Publications Except Requester Publications)

1. Publication Title
CHILD AND ADOLESCENT PSYCHIATRIC CLINICS OF NORTH AMERICA

2. Publication Number
011 – 368

3. Filing Date
9/18/2023

4. Issue Frequency
JAN, APR, JUL, OCT

5. Number of Issues Published Annually
4

6. Annual Subscription Price
$369

7. Complete Mailing Address of Known Office of Publication (Not printer) (Street, city, county, state, and ZIP+4®)
ELSEVIER INC.
230 Park Avenue, Suite 800
New York, NY 10169

Contact Person
Malathi Samayan
Telephone (Include area code)
91-44-4299-4507

8. Complete Mailing Address of Headquarters or General Business Office of Publisher (Not printer)
ELSEVIER INC.
230 Park Avenue, Suite 800
New York, NY 10169

9. Full Names and Complete Mailing Addresses of Publisher, Editor, and Managing Editor (Do not leave blank)

Publisher (Name and complete mailing address)
Dolores Meloni, ELSEVIER INC.
1600 JOHN F KENNEDY BLVD. SUITE 1600
PHILADELPHIA, PA 19103-2899

Editor (Name and complete mailing address)
Megan Ashdown, ELSEVIER INC.
1600 JOHN F KENNEDY BLVD. SUITE 1600
PHILADELPHIA, PA 19103-2899

Managing Editor (Name and complete mailing address)
PATRICK MANLEY, ELSEVIER INC.
1600 JOHN F KENNEDY BLVD. SUITE 1600
PHILADELPHIA, PA 19103-2899

10. Owner (Do not leave blank. If the publication is owned by a corporation, give the name and address of the corporation immediately followed by the names and addresses of all stockholders owning or holding 1 percent or more of the total amount of stock. If not owned by a corporation, give the names and addresses of the individual owners. If owned by a partnership or other unincorporated firm, give its name and address as well as those of each individual owner. If the publication is published by a nonprofit organization, give its name and address.)

Full Name	Complete Mailing Address
WHOLLY OWNED SUBSIDIARY OF REED/ELSEVIER, US HOLDINGS	1600 JOHN F KENNEDY BLVD. SUITE 1600 PHILADELPHIA, PA 19103-2899

11. Known Bondholders, Mortgagees, and Other Security Holders Owning or Holding 1 Percent or More of Total Amount of Bonds, Mortgages, or Other Securities. If none, check box → ☐ None

Full Name	Complete Mailing Address
N/A	

12. Tax Status (For completion by nonprofit organizations authorized to mail at nonprofit rates) (Check one)
The purpose, function, and nonprofit status of this organization and the exempt status for federal income tax purposes:
☒ Has Not Changed During Preceding 12 Months
☐ Has Changed During Preceding 12 Months (Publisher must submit explanation of change with this statement)

PS Form **3526**, July 2014 (Page 1 of 4 (see instructions page 4)) PSN: 7530-01-000-9931   PRIVACY NOTICE: See our privacy policy on www.usps.com.

---

13. Publication Title
CHILD AND ADOLESCENT PSYCHIATRIC CLINICS OF NORTH AMERICA

14. Issue Date for Circulation Data Below
JULY 2023

15. Extent and Nature of Circulation

		Average No. Copies Each Issue During Preceding 12 Months	No. Copies of Single Issue Published Nearest to Filing Date
a. Total Number of Copies (Net press run)		137	119
b. Paid Circulation (By Mail and Outside the Mail)	(1) Mailed Outside-County Paid Subscriptions Stated on PS Form 3541 (Include paid distribution above nominal rate, advertiser's proof copies, and exchange copies)	100	89
	(2) Mailed In-County Paid Subscriptions Stated on PS Form 3541 (Include paid distribution above nominal rate, advertiser's proof copies, and exchange copies)	0	0
	(3) Paid Distribution Outside the Mails Including Sales Through Dealers and Carriers, Street Vendors, Counter Sales, and Other Paid Distribution Outside USPS®	23	15
	(4) Paid Distribution by Other Classes of Mail Through the USPS (e.g., First-Class Mail®)	11	12
c. Total Paid Distribution (Sum of 15b (1), (2), (3), and (4))	▶	134	116
d. Free or Nominal Rate Distribution (By Mail and Outside the Mail)	(1) Free or Nominal Rate Outside-County Copies included on PS Form 3541	2	2
	(2) Free or Nominal Rate In-County Copies Included on PS Form 3541	0	0
	(3) Free or Nominal Rate Copies Mailed at Other Classes Through the USPS (e.g., First-Class Mail)	0	0
	(4) Free or Nominal Rate Distribution Outside the Mail (Carriers or other means)	1	1
e. Total Free or Nominal Rate Distribution (Sum of 15d (1), (2), (3) and (4))	▶	3	3
f. Total Distribution (Sum of 15c and 15e)	▶	137	119
g. Copies not Distributed (See Instructions to Publishers #4 (page 83))	▶	0	0
h. Total (Sum of 15f and g)	▶	137	119
i. Percent Paid (15c divided by 15f times 100)		97.63%	97.48%

* If you are claiming electronic copies, go to line 16 on page 3. If you are not claiming electronic copies, skip to line 17 on page 3.

PS Form **3526**, July 2014 (Page 2 of 4)

16. Electronic Copy Circulation

	Average No. Copies Each Issue During Preceding 12 Months	No. Copies of Single Issue Published Nearest to Filing Date
a. Paid Electronic Copies ▶		
b. Total Paid Print Copies (Line 15c) + Paid Electronic Copies (Line 16a) ▶		
c. Total Print Distribution (Line 15f) + Paid Electronic Copies (Line 16a) ▶		
d. Percent Paid (Both Print & Electronic Copies) (16b divided by 16c × 100) ▶		

☒ I certify that 50% of all my distributed copies (electronic and print) are paid above a nominal price.

17. Publication of Statement of Ownership
☒ If the publication is a general publication, publication of this statement is required. Will be printed in the OCTOBER 2023 issue of this publication.   ☐ Publication not required.

18. Signature and Title of Editor, Publisher, Business Manager, or Owner
Malathi Samayan   Date 9/18/2023

Malathi Samayan – Distribution Controller

I certify that all information furnished on this form is true and complete. I understand that anyone who furnishes false or misleading information on this form or who omits material or information requested on the form may be subject to criminal sanctions (including fines and imprisonment) and/or civil sanctions (including civil penalties).

PS Form **3526**, July 2014 (Page 3 of 4)   PRIVACY NOTICE: See our privacy policy on www.usps.com.

Moving?

Make sure your subscription moves with you!

To notify us of your new address, find your **Clinics Account Number** (located on your mailing label above your name), and contact customer service at:

Email: journalscustomerservice-usa@elsevier.com

800-654-2452 (subscribers in the U.S. & Canada)
314-447-8871 (subscribers outside of the U.S. & Canada)

Fax number: 314-447-8029

**Elsevier Health Sciences Division
Subscription Customer Service
3251 Riverport Lane
Maryland Heights, MO 63043**

*To ensure uninterrupted delivery of your subscription, please notify us at least 4 weeks in advance of move.